Liver Transplant: Reaching the Half Century

Guest Editors

CYNTHIA LEVY, MD
PAUL MARTIN, MD

CLINICS IN LIVER DISEASE

www.liver.theclinics.com

Consulting Editor
NORMAN GITLIN, MD

November 2011 • Volume 15 • Number 4

SAUNDERS an imprint of ELSEVIER, Inc.

W.B. SAUNDERS COMPANY

A Division of Elsevier Inc.

1600 John F. Kennedy Boulevard, Suite 1800 • Philadelphia, PA 19103-2899

http://www.theclinics.com

CLINICS IN LIVER DISEASE Volume 15, Number 4
November 2011 ISSN 1089-3261, ISBN-13: 978-1-4557-1108-6

Editor: Kerry Holland
Developmental Editor: Teia Stone

Clinics in Liver Disease (ISSN 1089-3261) is published quarterly by Elsevier Inc., 360 Park Avenue South, New York, NY 10010-1710. Months of issue are February, May, August, and November. Business and Editorial Offices: 1600 John F. Kennedy Blvd., Ste. 1800, Philadelphia, PA 19103-2899. Customer Service Office: 3251 Riverport Lane, Maryland Heights, MO 63043. Periodicals postage paid at New York, NY and additional mailing offices. Subscription prices are $251.00 per year (U.S. individuals), $124.00 per year (U.S. student/resident), $343.00 per year (U.S. institutions), $333.00 per year (foreign individuals), $171.00 per year (foreign student/ resident), $413.00 per year (foreign instituitions), $290.00 per year (Canadian individuals), $171.00 per year (Canadian student/resident), and $413.00 per year (Canadian institutions). Foreign air speed delivery is included in all *Clinics* subscription prices. All prices are subject to change without notice. **POSTMASTER:** Send address changes to *Clinics in Liver Disease*, Elsevier Health Sciences Division, Subscription Customer Service, 3251 Riverport Lane, Maryland Heights, MO 63043. **Customer Service: Telephone: 1-800-654-2452 (U.S. and Canada); 314-447-8871 (outside U.S. and Canada). Fax: 314-447-8029. E-mail: journalscustomer service-usa@elsevier.com (for print support); journalsonlinesupport-usa@elsevier.com (for online support).**

Reprints. For copies of 100 or more of articles in this publication, please contact the Commercial Reprints Department, Elsevier Inc., 360 Park Avenue South, New York, NY 10010-1710. Tel.: 212-633-3812; Fax: 212-462-1935; E-mail: reprints@elsevier.com.

Clinics in Liver Disease is covered in *MEDLINE/PubMed (Index Medicus)*, Science Citation Index Expanded, Journal Citation Reports/Science Edition, and Current Contents/Clinical Medicine.

Printed and bound by CPI Group (UK) Ltd, Croydon, CR0 4YY

Transferred to Digital Print 2011

Contributors

CONSULTING EDITOR

NORMAN GITLIN, MD, FRCP(LONDON), FRCPE(EDINBURGH), FACG, FACP
Formerly, Professor of Medicine, Chief of Hepatology, Emory University; Currently, Consultant, Atlanta Gastroenterology Associates, Atlanta, Georgia

GUEST EDITORS

CYNTHIA LEVY, MD
Associate Professor of Medicine, Division of Hepatology, Department of Medicine, University of Miami, Miami, Florida

PAUL MARTIN, MD, FRCP, FRCPI
Chief, Division of Hepatology, Department of Medicine, University of Miami, Miami, Florida

AUTHORS

SUMEET K. ASRANI, MD
Division of Gastroenterology and Hepatology, Mayo Clinic College of Medicine, Rochester, Minnesota

DIANE M. BISKOBING, MD
Associate Professor of Medicine, Division of Endocrinology, Virginia Commonwealth University, Richmond, Virginia

CORINNE BUCHANAN, MSN, ACNP-BC
Center for Liver Transplantation, Cedars Sinai Medical Center, Los Angeles, California

SUPHAMAI BUNNAPRADIST, MD
Kidney and Pancreas Transplant Program, Division of Nephrology, Department of Medicine, David Geffen School of Medicine at UCLA, Los Angeles, California

DANIEL E. CARL, MD
Assistant Professor of Medicine, Division of Nephrology, Virginia Commonwealth University, Richmond, Virginia

CLAUDIA A. COUTO, MD, PhD
Department of Internal Medicine, School of Medicine, Federal University of Minas Gerais, Belo Horizonte, Minas Gerais, Brazil

CATHERINE CRONE, MD
Associate Professor of Psychiatry, Clinical Professor of Psychiatry, Vice Chair, Department of Psychiatry at Inova Fairfax Hospital, George Washington University Medical Center, Inova Fairfax Hospital, Virginia Commonwealth University, Falls Church, Virginia

MARY AMANDA DEW, PhD
Professor of Psychiatry, Psychology, Epidemiology and Biostatistics, Associate Center Director and Director, Clinical Epidemiology Program, Research Methods and Biostatistics Core, Advanced Center for Interventions, and Services Research in Late Life Mood Disorders; Director, Quality of Life Research, Artificial Heart Program, Adult Cardiothoracic Transplantation, University of Pittsburgh School of Medicine and Medical Center, Pittsburgh, Pennsylvania

ANDREA DIMARTINI, MD
Associate Professor of Psychiatry, Associate Professor of Surgery, Consultation Liaison to the Liver Transplant Program, Starzl Transplant Institute, University of Pittsburgh Medical Center, Pittsburgh, Pennsylvania

ROBERTO J. FIRPI, MD
Division of Gastroenterology, Hepatology, and Nutrition, Department of Medicine, University of Florida College of Medicine, Gainesville, Florida

JOHN A. GOSS, MD
Director of Liver Center; Professor and Chief, Division of Abdominal Transplantation, Michael E. DeBakey Department of Surgery, The Liver Center, Baylor College of Medicine, Houston, Texas

THERESA R. HARRING, MD
Research Fellow, General Surgery Resident, Michael E. DeBakey Department of Surgery, Baylor College of Medicine, Houston, Texas

W. RAY KIM, MD
Division of Gastroenterology and Hepatology, Mayo Clinic College of Medicine, Rochester, Minnesota

MICHAEL J. KROWKA, MD
Professor of Medicine, Vice-Chair, Division of Pulmonary and Critical Care; Division of Gastroenterology and Hepatology, Mayo Clinic, Rochester, Minnesota

CHRISTINE LAU, MD
Kidney and Pancreas Transplant Program, Division of Nephrology, Department of Medicine, David Geffen School of Medicine at UCLA, Los Angeles, California

DAVID M. LEVI, MD, FACS
Professor of Clinical Surgery, DeWitt Daughtry Family Department of Surgery, University of Miami Miller School of Medicine; Miami Transplant Institute, Miami, Florida

CYNTHIA LEVY, MD
Associate Professor of Medicine, Department of Medicine, University of Miami, Miami, Florida

ALPNA R. LIMAYE, MD
Division of Gastroenterology, Hepatology, and Nutrition, Department of Medicine, University of Florida College of Medicine, Gainesville, Florida

PAUL MARTIN, MD, FRCP, FRCPI
Division of Hepatology, Department of Medicine, University of Miami, Miami, Florida

HOWARD C. MASUOKA, MD, PhD
Assistant Professor, Division of Gastroenterology and Hepatology, Indiana University School of Medicine, Indianapolis, Indiana

FLAVIA MENDES, MD
Division of Hepatology, Miami VA Medical Center, Miami, Florida

SEIGO NISHIDA, MD, PhD, FACS
Professor of Clinical Surgery, DeWitt Daughtry Family Department of Surgery, University of Miami Miller School of Medicine; Miami Transplant Institute, Miami, Florida

CHRISTINE A. O'MAHONY, MD
Assistant Professor, Division of Abdominal Transplantation, Michael E. DeBakey Department of Surgery, The Liver Center, Baylor College of Medicine, Houston, Texas

CHARLES B. ROSEN, MD
Professor of Surgery, Chair, Division of Transplantation Surgery and Mayo Clinic William J. von Liebig Transplant Center, Mayo Clinic College of Medicine, Rochester, Minnesota

R. TODD STRAVITZ, MD, FACP, FACG
Professor of Medicine and Medical Director of Liver Transplantation, Section of Hepatology, Division of Gastroenterology, Hepatology, and Nutrition, Hume-Lee Transplant Center, Virginia Commonwealth University, Richmond, Virginia

HUI-HUI TAN, MBBS, MRCP(UK)
Department of Gastroenterology and Hepatology, Singapore General Hospital, Singapore

TRAM T. TRAN, MD
Medical Director, Center for Liver Transplantation, Cedars Sinai Medical Center; Associate Professor of Medicine, Geffen UCLA School of Medicine, Los Angeles, California

Contents

Sumeet K. Asrani and W. Ray Kim

The Model for End-stage Liver Disease (MELD) score is the basis for allocation of liver allografts for transplantation in the United States. The MELD score, as an objective scale of disease severity, is also used in the management of patients with chronic liver disease in the nontransplant setting. Several models have been proposed to improve the MELD score. The authors believe that the MELD score is, by design, continually evolving and lends itself to continued refinement and improvement to serve as a metric to optimize organ allocation in the future.

Howard C. Masuoka and Charles B. Rosen

Cholangiocarcinoma (CCA) is a primary hepatic neoplasm that arises from malignant transformation of the biliary epithelium. Chronic biliary tree inflammation as occurs in primary sclerosing cholangitis (PSC) is a risk factor for the development of CCA. Surgical resection and liver transplantation following neoadjuvant therapy in patients with early extrahepatic CCA are the only potentially curative modalities. Biliary stenting, chemotherapy, radiation therapy, and photodynamic therapy are palliative treatment options for patients who are not surgical candidates. Liver transplantation following neoadjuvant therapy is an effective therapy for patients with hilar cholangiocarcinoma that is unresectable or arising in the setting of PSC.

David M. Levi and Seigo Nishida

The past 2 decades have witnessed an exponential increase in the incidence of hepatocellular carcinoma (HCC) in the United States and, concurrently, the development of liver transplantation as an effective modality in its treatment. "Early" HCC has been defined, allowing patients with unresectable HCC to be granted priority for transplant over the past decade. This situation has produced a dramatic increase in the number of transplants for HCC. The challenge has been how to expand the indications of liver transplant for HCC with improved cancer-free survival and fewer transplant-related complications without adversely affecting non-HCC transplant candidates.

Andrea DiMartini, Catherine Crone, and Mary Amanda Dew

In this article the epidemiology of substance use and substance disorders in the United States and their association with liver disease are reviewed.

The relevance of tobacco use and issues of candidacy as it pertains to substance use are discussed. The use of alcohol while on the waitlist and short sobriety are also addressed. The merits of monitoring of patients are discussed, and the outcomes of these patients after liver transplantation are examined. The article concludes with a summary of recommendations for clinicians working with these patients and possible future directions for both clinical care and research.

The management of hepatitis B in liver transplantation has evolved significantly over the past 2 decades. Introduction of hepatitis B immune globulin and subsequently nucleos(t)ide analogues has revolutionized transplantation for hepatitis B virus (HBV), increasing survival for patients transplanted for this indication. With the availability of new and potent antivirals for HBV, the need for liver transplant should continue to decrease in the coming years. Moreover, the newer antivirals with high resistance barriers will allow effective long-term viral prophylaxis and therefore, prevention of recurrence.

This article addresses the most common pulmonary issues that affect liver transplant candidates. Pretransplant diagnostic criteria of these pulmonary problems in liver transplant patients are reviewed. Successful pulmonary management schemes and caveats are described. Risks for liver transplant are emphasized.

Care of the liver transplant candidate is one of the most challenging, yet rewarding aspects of hepatology. Anticipation and intervention for the major complications of advanced liver disease increase the likelihood of survival until transplant.

Renal dysfunction is a frequent complication in patients with endstage liver disease awaiting orthotopic liver transplantation. Although the stereotypical form of renal dysfunction is the hepatorenal syndrome, common causes of acute kidney injury include prerenal azotemia and acute tubular necrosis in this population. Management involves hemodynamic support, renal replacement therapy, and mitigation of risk factors. Renal dysfunction in a cirrhotic patient usually implies a poor prognosis in the absence of liver transplantation. An important issue is the frequent need for kidney, in addition to liver, transplantation if renal insufficiency has been persistent in a decompensated cirrhotic.

Long-term survival of liver transplant recipients has become the rule rather than the exception. As a result, the medical complications of long-term survival, including atherosclerotic cardiovascular disease, metabolic bone disease, and de novo malignancy, have accounted for an increasing proportion of late morbidity and mortality. Risk factors for these complications begin before transplant and are potentially modifiable but are exacerbated by the requirement for immunosuppressive medications after transplantation. Surveillance and early intervention programs administered by transplant hepatologists and other medical subspecialists may improve long-term outcomes in liver transplant recipients by ameliorating risk factors for atherosclerosis, bone fractures, and cancer.

Recurrence of hepatitis C virus remains a near-universal phenomenon after liver transplantation (LT) and is responsible for the high morbidity and low survival seen in these patients. The severity of recurrent disease varies depending on multiple factors, only some of which are modifiable. Antiviral therapy is associated with improved outcomes, but viral clearance is only attainable in a small percentage of this patient population. This patient population is in need of new therapeutic options, and it remains to be seen whether direct-acting antiviral agents will be the answer to this ongoing therapeutic question.

Primary biliary cirrhosis (PBC), primary sclerosing cholangitis (PSC), and autoimmune hepatitis (AIH) each account for approximately 5% of liver transplants per year performed in the United States and Europe. Even though outcomes are excellent, with reported 5-year patient and graft survival exceeding 90% and 80%, 80% and 75%, 72% and 65% for PBC, PSC, and AIH, respectively, the issue of recurrent autoimmune liver disease after orthotopic liver transplantation is increasingly recognized as a cause of graft dysfunction, death, and need for retransplantation. This article reviews diagnostic criteria, epidemiology, risk factors, and outcomes of recurrent PBC, PSC, and AIH after liver transplantation.

Several criteria are used to differentiate between standard and extended allograft donors. These criteria include deceased after cardiac death, advanced donor age, steatosis, previous malignancy in the donor, hepatitis C virus-positive allografts, human T-cell lymphotropic virus-positive allografts, active infections in the donor, high-risk donors, split liver transplantations, and living donor liver transplantations. Review of the literature can lead each practitioner to incorporate extended criteria donors into their transplant program, thereby individualizing the use of these allografts, increasing the donor pool, and decreasing overall waitlist mortality.

RELATED INTEREST

Surgical Clinics of North America, August 2010 (Vol. 90, No. 4)
Liver Surgery: From Basics to Robotics
David A. Geller, MD, *Guest Editor*

THE CLINICS ARE NOW AVAILABLE ONLINE!

Access your subscription at:
www.theclinics.com

Preface

Liver Transplant: Reaching the Half Century

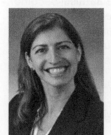 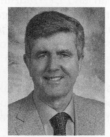

Cynthia Levy, MD   Paul Martin, MD
Guest Editors

Although the pioneering efforts of Dr Tom Starzl in liver transplant date back to the early 1960s, liver transplantation has become such a critical element in the management of patients with liver disease that it is sobering to reflect that its widespread use is still relatively recent after a NIH Consensus Conference in 1983 endorsed liver transplantation in patients with advanced liver disease. Similarly, the Model for End-stage Liver Disease (MELD) has become common parlance for assessing the severity of liver disease, although it was adopted by the United Network for Organ Sharing for organ allocation within the last 10 years. The role of liver transplantation for a number of controversial indications has become better defined during the same period of time including cholangiocarcinoma, hepatocellular carcinoma, and alcoholic liver disease. In this current issue of the *Clinics in Liver Disease*, with the aid of a distinguished group of authors, we provide an update on the current status of liver transplantation as it approaches the half century mark.

Drs Asrani and Kim provide a timely discussion on the profound impact of MELD in liver transplant. Dr Levi discusses the emergence of liver transplantation as a curative option for hepatocellular carcinoma and the importance of a multidisciplinary approach, while Drs Masuoka and Rosen address the role of transplant for cholangio-carcinoma. Drs Di Martini, Crone, and Dew discuss the challenging topic of alcohol and substance abuse in liver transplant candidates and provide excellent management recommendations. Dr Krowka has done extensive work on the impact and management of pulmonary complications of advanced liver disease and herein summarizes his thoughts and recommendations. As we contemplate transplantation in older and sicker patients, their preoperative management has become increasingly complex and time consuming, as described by Dr Tan, with the onset of renal dysfunction an ominous event in the progression of chronic liver disease, as addressed by Drs Lau and Bunnapradist. However, despite our best efforts, patients continue to succumb to their liver disease while listed for liver transplant. Drs Harring, O'Mahony,

Clin Liver Dis 15 (2011) xi–xii
doi:10.1016/j.cld.2011.09.001

and Goss provide a thorough discussion on strategies utilized to expand the donor pool with extended donors to decrease waitlist mortality.

Although liver transplant is curative for some transplant recipients, recurrent disease is a major threat to graft and patients. Drs Limaye and Firpi discuss the impact of HCV recurrence, its predictors, and the role of early versus late antiviral treatment. Conversely, prevention of recurrent hepatitis B has been one of the major triumphs in liver transplant, as described by Ms Buchanan and Dr Tran. It has also become apparent that autoimmune liver diseases can recur, potentially threatening the graft, as addressed by Drs Mendes and Couto. Finally, Drs Stravitz, Carl, and Biskobing provide a detailed discussion on the importance of paying meticulous attention to co-morbidities, which are common in liver transplant recipients to sustain continued excellent long-term survival for all recipients.

We would like to thank all our contributors for sharing their expertise with us to provide this update on liver transplant as it reaches its half century. We would also like to thank Kerry Holland for her efforts to bring this *Clinics* to press and Dr Norman Gitlin for entrusting this issue to us.

Cynthia Levy, MD

Paul Martin, MD
Division of Hepatology
Department of Medicine
University of Miami
1500 NW 12th Avenue, Suite 1101
Miami, FL 33136, USA

E-mail addresses:
Clevy@med.miami.edu (C. Levy)
Pmartin2@med.miami.edu (P. Martin)

Model for End-Stage Liver Disease: End of the First Decade

Sumeet K. Asrani, MD, W. Ray Kim, MD*

KEYWORDS

• MELD • Organ allocation • Waiting-list mortality
• Mathematical models • Prognosis • Survival

In February 2002 the Model for End-stage Liver Disease score (MELD) was adopted as the basis for allocation of allografts for liver transplantation (LT) in the United States. Implementation of the MELD score led to a reduction in waiting-list registration and waiting-list mortality and an increase in deceased donor transplants.[1] Despite transplanting sicker patients (higher MELD scores), there has been no appreciable decrement in survival after LT.[2] Further, as a common metric of underlying severity, the MELD score has been used in the management of patients with a wide spectrum of liver disease.[3] The MELD score is a working model and has served as a template for further refinement to achieve the goal of equitable distribution of a scarce resource.[4,5] This article highlights the strengths of the current MELD score, addresses its limitations, and discusses proposed modifications to successfully enrich a MELD-based allocation system for the next decade of LT.

DEVELOPMENT OF THE MELD SCORE

The recognition of several limitations of the existing liver allocation policy in the late 1990s provided a strong impetus to devise a more equitable and efficient system. Transplant candidates were categorized into 4 broad United Network for Organ Sharing (UNOS) statuses, which were in part defined by arbitrary descriptors of disease severity (eg, intensive care admission). For patients not in intensive care, the Child-Turcotte-Pugh score was used to measure disease severity. However, the score consisted of variables that were subjective (eg, ascites, encephalopathy) or influenced by interlaboratory variability (eg, prothrombin time, albumin) and lacked

Financial disclosure: None of the authors have conflicts of interest or any specific financial interests relevant to the subject of this article. This study was supported by a grant from the NIH (R01DK-34238) and a NIH digestive diseases training grant (T32 DK07198).
Division of Gastroenterology and Hepatology, Mayo Clinic College of Medicine, 200 First Street SW, Rochester, MN 55905, USA
* Corresponding author.
E-mail address: kim.ray@mayo.edu

Clin Liver Dis 15 (2011) 685–698
doi:10.1016/j.cld.2011.08.009
1089-3261/11/$ – see front matter © 2011 Elsevier Inc. All rights reserved.

statistical validity (eg, equal weights to all elements such as mild hyperbilirubinemia vs grade II hepatic encephalopathy). Because of the inability of this transplant status system to accurately stratify patients according to their level of sickness, there were a large number of patients within a given status for whom waiting time was used to determine priorities in allocation. Sicker candidates who were listed late in the course of disease progression were disadvantaged because they had not accrued enough waiting time despite their high risk of mortality. In this system, waiting-list mortality continued to increase.[6–8] In studies that correlated waiting time and risk of mortality, waiting time was shown to be a poor metric for disease severity.[9] In 1999, the Institute of Medicine and the US Department of Health and Human Services issued a mandate to the liver transplant community to design an organ allocation system that de-emphasized waiting time and set allocation priorities based on the severity of liver disease and risk of mortality.[10]

The MELD score was initially created to predict survival in patients with complications of portal hypertension undergoing elective placement of transjugular intrahepatic portosystemic shunts (TIPS).[11] The model was subsequently validated as a predictor of survival in several independent cohorts of patients with varying levels of liver disease severity (eg, hospitalized and ambulatory patients), as well as patients of geographically and temporally diverse origin.[12] In a prospective study of candidates on the waiting list, MELD was an excellent predictor of waiting-list mortality. The concordance (c-statistic), with 3-month mortality as the end point, for the MELD score was 0.83 indicating that when a pair of patients is randomly drawn out of the study population, 83% of the time the model correctly predicts the first patient to die.[3]

Although the original derivation of the model included the cause of liver disease, subsequent studies de-emphasized the importance of the cause of liver disease.[3] Further, early studies showed that individual complications of portal hypertension, such as spontaneous bacterial peritonitis, encephalopathy, variceal bleeding, or ascites, did not provide further prognostic information when added to MELD.[12] Thus, when the MELD score was selected as the metric for the new allocation policy, the cause of liver disease was removed from the score. In addition, several changes were introduced to the score.[13] They included lower bounds for serum creatinine, bilirubin, and International Normalized Ratio (INR) fixed at 1 to avoid negative scores and an upper bound of serum creatinine at 4 mg/dL, including patients on hemodialysis. Although these modifications were made empirically, they were widely accepted and our recent study largely supported those upper and lower bounds (see later discussion).

Strengths of the MELD score include that it is an objective metric using a continuous scale that lends itself to ranking patients based on disease severity. It incorporates laboratory parameters that are easily available and reproducible. Its validity as a robust mathematical model to assess mortality risk in patients with end-stage liver disease has been shown in many studies.[3] MELD has been shown to be superior to clinical judgment in identifying patients at risk of mortality.[14]

COMPONENTS OF THE MELD SCORE
Bilirubin

In patients with end-stage liver disease, serum bilirubin concentration is a well-established marker of the hepatic synthetic function, although, in the strictest sense, it represents excretory function. Of the 3 MELD variables, serum bilirubin is the most important. It has a linear relationship with 90-day mortality in patients waiting for LT (Fig. 1), despite lack of consideration for interlaboratory variability in the measurement of serum bilirubin.[15]

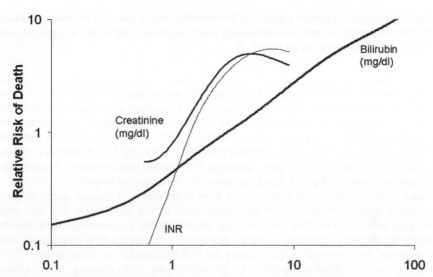

Fig. 1. The relation between risk of 90-day mortality and individual MELD variables after adjustment for the other components.

In the MELD score, the serum total bilirubin concentration is used for the bilirubin variable. In theory, direct bilirubin is a better physiologic marker of liver function than total bilirubin, because the indirect fraction of bilirubin is susceptible to other processes in the body, such as hemolysis and genetic variability in the bilirubin metabolism. However, in our evaluation of direct bilirubin as an alternative to total bilirubin, we did not find the former to be a superior predictor than the latter (Kim WR, unpublished data, 2010).

Creatinine

It is common to see a substantial degree of variability in renal function in patients with end-stage liver disease. More importantly, diminished renal function is an important predictor of survival in those patients.[16–19] Incorporation of serum creatinine in the MELD score as a predictor of survival affords considerable advantage compared with other measures of liver disease such as the Child-Pugh score. In **Fig. 1**, serum creatinine has a sigmoid pattern in that the increase in mortality is linear within a range of creatinine, in partial support of the current lower and upper bounds of 1 and 4, respectively.

However, accuracy of noninvasive measurement of renal function, including serum creatinine, has been shown to be suboptimal among cirrhotic patients.[20–22] Measured glomerular filtration rate (GFR; eg, by iothalamate clearance measurement) is better at assessing prognosis than creatinine and mathematical equations containing creatinine.[20,21] A multivariable model that incorporates calculated GFR and/or serum sodium is superior to the MELD score (see later discussion for MELD with serum sodium [MELDNa]).[22]

There has been a recent push for standardizing creatinine measurement in laboratories. The traditional colorimetric alkaline picric Jaffe method has several limitations, one of which is interference with bilirubin in high concentrations.[23] In patients with high serum bilirubin (>25 mg/dL), serum creatinine can be overestimated, leading to imprecise calculation of the MELD score. Accordingly, the new standard is an enzymatic method for measuring serum creatinine. Preferential use of the new method and standardization of measurement processes has been proposed, especially in patients with serum bilirubin greater than 25 mg/dL.[3]

INR

Prothrombin time and the INR reflect coagulopathy associated with synthetic dysfunction in patients with end-stage liver disease. The liver plays an important role in the coagulation pathways by generating most of the clotting factors. In patients with end-stage liver disease, decreased production of factors along the intrinsic pathway prolongs prothrombin time. **Fig. 1** shows that, after adjusting for bilirubin and creatinine, INR is associated with a steep increase in mortality risk. However, once it reaches approximately 3, the risk does not seem to increase any further.

A well-known limitation of prothrombin time is variability in assays depending on the reagent and/or measurement technique used in the laboratory. The INR was developed to overcome this limitation by standardizing prothrombin time results primarily for patients receiving warfarin. However, when applied to individuals with liver disease, this method of calculation for INR proves to be suboptimal.[24,25] In studies in which plasma samples of patients with liver disease were tested using different prothrombin reagents, there was a substantial degree of variation in INR values.[26,27] In contrast, if calibration is done using standards derived for patients with liver disease, interassay and interlaboratory variability could be reduced significantly.

Based on these data, incorporation of a liver-specific INR may improve the predictive ability of the current MELD. However, there are many practical issues that would need to be addressed.[28] Manufacturers of INR reagents would need to determine 2 separate measurements for derivation of the INR, leading to increased costs and confusion, and the potential for laboratory error. In addition, implementation and monitoring for standardization across laboratories are expected to be costly and unlikely to be funded given the low prevalence of end-stage liver disease. Thus, despite the theoretic advantages of INR calibrated for patients with liver disease, practical challenges to the application of this important concept are not easily surmountable at this time.[25]

Application of MELD scores in patients on anticoagulation therapy presents a challenge. If a high MELD score is mostly driven by an artificially high INR, the true MELD may be low (eg, <15), making the transplantation less beneficial to the patient (see later discussion).[29] Heuman and colleagues[30] examined a model without INR (MELD-XI) for liver transplantation candidates on stable oral anticoagulation. The model was still less accurate than MELD, suggesting that, even in those patients, INR carries prognostic information.

In summary, there remains a strong need for a reproducible and accurate measure of coagulopathy in patients with liver disease, which may replace INR in MELD, making it even more accurate.[31] However, at the present time, INR remains a practically useful and statistically significant correlate of mortality risk in patients with end-stage liver disease.[32] It is also widely available and is likely continue to be used as an indicator of survival in patients with end-stage liver disease and as a component of the MELD score.[3]

APPLICATION OF MELD IN LIVER TRANSPLANTATION

Coinciding with the implementation of MELD-based liver allocation, there was an immediate 12% reduction in LT waiting-list registrations, especially in candidates with MELD scores of less than 10.[2] More importantly, there was a 3.5% reduction in waiting-list death rate,[2,22,33] accompanied by a decrease in median waiting time from 656 days to 416 days.[8] More recent data showed longer term benefits of the MELD system: between 2002 and 2008, the number of waiting-list candidates decreased by 3.4%, whereas the annual dropout rate from the waiting list remained stationary.[34] Waiting time also decreased, with a higher proportion of candidates being transplanted within 30 days (23% in 2001 to 37% in 2008). Thus, the MELD score has been a pivotal element of the current allocation system, contributing to more effective allocation of the scarce donor organs and to a significant increase in the probability of receiving an LT.[2,35]

An initial concern in implementing the MELD-based allocation system was that selection of patients with high MELD scores undermines the outcome following LT. However, data have shown that the 1-year patient and graft survival did not change between the pre-MELD and post-MELD eras, although the mean MELD score at LT did increase from 17 to 21.[2,36,37] Furthermore, when the survival outcomes were controlled for appropriate covariates, adjusted 1-year graft survival improved from 79.5% to 85.6%, and patient survival from 85.4% to 89.4%, between 1998 and 2007. Similar benefits from implementation of the MELD score have been shown outside the United States.[38–40]

There are several basic features of the MELD score that need to be recognized. First, the MELD score was created in a carefully screened population that was devoid of acute, reversible complications (eg, infection or volume depletion). Hence, it may not accurately capture the risk of mortality in acutely decompensated cirrhotic patients.[3] Second, although the MELD score applies to most patients with chronic liver disease, it does not address mortality associated with rare complications of end-stage liver disease (eg, portopulmonary hypertension).[8] To assign appropriate priority in these patients beyond their native MELD score, exception scores have been increasingly used: between 2002 and 2008, MELD exception on the waiting list increased from 382 to 890. Similarly, the original MELD score derivation excluded persons with hepatocellular carcinoma (HCC). As the incidence of HCC in the US continues to increase, the number of LT candidates receiving the standard exception score for HCC has been increasing.[34] The LT community is still deciding how to assign appropriate exception scores for HCC to ensure equitability between patients with HCC and those with a high biologic MELD score.[34,41–44] Lastly, pretransplant patient status in general, and the MELD score in particular, have a limited ability to predict posttransplant mortality as a result of factors such as donor characteristics, transplant factors, and random postoperative complications that have little to do with pretransplant patient condition.

Renal Dysfunction

Patients with renal dysfunction (serum creatinine $\geq$1.5 mg/dL) at the time of LT increased from 26.1% in 2002 to 29.8% in 2008.[34] However, implementation of the MELD allocation system has not been associated with an increased mortality or occurrence of stage 3 of 4 chronic kidney disease in the first 2 years after LT.[45,46] Since introduction of MELD, kidney transplantation, preoperative creatinine, and number of patients requiring preoperative hemodialysis have increased. These patients are older, more ethnically diverse, and have received organs from older donors[47,48] Despite this, patient survival within the first 2 to 3 years did not differ compared with the pre-MELD era.[47,48]

These trends were also accompanied by an increase in the number of simultaneous liver-kidney transplantations (SLKs), from 100 in 1999 to 379 in 2008. This may be driven by an increased awareness of the impact of renal dysfunction on postoperative mortality.[34] Strategies for optimal utilization of SLK continue to evolve and remain to be established in an evidence-based fashion.[16,17]

Benefit of LT

The MELD score has enabled the transplant community to objectively assess the benefit of LT. In their seminal paper, Merion and colleagues[49] considered the survival benefit of LT. They showed that the benefit of LT at 1 year was highest among those with MELD scores greater than 18. Recipient mortality was higher among candidates with low MELD scores. For example, for patients with MELD scores between 6 and 11, the risk of mortality was 3.6 times higher by undergoing LT rather than remaining on the waiting list (hazard ratio [HR] 3.6; P<.01). For MELD 12 to 14, the risk remained significantly increased (HR 2.4; P<.01). Subsequently, these findings led to a change in allocation policy: an organ would need to be shared within the larger region before use for a local candidate with an MELD score less than 15 (SHARE 15).[49]

This concept was further expanded by Volk and colleagues,[50] who studied matching between donor and recipient in the MELD era. With the MELD system, a donated organ is prioritized to the candidate with the highest MELD score. At the time of the organ offer, whether it is accepted for the given candidate remains at the discretion of the surgeon, who makes the decision trying to achieve the best post-LT outcome possible. The study by Volk and colleagues[50] showed that the overall quality of organs (as quantified by the donor risk index [DRI]) decreased in the post-MELD era, as more marginal organs were used as a result of continued organ shortage. More importantly, these higher-risk organs were being transplanted in the less urgent patients (low MELD) leading to poor outcomes in these candidates. It is feared that this practice has reduced posttransplant survival in recent years among patients with low MELD scores. Similarly, Schaubel and colleagues[51] showed that high-DRI organs were more often transplanted into low-MELD recipients. Compared with waiting for a low-DRI organ, the recipients in the lowest MELD categories (MELD 6–8) who received high-DRI organs experienced significantly higher mortality (HR 3.7; P<.01). These studies highlight the advantage of the MELD score, which has provided a tool with which to critically examine the organ allocation and acceptance practice as well as to shape the distribution policy to optimize the overall outcome after LT.[52,53]

Gender and the MELD Score

Female gender has been associated with an approximate 15% increased risk of death on the waiting list and a 12% decrease in the probability of receiving an LT.[54–56] It is believed that women may be disadvantaged in the MELD system because serum creatinine is used in the MELD equation.[57] As a function of less muscle mass, serum creatinine may underestimate the severity of renal dysfunction in women. Hence, an inaccurate representation of their renal dysfunction may disadvantage women, with lower rates of LT and higher waiting-list mortality.[58]

The relationship between MELD and mortality in women and men remains to be fully characterized.[54,56,59] Myers and colleagues[56] examined the UNOS database (2002–2007) and showed that women had a lower serum creatinine but also a lower estimated GFR (eGFR) across most strata of the MELD score. In addition, women also tended to have greater hepatic dysfunction as characterized by bilirubin and INR across MELD categories. In their primary analysis, after adjusting for serum creatinine, female gender was associated with a 13% increased risk of death within 90 days. Higher rates of mortality were seen between MELD scores of 21 and 35. However, in separate models adjusting for MELD and serum sodium, the difference in mortality was reduced to 7% and was no longer significant. Using eGFR as defined by the

Modification of Diet in Renal Disease (MDRD) equation conferred a 15% survival advantage to women.[56]

There may be other confounders that may explain the gender-based difference in waiting-list outcomes.[60] Recently, Lai and colleagues[54] examined the UNOS database (2002–2008) and reported that a 19% increased risk of mortality among women was decreased to 5% and was no longer significant after consideration of pertinent covariates such as body size, especially height. However, transplantation rates remained lower among women, even after adjustment for height (HR 0.88; 95% confidence interval 0.82–0.92; P<.001).

The extent to which serum creatinine is responsible for the gender disparity in waiting-list outcome can only be examined by a study that includes direct measurement of GFR. The increased mortality seen in women may be multifactorial; data so far suggest that smaller body size in women, leading to lower serum creatinine and thus MELD and limiting their access only to smaller organs, may explain a large part of the observation. Women also tended to present with worse overall hepatic dysfunction, increasing the urgency for LT. As discussed later, revising the lower bound of creatinine to 0.8 or addition of serum sodium may attenuate this difference in mortality.[22,32] Serum or urine biomarkers to accurately represent renal function in patients with end-stage liver disease may provide further improvement.[22]

MELD and Retransplantation

Since implementation of MELD, the number of transplant recipients increased (4969 in 2002 and 6069 in 2008) with a decrease in retransplantation rates. For hepatitis C virus (HCV) negative recipients, the rate of retransplantation decreased from 12% to 9%, and, for those with HCV, from 8% to 5%.[34] This raises a question whether the MELD score systematically disadvantages LT candidates who are waiting for repeat transplantation. We addressed this question in a recent study. The current MELD-based allocation system seemed to serve primary and retransplantation candidates equitably.[35] As expected, retransplantation candidates are listed at higher MELD scores (21 vs 15). In the MELD score ranges in which most LT is performed, there is no large difference in waiting-list mortality for a given MELD score. The mortality risk does not increase as fast in retransplant candidates compared with primary liver transplant at high MELD scores (eg >35); in the very low MELD score ranges, the mortality trend is reversed.[35]

APPLICATION OF MELD SCORE IN NON–LIVER TRANSPLANT SETTINGS

The MELD score, as an objective scale of disease severity, has been used in the management of patients with chronic liver disease in the nontransplant setting. Although the initial assessment of the score was limited to survival within 90 days, the MELD score is a predictor of long-term survival in patients with decompensated cirrhosis.[61] The application of MELD in persons with chronic liver disease has included prognosis and treatment of variceal bleeding, infection, alcoholic hepatitis, surgical resection of hepatocellular carcinoma, placement of TIPS, and management of fulminant hepatic failure and renal failure.[3,62–64] The MELD score is a predictor of nontransplant surgical mortality in patients with cirrhosis.[65,66]

IMPROVING MELD

Several models have been proposed to refine and improve the MELD score. These models includes measurement of serial MELD scores, addition of variables (eg, serum sodium), or reweighting components of the MELD score.

Delta MELD

The usefulness of a change in MELD (delta MELD) in predicting waiting-list mortality has been studied with disparate results.[67–70] It may make intuitive sense that patients with an acutely increasing MELD may have worse outcomes than those with a stable score. In univariate analysis, a change in MELD is predictive of mortality. However, the increase in MELD is confounded by (1) patients with a sharp increase in MELD tending to have a high MELD score currently, and (2) in retrospective analysis, patients who are acutely worsening have frequent laboratory testing, which may represent the clinician's clinical judgment of the worsening patient's condition. These concerns were born out in multivariable analysis in which, once the current MELD and the number of MELD scores available were taken into account, delta MELD was no longer significant.[71]

Incorporation of Serum Sodium

Serum sodium concentration, as a reflection of activation of neurohumoral systems and water retention, has been recognized as an important prognostic factor in patients with liver cirrhosis.[72–75] Hyponatremia is associated with neurologic dysfunction, refractory ascites, hepatorenal syndrome, and death from liver disease.[76,77] Hyponatremia, with lower sodium values portending worse outcomes, has been shown to be an independent predictor of survival at 3 and 12 months.[78,79]

Given the important prognostic value of sodium, its role has been evaluated as an adjunct to the MELD score in prediction of mortality in patients with end-stage liver disease. After controlling for MELD, serum sodium was associated with a higher risk of mortality: each 1 mmol/L decrease in the serum sodium concentration for values between 125 and 140 mmol/L was associated with 5% increase in mortality (P<.001).[78] This effect was greater in patients with lower MELD scores. For 23% of the patients, the difference between the MELDNa and MELD scores was large enough to have affected allocation priority. About 7% of the deaths on the waiting list could have been prevented by using MELDNa rather than MELD. In addition to waiting-list mortality, serum sodium and MELD have been shown to be closely correlated with dropout rates among patients awaiting LT.[80]

We believe that an underlying event that decreases survival in hyponatremic patients is worsening renal function. As discussed earlier, serum creatinine is an imperfect gauge of renal function and hyponatremia may reflect an aspect of renal function that is not effectively captured by serum creatinine.[22] Hyponatremia may be an earlier and more sensitive marker than creatinine to detect renal impairment and/or circulatory dysfunction in patients with advanced cirrhosis.[81] In predicting mortality, survival models that include directly measured GFR are superior to those with serum creatinine or creatinine-based GFR estimates.[22] Once an accurate measure of GFR is taken into account, serum sodium is no longer significant.

Like other elements of the MELD score, serum sodium assessment is a widely measured objective and easily available. Potential limitations of the use of serum sodium include variability that may be altered by volume status and free-water intake, making it potentially subject to willful manipulation. However, altering serum sodium to a degree that significantly alters organ allocation is difficult.[32,78,79,82] It remains unknown whether correction of severe hyponatremia into the normal range (eg, by use of vaptans) restores the risk of mortality attributable to serum sodium. Based on our hypothesis that the underlying process of hyponatremia is progressive renal dysfunction, we predict that the effects of hyponatremia are not easily ameliorated by simple correction of serum sodium. Whether transplanting patients with hyponatremia would simply shift the mortality from the waiting list to after transplantation is also a potential concern. Although data about the impact of pretransplant hyponatremia on posttransplant outcome are conflicting, the largest US study showed that hyponatremia (of any degree) did not have a detrimental impact on survival 90 days after LT (HR 1.00; $P = .99$). Thus, incorporating serum sodium in the organ allocation process may not adversely affect the overall outcome after LT.[22]

Reweighting Components of MELD

Given the origin of the MELD score in patients undergoing TIPS, reweighting the components of the MELD score using a contemporary cohort of LT candidates may improve prediction of waiting-list mortality.[83] Recently, Leise and colleagues[32] examined (1) whether the mortality prediction by MELD could be improved by optimizing the coefficients of MELD based on patients on waiting lists, and (2) whether addition of serum sodium remains important once the coefficients for the components of MELD have been optimized. Based on the UNOS data, a model was developed and validated that includes updated coefficients and amended upper and lower limit bounds with and without serum sodium. This model has statistically significant gain in its ability to rank LT candidates based on their risk of mortality and hence their chance of receiving an LT (**Box 1**). The model's discrimination was also superior in candidates listed at a MELD score greater than or equal to 15. Implementation of the new score would affect 3.3% of all waiting-list registrants and 12.0% of all transplants, with 9% fewer deaths.

The existing upper and lower bounds of each variable set by the UNOS were empiric and not evidence based. We reexamined these bounds in an iterative fashion with final determination of the bounds based on statistical relevance (goodness of fit) as well as physiologic interpretation (eg, the upper limit of normal) of the cutoff values. A lower limit for serum creatinine (0.8) would effectively capture persons with renal dysfunction that is not adequately represented by a falsely low serum creatinine because of decreased muscle mass. An upper limit cutoff of 3.0 fits the data better and allays the purported emphasis on renal dysfunction and transplantation of patients with intrinsic liver disease. A cutoff for INR would limit the impact of outliers, many of

---

Box 1
Proposed modification of MELD score and MELDNa score to update coefficients, change upper and lower bounds, and incorporate serum sodium levels using waiting-list data from adult primary liver transplantation candidates from the Organ Procurement and Transplantation Network (2005–2008)

ReFit MELD = $4.082 \times \log_e(\text{bilirubin}) + 8.485 \times \log_e(\text{creatinine}) + 10.671 \times \log_e(\text{INR}) + 7.432$

Bilirubin = bilirubin bounded below by 1 mg/dL; creatinine = creatinine bounded by 0.8 mg/dL below and 3 mg/dL above; INR = INR bounded by 1 below and 3 above. Renal replacement therapy = 3 mg/dL.

ReFit MELDNa = $4.258 \times \log_e(\text{bilirubin}) + 6.792 \times \log_e(\text{creatinine}) + 8.290 \times \log_e(\text{INR}) + 0.652 \times (140-\text{Na}) - 0.194 \times (140-\text{Na}) \times \text{bilirubin} + 6.327$

bilirubin = bilirubin bounded below by 1 mg/dL and above by 20 mg/dL; creatinine = creatinine bounded by 0.8 mg/dL below and 3 mg/dL above; INR =INR bounded by 1 below and 3 above. Renal replacement therapy = 3 mg/dL; sodium (Na) = Na bounded by 125 mEq/L below and 140 mEq/L above.

Abbreviation: Na, serum sodium.

whom may be taking warfarin. The impact of hyponatremia is greatest in persons with a low bilirubin; hence, to reflect the interaction between sodium and bilirubin, an upper limit of bilirubin (20 mg/dL) is introduced.

SUMMARY

The MELD score has been an important contribution to hepatology given its ability to accurately gauge the severity of liver disease and effectively assess the risk of mortality and determine organ allocation priority in patients wait-listed for LT in the United States as well as many countries around the world. It has become part of the hepatologists vocabulary because MELD score conveys a succinct picture of the health status of a patient with end-stage liver disease. By design, it is continually evolving; it lends itself to continued refinement and improvement in a data-driven fashion. We believe that the MELD score will be used as a template to improve on as an objective gauge of disease severity and a metric to optimize allocation of scarce donor organs for liver transplantation for the next decade and beyond.

REFERENCES

1. Olthoff KM, Brown RS Jr, Delmonico FL, et al. Summary report of a national conference: evolving concepts in liver allocation in the MELD and PELD era. December 8, 2003, Washington, DC, USA. Liver Transpl 2004;10(10 Suppl 2): A6–22.
2. Freeman RB, Wiesner RH, Edwards E, et al. Results of the first year of the new liver allocation plan. Liver Transpl 2004;10(1):7–15.
3. Kamath PS, Kim WR. The Model for End-stage Liver Disease (MELD). Hepatology 2007;45(3):797–805.
4. Freeman RB Jr. Model for End-stage Liver Disease (MELD) for liver allocation: a 5-year score card. Hepatology 2008;47(3):1052–7.
5. Lake JR. MELD–an imperfect, but thus far the best, solution to the problem of organ allocation. J Gastrointestin Liver Dis 2008;17(1):5–7.
6. Freeman RB Jr. Is waiting time a measure of access to liver transplantation? Is shorter necessarily better? Hepatology 2007;46(2):602–3.
7. Freeman RB Jr. The Model for End-stage Liver Disease comes of age. Clin Liver Dis 2007;11(2):249–63.
8. Wiesner R, Lake JR, Freeman RB, et al. Model for End-stage Liver Disease (MELD) exception guidelines. Liver Transpl 2006;12(12 Suppl 3):S85–87.
9. Freeman RB Jr, Edwards EB. Liver transplant waiting time does not correlate with waiting list mortality: implications for liver allocation policy. Liver Transpl 2000; 6(5):543–52.
10. Assessing current policies and the potential impact of the DHHS Final Rule. In: Committee on Organ Procurement and Transplantation Policy O, Transplantation. Pa, editors. Washington, DC: National Academy Press; 1999.
11. Malinchoc M, Kamath PS, Gordon FD, et al. A model to predict poor survival in patients undergoing transjugular intrahepatic portosystemic shunts. Hepatology 2000;31:864–71.
12. Kamath PS, Wiesner RH, Malinchoc M, et al. A model to predict survival in patients with end-stage liver disease. Hepatology 2001;33(2):464–70.
13. Freeman RB Jr, Wiesner RH, Harper A, et al. The new liver allocation system: moving toward evidence-based transplantation policy. Liver Transpl 2002;8(9): 851–8.

14. Fink MA, Angus PW, Gow PJ, et al. Liver transplant recipient selection: MELD vs. clinical judgment. Liver Transpl 2005;11(6):621–6.
15. Gish RG. Do we need to MEND the MELD? Liver Transpl 2007;13(4):486–7.
16. Charlton MR, Wall WJ, Ojo AO, et al. Report of the first international liver transplantation society expert panel consensus conference on renal insufficiency in liver transplantation. Liver Transpl 2009;15(11):S1–34.
17. Eason JD, Gonwa TA, Davis CL, et al. Proceedings of Consensus Conference on Simultaneous Liver Kidney Transplantation (SLK). Am J Transplant 2008;8(11): 2243–51.
18. Sharma P, Welch K, Eikstadt R, et al. Renal outcomes after liver transplantation in the Model for End-stage Liver Disease era. Liver Transpl 2009;15(9):1142–8.
19. Nair S, Verma S, Thuluvath PJ. Pretransplant renal function predicts survival in patients undergoing orthotopic liver transplantation. Hepatology 2002;35(5):1179–85.
20. Francoz C, Glotz D, Moreau R, et al. The evaluation of renal function and disease in patients with cirrhosis. J Hepatol 2010;52(4):605–13.
21. Francoz C, Prie D, Abdelrazek W, et al. Inaccuracies of creatinine and creatinine-based equations in candidates for liver transplantation with low creatinine: impact on the Model for End-stage Liver Disease score. Liver Transpl 2010;16(10): 1169–77.
22. Lim YS, Larson TS, Benson JT, et al. Serum sodium, renal function, and survival of patients with end-stage liver disease. J Hepatol 2010;52(4):523–8.
23. Cholongitas E, Marelli L, Kerry A, et al. Different methods of creatinine measurement significantly affect MELD scores. Liver Transpl 2007;13(4):523–9.
24. Arjal R, Trotter JF. International normalized ratio of prothrombin time in the Model for End-stage Liver Disease score: an unreliable measure. Clin Liver Dis 2009; 13(1):67–71.
25. Trotter JF, Olson J, Lefkowitz J, et al. Changes in International Normalized Ratio (INR) and Model for Endstage Liver Disease (MELD) based on selection of clinical laboratory. Am J Transplant 2007;7(6):1624–8.
26. Bellest L, Eschwege V, Poupon R, et al. A modified International Normalized Ratio as an effective way of prothrombin time standardization in hepatology. Hepatology 2007;46(2):528–34.
27. Tripodi A, Chantarangkul V, Primignani M, et al. The International Normalized Ratio calibrated for cirrhosis [INR(liver)] normalizes prothrombin time results for Model for End-stage Liver Disease calculation. Hepatology 2007;46(2):520–7.
28. Porte RJ, Lisman T, Tripodi A, et al. The International Normalized Ratio (INR) in the MELD score: problems and solutions. Am J Transplant 2010;10(6):1349–53.
29. Biggins SW, Bambha K. MELD-based liver allocation: who is underserved? Semin Liver Dis 2006;26(3):211–20.
30. Heuman DM, Mihas AA, Habib A, et al. MELD-XI: a rational approach to "sickest first" liver transplantation in cirrhotic patients requiring anticoagulant therapy. Liver Transpl 2007;13(1):30–7.
31. Marlar RA. Determining the Model for End-stage Liver Disease with better accuracy: neutralizing the international normalized ratio pitfalls. Hepatology 2007; 46(2):295–6.
32. Leise MD, Kim WR, Kremers WK, et al. A revised Model for End-stage Liver Disease optimizes prediction of mortality among patients awaiting liver transplantation. Gastroenterology 2011;140(7):1952–60.
33. Austin MT, Poulose BK, Ray WA, et al. Model for End-stage Liver Disease: did the new liver allocation policy affect waiting list mortality? Arch Surg 2007;142(11): 1079–85.

34. Thuluvath PJ, Guidinger MK, Fung JJ, et al. Liver transplantation in the United States, 1999-2008. Am J Transplant 2010;10(4 Pt 2):1003–19.

35. Kim HJ, Larson JJ, Lim YS, et al. Impact of MELD on waitlist outcome of retransplant candidates. Am J Transplant 2010;10(12):2652–7.

36. Freeman RB, Harper A, Edwards EB. Excellent liver transplant survival rates under the MELD/PELD system. Transplant Proc 2005;37(2):585–8.

37. Kanwal F, Dulai GS, Spiegel BM, et al. A comparison of liver transplantation outcomes in the pre- vs. post-MELD eras. Aliment Pharmacol Ther 2005;21(2): 169–77.

38. Benckert C, Quante M, Thelen A, et al. Impact of the MELD allocation after its implementation in liver transplantation. Scand J Gastroenterol 2011;46(7–8): 941–8.

39. Nagler E, Van Vlierberghe H, Colle I, et al. Impact of MELD on short-term and long-term outcome following liver transplantation: a European perspective. Eur J Gastroenterol Hepatol 2005;17(8):849–56.

40. Palmiero HO, Kajikawa P, Boin IF, et al. Liver recipient survival rate before and after Model for End-stage Liver Disease implementation and use of donor risk index. Transplant Proc 2010;42(10):4113–5.

41. Pomfret EA, Washburn K, Wald C, et al. Report of a national conference on liver allocation in patients with hepatocellular carcinoma in the United States. Liver Transpl 2010;16(3):262–78.

42. Thuluvath PJ, Maheshwari A, Thuluvath NP, et al. Survival after liver transplantation for hepatocellular carcinoma in the Model for End-stage Liver Disease and pre-Model for End-stage Liver Disease eras and the independent impact of hepatitis C virus. Liver Transpl 2009;15(7):754–62.

43. Washburn K. Model for End Stage Liver Disease and hepatocellular carcinoma: a moving target. Transplant Rev (Orlando) 2010;24(1):11–7.

44. Washburn K, Edwards E, Harper A, et al. Hepatocellular carcinoma patients are advantaged in the current liver transplant allocation system. Am J Transplant 2010;10(7):1643–8.

45. Davis CL. Impact of implementation of the MELD scoring system on the prevalence and incidence of chronic renal disease following liver transplantation. Liver Transpl 2006;12(5):707–9.

46. Machicao VI, Srinivas TR, Hemming AW, et al. Impact of implementation of the MELD scoring system on the prevalence and incidence of chronic renal disease following liver transplantation. Liver Transpl 2006;12(5):754–61.

47. Davis CL. Kidney failure in liver transplantation: it is time for action. Am J Transplant 2006;6(11):2533–4.

48. Gonwa TA, McBride MA, Anderson K, et al. Continued influence of preoperative renal function on outcome of orthotopic liver transplant (OLTX) in the US: where will MELD lead us? Am J Transplant 2006;6(11):2651–9.

49. Merion RM, Schaubel DE, Dykstra DM, et al. The survival benefit of liver transplantation. Am J Transplant 2005;5(2):307–13.

50. Volk ML, Lok AS, Pelletier SJ, et al. Impact of the Model for End-stage Liver Disease allocation policy on the use of high-risk organs for liver transplantation. Gastroenterology 2008;135(5):1568–74.

51. Schaubel DE, Sima CS, Goodrich NP, et al. The survival benefit of deceased donor liver transplantation as a function of candidate disease severity and donor quality. Am J Transplant 2008;8(2):419–25.

52. Hameed B, Lake JR. Using higher risk organs for liver transplantation: in whom and at what price? Gastroenterology 2008;135(5):1452–4.

53. Brown RS Jr, Lake JR. The survival impact of liver transplantation in the MELD era, and the future for organ allocation and distribution. Am J Transplant 2005; 5(2):203–4.
54. Lai JC, Terrault NA, Vittinghoff E, et al. Height contributes to the gender difference in wait-list mortality under the MELD-based liver allocation system. Am J Transplant 2010;10(12):2658–64.
55. Moylan CA, Brady CW, Johnson JL, et al. Disparities in liver transplantation before and after introduction of the MELD score. JAMA 2008;300(20):2371–8.
56. Myers RP, Shaheen AA, Aspinall AI, et al. Gender, renal function, and outcomes on the liver transplant waiting list: assessment of revised MELD including estimated glomerular filtration rate. J Hepatol 2011;54(3):462–70.
57. Cholongitas E, Thomas M, Senzolo M, et al. Gender disparity and MELD in liver transplantation. J Hepatol 2011;55(2):500–1.
58. Cholongitas E, Marelli L, Kerry A, et al. Female liver transplant recipients with the same GFR as male recipients have lower MELD scores–a systematic bias. Am J Transplant 2007;7(3):685–92.
59. Leise MD, Larson JJ, Benson J, et al. Sexism in liver transplantation? The impact of gender specific creatinine values on waitlist mortality. Hepatology 2010; 52(S1):177.
60. Durand F, Valla D. Assessment of prognosis of cirrhosis. Semin Liver Dis 2008; 28(1):110–22.
61. D'Amico G, Garcia-Tsao G, Pagliaro L. Natural history and prognostic indicators of survival in cirrhosis: a systematic review of 118 studies. J Hepatol 2006;44(1): 217–31.
62. Yantorno SE, Kremers WK, Ruf AE, et al. MELD is superior to King's college and Clichy's criteria to assess prognosis in fulminant hepatic failure. Liver Transpl 2007;13(6):822–8.
63. Kremers WK, van IM, Kim WR, et al. MELD score as a predictor of pretransplant and posttransplant survival in OPTN/UNOS status 1 patients. Hepatology 2004; 39(3):764–9.
64. Alessandria C, Ozdogan O, Guevara M, et al. MELD score and clinical type predict prognosis in hepatorenal syndrome: relevance to liver transplantation. Hepatology 2005;41(6):1282–9.
65. Northup PG, Wanamaker RC, Lee YD, et al. Model for end-stage liver disease (MELD) predicts nontransplant surgical mortality in patients with cirrhosis. Ann Surg 2005;242(2):244–51.
66. Teh SH, Nagorney DM, Stevens SR, et al. Risk factors for mortality after surgery in patients with cirrhosis. Gastroenterology 2007;132(4):1261–9.
67. Bambha K, Kim WR, Kremers W, et al. Predicting survival among patients listed for liver transplantation: an assessment of serial MELD measurements. Am J Transplant 2004;4(11):1798–804.
68. Huo TI, Wu JC, Lin HC, et al. Evaluation of the increase in Model for End-stage Liver Disease (DeltaMELD) score over time as a prognostic predictor in patients with advanced cirrhosis: risk factor analysis and comparison with initial MELD and Child-Turcotte-Pugh score. J Hepatol 2005;42(6):826–32.
69. Kamath PS, Kim WR. Is the change in MELD score a better indicator of mortality than baseline MELD score? Liver Transpl 2003;9(1):19–21.
70. Merion RM, Wolfe RA, Dykstra DM, et al. Longitudinal assessment of mortality risk among candidates for liver transplantation. Liver Transpl 2003;9(1):12–8.
71. D'Amico G. Developing concepts on MELD: delta and cutoffs. J Hepatol 2005; 42(6):790–2.

72. Biggins SW, Kim WR, Terrault NA, et al. Evidence-based incorporation of serum sodium concentration into MELD. Gastroenterology 2006;130(6):1652–60.
73. Biggins SW, Rodriguez HJ, Bacchetti P, et al. Serum sodium predicts mortality in patients listed for liver transplantation. Hepatology 2005;41(1):32–9.
74. Heuman D, Abou-assi SG, Habib A, et al. Persistent ascites and low serum sodium identify patients with cirrhosis and low MELD scores who are at high risk for early death. Hepatology 2004;40(4):802–10.
75. Ruf AE, Kremers W, Chavez LL, et al. Addition of serum sodium into the MELD score predicts waiting list mortality better than MELD alone. Liver Transpl 2005; 11(3):336–43.
76. Gines P, Guevara M. Hyponatremia in cirrhosis: pathogenesis, clinical significance, and management. Hepatology 2008;48(3):1002–10.
77. Gines P, Schrier RW. Renal failure in cirrhosis. N Engl J Med 2009;361(13): 1279–90.
78. Kim WR, Biggins SW, Kremers WK, et al. Hyponatremia and mortality among patients on the liver-transplant waiting list. N Engl J Med 2008;359(10):1018–26.
79. Londono MC, Cardenas A, Guevara M, et al. MELD score and serum sodium in the prediction of survival of patients with cirrhosis awaiting liver transplantation. Gut 2007;56(9):1283–90.
80. Biselli M, Gitto S, Gramenzi A, et al. Six score systems to evaluate candidates with advanced cirrhosis for orthotopic liver transplant: which is the winner? Liver Transpl 2010;16(8):964–73.
81. Wiesner RH. Evidence-based evolution of the MELD/PELD liver allocation policy. Liver Transpl 2005;11(3):261–3.
82. Gerbes AL, Huber E, Gulberg V. Terlipressin for hepatorenal syndrome: continuous infusion as an alternative to I.V. bolus administration. Gastroenterology 2009;137(3): [author reply: 1179–81].
83. Sharma P, Schaubel DE, Sima CS, et al. Re-weighting the Model for End-stage Liver Disease score components. Gastroenterology 2008;135(5):1575–81.

Transplantation for Cholangiocarcinoma

Howard C. Masuoka, MD, PhD[a], Charles B. Rosen, MD[b],*

KEYWORDS

- Cholangiocarcinoma • Klatskin tumor • Liver transplantation
- Living donor liver transplantation • Neoadjuvant therapy
- Biliary stricture • Biliary stenting • Acute cholangitis

Cholangiocarcinoma (CCA) is a primary hepatic neoplasm that arises from the malignant transformation of cholangiocytes, the epithelial cells that line the biliary tree. Most tumors are classified as adenocarcinoma. CCA is the second most common primary hepatic malignancy and it is increasing in incidence globally.[1–4] Nevertheless, CCA remains a rare malignancy with 3500 to 5000 cases diagnosed annually in the United States and an incidence of approximately 0.85 per 100,000.[5]

RISK FACTORS

Although most cases of CCA arise in patients without an identifiable risk factor (ie, de novo CCA), several risk factors for the development of CCA have been identified, with chronic biliary inflammation being a common feature shared by many of them. Primary sclerosing cholangitis (PSC) is the most common identifiable risk factor in Western countries. The incidence of CCA in patients with PSC is 0.6% to 1.5% per year.[6,7] The lifetime risk of developing CCA in patients with PSC is between 7% and 17%, depending on the series.[6–9] Interestingly, the risk of developing CCA is not associated with the duration or severity of PSC or the presence of inflammatory bowel disease.[10] Chronic infection with the Asian liver flukes *Opisthorchis viverrini* and *Clonorchis sinensis* are risk factors for the development of CCA.[11] The high prevalence of *O viverrini* infection in Northeast Thailand is likely responsible for the highest incidence of CCA in the world (96/100,000 in men and 38/100,000 in women).[12] Patients who received Thorotrast, a radiograph contrast agent used in the 1930s to 1950s that contains the radioactive compound thorium dioxide, are at an increased risk for the development of several cancers, including CCA, decades after exposure. CCA is one of the cancers that occur at an increased frequency in patients with Lynch syndrome.[13] Biliary papillomatosis, a condition characterized by multiple papillary

[a] Division of Gastroenterology and Hepatology, Indiana University School of Medicine, 541 North Clinical Drive/CL 500, Indianapolis, IN 46202, USA
[b] Division of Transplantation Surgery and Mayo Clinic William J. von Liebig Transplant Center, Mayo Clinic College of Medicine, 200 First Street Southwest, Rochester, MN 55905, USA
* Corresponding author.
E-mail address: rosen.charles@mayo.edu

Clin Liver Dis 15 (2011) 699–715
doi:10.1016/j.cld.2011.08.004
1089-3261/11/$ – see front matter © 2011 Elsevier Inc. All rights reserved.

adenomas in the biliary tree, carries a significant risk for the development of papillary adenocarcinoma and mucinous carcinoma forms of CCA.[14] Choledochal cysts carry a significant risk for the development of CCA by adulthood.[15,16] Cirrhosis from common causes, such as chronic hepatitis C and steatohepatitis, also carries an increased risk for CCA.[17]

PATHOPHYSIOLOGY AND CLASSIFICATION

Greater than 90% of CCAs are adenocarcinomas.[18] Typically CCA is a well-differentiated to moderately differentiated adenocarcinoma with a prominent, dense, desmoplastic stroma (**Fig. 1**). This stroma leads to annular thickening of the bile duct caused by the infiltration and fibrosis of the periductal tissues. The large amount of fibrous stroma greatly increases the difficulty in confirming CCA by cytology and biopsy. Uncommon histologic variants include papillary adenocarcinoma, squamous cell, mucinous, lymphoepitheliomalike, and anaplastic carcinoma.[18,19] Tumor cells are frequently positive for the immunohistochemical markers cytokeratins-7 and -20, alpha-v beta-6 integrin, cytoplasmic carcinoembryonic antigen, mucins, and epidermal growth factor receptor (EGFR).[20–22]

CCA is classified as either intrahepatic or extrahepatic based on its location in the biliary tree. This classification is relevant given the typically different presentations and management of intrahepatic versus extrahepatic CCA.

Intrahepatic CCA originates in a bile duct within the hepatic parenchyma. Intrahepatic CCA is typically a mass-forming neoplasm and is often confused with metastatic

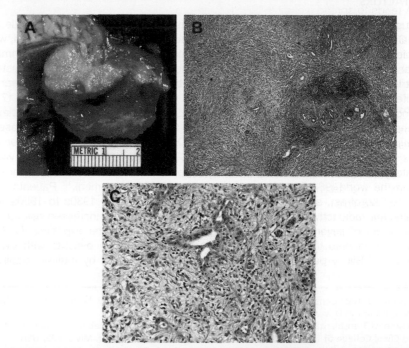

Fig. 1. Gross and microscopic pathology of CCA. (*A*) Gross pathology of CCA present in the distal common bile duct. (*B*) Microscopic pathology of CCA. CCA is present on the left portion of the image, benign peribiliary glands are located on the right, and normal liver tissue is in the upper portion of the image. (*C*) Higher power view of CCA. (*Courtesy of* Dr Thomas C. Smyrk, Mayo Clinic.)

adenocarcinoma of unknown primary. As with other intrahepatic malignancies, intrahepatic CCA typically has an insidious presentation consisting of mild abdominal pain, weight loss, nausea, and anorexia. Jaundice is rare but it can occur with advanced tumors that grow into the liver hilus and obstruct the biliary confluence. Intrahepatic CCA usually presents late, and patients frequently have evidence of extrahepatic metastases on imaging.

Extrahepatic CCA involves the bile ducts outside of the hepatic parenchyma. Extrahepatic CCA is more common than intrahepatic CCA and accounts for approximately two-thirds of all CCA. Approximately 60% of extrahepatic CCA involve the hepatic hilum (ie, so-called hilar CCA or Klatskin tumors), making it the most common type of CCA.[23] Extrahepatic CCA has been classified by the Bismuth-Corlette classification (**Fig. 2**) based on the tumor involvement of the common hepatic duct, biliary confluence, and right or left ductal systems.[24] These tumors frequently present with obstructive symptoms, such as jaundice, dark urine, pale stools, pruritus, malaise, abdominal pain, and weight loss. It is uncommon for patients to develop cholangitis because of the insidious nature of the obstruction. Those at risk for cholangitis often have underlying PSC or have undergone instrumentation of the biliary tree. Laboratory tests frequently demonstrate a cholestatic picture with increased total and direct bilirubin, alkaline phosphatase, and gamma-glutamyltransferase. If the tumor has only unilateral involvement of the biliary system, it will often be asymptomatic until it progresses to obstruct the contralateral biliary system or has become quite large. CCA should always be considered in patients with PSC who develop rapid decompensation of their disease.

CCA tends to spread along the bile duct and to adjacent structures. Metastasis to distant sites is uncommon early in the disease course. Although compression of local vascular structures is frequently seen, extension into vessels and tumor thrombus are rare. Metastasis to regional lymph nodes is common and is an adverse prognostic survival factor. Late metastatic spread typically involves distant lymph nodes and the peritoneum, with metastasis to the lung and bone being less common.

Diagnosis

Diagnosis of CCA can be difficult because of subtle or nonspecific imaging findings. The desmoplastic nature of this tumor makes obtaining a definitive tissue diagnosis difficult. Diagnosing CCA is especially challenging in patients with underlying biliary tract diseases, such as PSC. Rapid decompensation of previously stable disease, especially in the setting of a dominant stricture, should prompt consideration of CCA as the possible underlying cause. Criteria for diagnosis of CCA are listed in **Box 1**.

In patients with CCA presenting with obstructive jaundice, ultrasonography is usually the best initial imaging modality. It will typically demonstrate intrahepatic bile duct dilation. Ultrasonography can also demonstrate intrahepatic metastases, occlusion of hepatic arteries and portal veins, or enlargement of lymph nodes that are concerning for metastatic disease. Cross-sectional imaging, such as a computerized tomography (CT), is typically obtained to provide anatomic details needed for the determination of resectability. Local invasion, the relationship of the tumor to the hilar vessels, lobar atrophy, regional and distant lymph node enlargement, and distant metastases can all be readily appreciated with CT.

Imaging of the biliary system is critical in defining the location and extent of the tumor. Endoscopic retrograde cholangiopancreatography (ERCP) provides the most detailed visualization of the biliary strictures and permits brush cytology and biopsies of the bile ducts. Magnetic resonance imaging (MRI) with concurrent magnetic resonance cholangiopancreatography (MRCP) can also be used. Although MRCP is

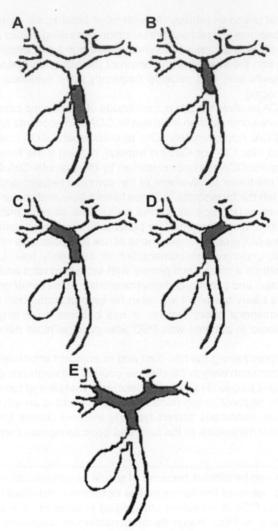

Fig. 2. Bismuth-Corlette classification of hilar CCA. (*A*) CCA is classified as Bismuth-Corlette type I CCA if there is only involvement of the common hepatic duct at least 2 cm below the confluence of the left and right hepatic ducts, (*B*) type II if there is involvement of the common hepatic duct less than 2 cm from the biliary confluence without invasion above the confluence, type IIIa and type IIIb if there is involvement of the biliary confluence and the right (*C*) or left (*D*) bile duct, respectively, and (*E*) type IV if there is involvement of the biliary confluence along with secondary biliary radicals or multiple discontinuous sites in the right and left ductal systems.

unable to obtain cells for cytologic examination, it has the advantages of being much less invasive and able to define biliary anatomy beyond strictures too narrow to pass via ERCP (**Fig. 3**). MRI provides cross-sectional imaging that provides additional information regarding the biliary tree and the involvement of surrounding structures (ie, segmental bile duct dilatation, atrophy, intrahepatic metastasis, and vascular encasement). Therefore, MRI/MRCP has become the imaging modality of choice for this neoplasm.

Box 1
Diagnostic criteria for CCA

1. Definitive diagnostic criteria

   a. Biopsy (transluminal) positive for cancer

   b. Positive or suspicious cytology on brush cytology

   c. Mass lesion on cross-sectional imaging

   d. Malignant-appearing stricture and Cancer Antigen 19-9 (CA 19-9), >100 U/ml, or fluorescence in situ hybridization (FISH) polysomy

2. Indeterminate diagnostic criteria

   a. FISH trisomy (7 or 3)

   b. Dysplasia

   c. FISH polysomy in absence of malignant-appearing stricture

   d. Malignant-appearing stricture in absence of mass lesion, positive cytology, biopsy, elevated CA 19.9, or FISH polysomy

---

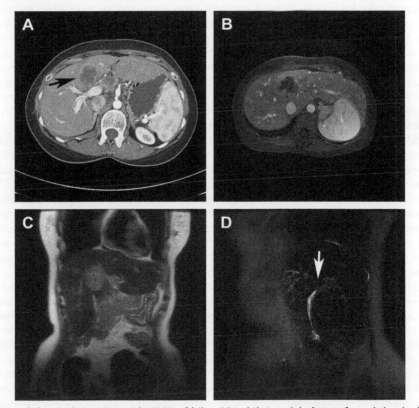

Fig. 3. Abdominal CT, MRI, and MRCP of hilar CCA. (*A*) Arterial phase of an abdominal CT demonstrating a hilar CCA that appears as a low-density peripherally enhancing mass at the junction of the right and left main hepatic ducts (*black arrow*). (*B*) MRI of the same patient following contrast administration. (*C*) Coronal view of MRI from this patient. (*D*) MRCP on the same patient demonstrating a stricture at the hilum seen as a filling defect (*white arrow*) with associated intrahepatic ductal dilatation.

Abdominal imaging by CT or MRI can aid in the diagnosis of CCA and is a critical component in the evaluation of the resectability of CCA. Frequently, these studies do not demonstrate a mass, especially in patients with CCA occurring in the setting of PSC. On abdominal CT, CCA occasionally seems to be a hypodense lesion with delayed venous phase enhancement after intravenous contrast administration. On MRI, CCA seems hypointense on T1-weighted images, hyperintense on T2-weighted images, and enhances with MRI contrast. Visualization of CCA by MRI is usually improved with the infusion of superparamagnetic iron (eg, ferumoxides, such as Feridex) that results in the darkening of the surrounding hepatic parenchyma and enhanced visualization of the CCA with delayed gadolinium images. Unilateral lobular bile duct obstruction often results in atrophy of the affected hepatic lobe with hypertrophy of the unaffected lobe, a phenomenon known as the atrophy-hypertrophy complex. The presence of atrophy alone suggests vascular encasement of the affected lobe by CCA.

Suspicious biliary lesions should be sampled by ERCP with biliary brushings and intraductal biopsy for histologic and cytologic analysis. A percutaneous cholangiogram can be used if the lesion cannot be accessed via ERCP. When possible, ERCP is preferred to percutaneous transhepatic cholangiography because of the increased risks for seeding of the tumor along the percutaneous tract. The sensitivity of routine cytology ranges from almost 20% to 60% and the specificity varies from 61% to 100% depending on the series.[25] Fluorescent in situ hybridization (FISH) is an advanced cytologic test for aneuploidy that aids early diagnosis of CCA, especially in high-risk patients.[26] FISH uses fluorescent probes to detect chromosomal amplification or loss. The addition of this technique to routine cytology increases the sensitivity without compromising the specificity for the diagnosis of CCA. In the authors' experience, FISH analysis permits the detection of an additional 14% of CCA in patients with PSC who had normal cytology.

Endoscopic ultrasound (EUS)-guided sampling of regional lymph nodes is useful in determining the resectability of CCA. In a small series of patients with CCA, EUS with fine-needle aspiration of visualized regional lymph nodes demonstrated nodal metastases in 17% of patients without lymphadenopathy by prior imaging studies.[27] It cannot be overemphasized that EUS-guided or percutaneous biopsy or fine-needle aspiration of hilar masses or biliary strictures is not recommended for patients with disease that might be amenable to potentially curative treatment. These transperitoneal procedures cause tumor seeding. Indeed, diagnostic biopsy or aspiration with either of these approaches is now one of the exclusion criteria for transplantation under the Mayo CCA liver transplantation protocol.

Tumor markers, although nonspecific, can aid in the diagnosis of CCA. CA 19-9 has proven the most useful. CA 19-9 detects circulating high-molecular-weight mucin glycoproteins coated with sialylated blood group epitopes (ie, sialyl Lewis). It is important to bear in mind that other malignancies and bacterial cholangitis can result in an increase in CA 19-9. Also, approximately 7% of the population is Lewis negative and will always have an undetectable CA 19-9 even in the presence of malignancy.[28] A serum CA 19-9 of greater than 100 U/mL is 89% sensitive and 86% specific for CCA in patients with PSC who do not have cholangitis but it has a sensitivity of only 53% in patients without PSC.[29]

Staging

The staging systems for CCA are still undergoing refinement because of the different pathobiology of intrahepatic and extrahepatic tumors and the trends in staging systems to better reflect the eligibility for surgical resection.

For intrahepatic CCA, stage I disease is defined as a solitary tumor without vascular invasion, stage II disease as a solitary tumor with vascular invasion, stage IIIA disease as multiple tumors with or without vascular invasion, stage IIIB disease as any tumor with regional lymph node metastasis, and stage IV disease as any tumor with distant metastases. This system correlates with survival after hepatic resection. The median 3-year survival rate following resection in one series was 74% for stage I, 48% for stage II, 18% for stage IIIA, and 7% for stage IIIB CCA.[30]

Because the only effective treatment of extrahepatic CCA is resection or liver transplantation, the staging system for extrahepatic CCA has evolved toward one that determines resectability. The T-stage modification of the Memorial Sloan-Kettering staging system for hilar tumors is based on the involvement of biliary and vascular structures and correlates with the resectability of hilar tumors.[31] In this system, T1 tumors involve the biliary confluence and may also have unilateral extension to second-order biliary radicles. T2 tumors have ipsilateral portal vein involvement and may have ipsilateral hepatic lobar atrophy. T3 tumors have unilateral extension to second-order biliary radicles with contralateral portal vein involvement or contralateral hepatic lobar atrophy or main or bilateral portal venous involvement.

A new staging system has been proposed by an international group of hepatobiliary and transplant surgeons and hepatologists. This system combines the strengths of other systems and provides a comprehensive description of CCA such that investigators will be able to compare results of different treatment modalities at a multitude of centers. A registry using this system is under development.[32]

Management of Biliary Strictures

Dilation and stenting of biliary strictures should be done to alleviate obstruction and treat cholangitis. If neither of these is present, placement of a prophylactic stent is not recommended. Drainage of ducts from the dominant hepatic lobe is typically sufficient to alleviate biliary obstruction. In most instances, drainage of both ductal systems is not necessary. For patients who may be transplant or resection candidates, the authors recommend placement of plastic rather than metallic biliary stents because the former can be easily removed at the time of the surgical procedure. Plastic biliary stents will typically remain patent for 8 to 12 weeks depending on their diameter. Exchange of the biliary stent is either performed at a predetermined interval or based on the signs of stent obstruction (jaundice, increasing liver function tests in an obstructive pattern, or acute cholangitis) depending on patient preference and the availability of ERCP. In patients with a biliary stent, it has been the authors' practice to provide these patients with a prescription for a 7-day course of oral antibiotics, such as a fluoroquinolone, to be taken if they develop acute cholangitis. Antibiotics will usually temporize the situation and allow an ERCP to be scheduled on an urgent rather than emergency basis. Percutaneous transhepatic cholangiography can also be used to manage biliary strictures. The authors recommend this approach only if ERCP is unsuccessful or contraindicated because they have observed several cases of seeding of tumor along the percutaneous tract. Such seeding is usually not evident until the staging laparotomy or in the posttransplant period.

Treatment

CCA continues to be a significant treatment challenge. To date, there are no nonsurgical therapies that are curative or even offer a substantial increase in patient survival. Surgical resection and neoadjuvant therapy with orthotropic liver transplantation in carefully selected patients are the only potentially curative treatment options.

CHEMOTHERAPY

Several chemotherapeutic regimens have been used in the treatment of CCA. However, the currently available chemotherapeutic or radiation therapy regimens only affect a modest improvement in patient survival. Most studies are difficult to interpret because of the small numbers of patients in each series and the inclusion of other neoplasms, such as gallbladder, pancreas, or hepatocellular carcinoma, which likely have a different response. Several regimens have used infusional 5-fluorouracil (5-FU) or gemcitabine alone or in combination with other agents. Studies are ongoing but the most promising regimen so far has been gemcitabine combined with cisplatin. One series had a median overall survival of 11.7 months in the cisplatin-gemcitabine group compared with 8.1 months in the gemcitabine monotherapy group.[33] Chemotherapy combined with radiation therapy has also been used in small series. The use of the multi-kinase inhibitors, Sorafenib and Sunitinib, are also potential therapies that are under investigation for CCA.[34] Targeted therapies, such as antibodies to vascular endothelial growth factor and EGFR, are currently in trials and are exciting potential therapies as first-line therapy in combination with established chemotherapy regimens or as salvage therapy.[35,36]

Because biliary obstruction is a major cause of morbidity and mortality in these patients, biliary stenting is commonly required in patients with extrahepatic CCA. Palliative biliary stenting reduces morbidity and results in modestly improved survival for patients with unresectable CCA from 3 months to 6 months.[37] The choice of biliary stent type depends on potential therapeutic interventions and patient life expectancy. Typically the authors use metallic biliary stents in patients who are not candidates for surgery or photodynamic therapy (PDT) and who have a life expectancy of greater than 2 months given the longer period of patency of these stents.

PDT is another palliative therapy that has shown some promise in the treatment of CCA. PDT involves the systemic infusion of a photosensitizing agent followed by the endoscopic biliary application of laser light at the appropriate wavelength resulting in selective tumor toxicity. PDT can typically be repeated every 3 months. If candidates for PDT require biliary stenting, the authors recommend the placement of plastic rather than metal stents. PDT has been demonstrated to increase median survival in unresectable extrahepatic CCA to 16 to 21 months compared with 3 to 7 months with biliary stenting alone.[38] However, PDT is only available at a limited number of centers and the improvement in survival is likely primarily caused by better treatment of biliary obstruction.

Locoregional therapy with transarterial chemoembolization has shown promise in treating patients with intrahepatic CCA without extrahepatic metastasis. In one series, the median survival from time of diagnosis was 20 months, with 1-, 2-, and 3-year survival of 75%, 39%, and 17%, respectively.[39] Radioembolization with yttrium-90 has also been used in the treatment of in intrahepatic CCA, although studies have not yet been published on the effectiveness of this therapy in CCA. Following locoregional therapy, patients are subsequently treated with systemic chemotherapy if they are candidates based on certain factors, such as performance status.

SURGICAL RESECTION

Surgical resection provides the only potential curative therapy for CCA. Unfortunately, CCA usually presents late in the disease course, and most patients have unresectable disease at presentation. Criteria for unresectability include distant lymph node or liver metastases; predicted inadequate function in the liver remnant; and bilobar involvement, including bilateral hepatic duct involvement of the secondary biliary radicals or atrophy of one lobe of the liver with encasement of the contralateral portal venous branch. Regional lymph node involvement is not a contraindication to resection. In the case of inadequate liver remnant, ipsilateral portal vein embolization can occasionally be used to induce compensatory contralateral lobe hypertrophy to provide adequate liver mass for survival in the immediate postoperative period. Hypertrophy typically requires 4 to 6 weeks to occur. Adequate biliary drainage is a requisite for hypertrophy of the contralateral lobe. It is important to bear in mind that PSC is a contraindication to surgical resection because of the survival rate of less than 5% at 3 years.[9,40]

The extent of surgical resection is determined by the need for a negative surgical margin and anatomy. For hilar CCA, the Bismuth-Corlette classification (see **Fig. 2**) is a useful guide to determine resectability. Bismuth-Corlette type I CCA (common hepatic duct at least 2 cm below the biliary confluence) only requires resection of the extrahepatic biliary tree, the gallbladder, and regional lymph nodes. Bismuth-Corlette type II CCA (common hepatic duct less than 2 cm from the biliary confluence) frequently requires the resection of a portion of the caudate (hepatic segment 1) or segment IV-A because of their proximity to the hilus. Bismuth-Corlette type IIIa and type IIIb (biliary confluence and the right or left bile duct, respectively) require hepatic lobectomy, including the caudate with resection of the extrahepatic biliary tree, gallbladder, and regional lymph nodes. Following resection, bilioenteric continuity is established via a hepaticojejunostomy.

It is the authors' practice to perform a staging laparoscopy in patients being considered for resection, typically before portal vein embolization or immediately before resection. Laparoscopy identifies peritoneal carcinomatosis or small intrahepatic metastases in up to 36% of patients previously thought to be resectable based on cross-sectional imaging.[41] Further evaluation for metastatic disease, including distant lymph node metastases, is performed during the laparotomy before hepatic resection. If metastatic disease is detected beyond the regional lymph nodes, resection is not performed and nonsurgical treatments are pursued.

The survival rate following resection varies widely in reported series likely because of the differences in patient selection and surgical technique. Depending on the series, survival following resection of CCA is approximately 53% to 83% at 1 year, 30% to 63% at 2 years, 16% to 48% at 3 years, and 16% to 44% at 5 years.[42–44] The median survival is 12 to 44 months compared with 5 months in unresected patients.[45] Overall, there has been a trend toward improved survival during the last 2 decades, likely because of the careful exclusion of patients with metastatic disease or PSC combined with more aggressive surgical resection. In particular, the addition of caudate resection to segmental hepatectomy for the resection of hilar CCA has improved long-term survival. A positive resection margin, lymph node metastasis, multiple tumors, tumor size, vascular invasion, and lymphatic invasion have been identified as risk factors for recurrence.[46,47] Importantly, patients with positive surgical margins have survival comparable with those receiving only palliative therapy.[31,48] Thus, there is no role for palliative resection. Obtaining a tumor-free margin can be difficult because the microscopic ductal spread is typically far more extensive than the macroscopic borders of the tumor. Locations of recurrence are typically biliary, hepatic, retroperitoneal or hilar lymph nodes, and peritoneal sites.

The role of biliary stenting in candidates for surgical resection remains complex and controversial. Adequate biliary drainage of the remnant liver is needed to ensure liver regeneration. However, excessive stenting of poorly drained segments promotes cholangitis and is associated with adverse postoperative infectious complications. Ultimately, biliary stenting is best undertaken with a team approach, including the endoscopist and surgeon.

Adjuvant chemotherapy and radiation therapy have not been clearly demonstrated to improve survival following resection. Some studies have demonstrated improved survival with adjuvant chemotherapy, whereas others have shown no benefit.[44,49] Adjuvant external beam radiation has not been shown to improve survival and may even lead to hepatic decompensation.[50] Further randomized trials are ongoing to help determine if there is a role for combined adjuvant chemotherapy and radiation. Similarly, the role for neoadjuvant chemotherapy and radiation therapy in a select group of patients before resection is yet to be determined.

LIVER TRANSPLANTATION

Initial experiences with orthotropic liver transplantation (OLT) for unresectable CCA were disappointing because of the frequent recurrence of CCA. The 5-year survival rate was only 5% to 15% in these early studies.[51,52] However, there were some long-term survivors among patients with negative surgical resection margins and negative regional lymph nodes.[53] This finding prompted the development of a protocol at the University of Nebraska and Mayo Clinic for neoadjuvant chemoradiation followed by OLT in highly selected patients with early stage, unresectable hilar CCA (**Fig. 4**). The success of this protocol is attributable to patient selection, neoadjuvant therapy with external beam radiation and intrabiliary radiation, and operative staging of all patients before liver transplantation.

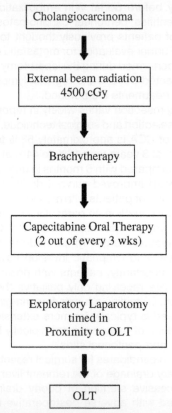

Cholangiocarcinoma

↓

External beam radiation
4500 cGy

↓

Brachytherapy

↓

Capecitabine Oral Therapy
(2 out of every 3 wks)

↓

Exploratory Laparotomy
timed in
Proximity to OLT

↓

OLT

Fig. 4. The Mayo Clinic protocol for liver transplantation with neoadjuvant chemotherapy and radiation therapy for hilar CCA.

Only patients that meet selective criteria are considered for liver transplantation under the CCA protocol. Patients must meet one of the definitive diagnostic criteria for CCA as listed in **Box 1**. These criteria include: (1) brush cytology or transluminal biopsy positive for adenocarcinoma, (2) an ERCP demonstrating a malignant-appearing stricture along with polysomy on FISH analysis on brushings of the stricture or a serum CA 19-9 of greater than 100 U/mL in the absence of cholangitis, or (3) a malignant-appearing stricture with an associated mass lesion on cross-sectional imaging.

Patients are not eligible for the protocol if they only meet indeterminate diagnostic criteria. (ie, have only dysplasia, trisomy on FISH, polysomy on FISH in the absence of a malignant-appearing stricture, or a malignant-appearing stricture with normal brushings and no mass). Such patients are suspected of having CCA and are followed closely with repeat ERCP with biliary brushings for cytology and FISH, cross-sectional imaging, and laboratory testing. It should be noted that liver transplantation is contra-indicated in patients with intrahepatic CCA because of the extremely high recurrence rates and lack of effective neoadjuvant or adjuvant therapy. Patients are also excluded if they have extrahepatic CCA with intrahepatic metastasis; evidence of extrahepatic disease, including local lymph node metastasis; prior attempts at resection; prior treatment with chemotherapy or radiation; or have undergone transperitoneal, percu-taneous, or EUS-guided fine-needle aspiration, or biopsy of the primary tumor. Vascular compression, including the encasement of 1 or more of the hilar vessels, is common with CCA and is not a contraindication because actual vascular invasion is extremely rare with this tumor. Preoperative staging to evaluate for extrahepatic metastases includes a CT scan of the chest and abdomen, bone scan, and EUS with biopsies of regional lymph nodes.

All patients are treated with continuous infusion 5-FU combined with external beam radiation therapy administered over a 4-week period. This treatment is followed 2 weeks later by brachytherapy in 4 sessions over 2 days via transcatheter radiation to the tumor. Patients are then maintained on a protracted course of oral chemo-therapy with capecitabine (Xeloda). Capecitabine is given as 3-week cycles with 2 weeks on and 1 week off therapy. Close to the expected time of transplantation and at least 2 weeks after brachytherapy, all patients undergo a pretransplant staging exploratory laparotomy to evaluate for metastatic disease. Regional lymph nodes are biopsied during the procedure even if they seem benign.[54]

The outcome for patients receiving OLT has been nearly as high as the survival for patients undergoing liver transplantation for benign disease. The first reported series of 11 patients transplanted for CCA following neoadjuvant therapy demonstrated 45% tumor-free survival with a median follow-up of 7.5 years.[55] In a subsequent series, survival following liver transplantation was 82% at 5 years.[54,56] From 1993 to March 2007, 131 patients were enrolled in the CCA protocol at Mayo Clinic. Following neo-adjuvant chemoradiation, 21% of these patients were found to have metastases at operative staging and did not undergo OLT. Eighty-one patients underwent OLT with 72% 5-year survival. These results are significantly better than results for patients who underwent resection and are comparable with those for patients undergoing liver transplantation for other indications. Results have been satisfactory with both deceased and living donor transplants.

Pretransplant Management

There are several issues in the pretransplant management of patients with CCA that are unique to this condition and deserve special attention.

Biliary obstruction is the major cause of morbidity in this patient population. Endoscopic biliary stenting is the preferred modality for biliary drainage given its negligible morbidity and mortality. Adequate drainage of a single functional hepatic lobe (30% of total liver volume) is sufficient to relieve cholestasis. Therefore, drainage of only one lobe is usually sufficient to relieve jaundice. More aggressive stenting is associated with an increased incidence of bacterial cholangitis and does not improve outcomes.[57] Metal stents are recommended only for patients who are not candidates for resection or liver transplantation. Percutaneous drainage can also be performed, especially when endoscopic intervention fails but it has the disadvantage of external drains, the risk of bile leakage, and the potential for tumor seeding along the percutaneous tract. Surgical biliary bypass is associated with high perioperative morbidity and mortality and is rarely necessary.

Acute cholangitis is a significant problem in this patient population and can carry significant morbidity and mortality if not treated appropriately and in a timely fashion. Typically, acute cholangitis does not become a significant issue until patients have undergone instrumentation of the biliary system. Adequate biliary drainage of an infected biliary segment is the cornerstone of treating acute cholangitis. It is important to emphasize that treatment with antibiotics in patients without subsequent adequate biliary drainage can result in the development of highly resistant bacteria and the formation of intrahepatic abscesses. Also, obstruction of up to half of the biliary system can occur even without a significant elevation of bilirubin, so a normal bilirubin should not be taken as an indication of adequate biliary drainage. The authors have found treatment with a course of a fluoroquinolone to provide adequate antibiotic coverage in most patients. Patients who develop a breakthrough of acute cholangitis symptoms while on antibiotic treatment are suspected of having antibiotic-resistant organisms. In such patients, the antibiotic coverage is broadened by treatment with piperacillin/tazobactam or a carbapenem. The addition of metronidazole or other coverage targeted at anaerobic organisms is rarely needed. It is the authors' practice to administer prophylactic antibiotics immediately before ERCP and for 3 to 5 days following the procedure. The authors typically provide patients who have a biliary stent in place or who have a history of acute cholangitis with a prescription for antibiotics to be taken at the onset of episodes of acute cholangitis. Prompt initiation of an antibiotic will usually temporize the situation and allow an ERCP to be scheduled on an urgent rather than emergency basis.

Cholecystitis can develop in patients either because of tumor involvement of the cystic duct origin or compression by biliary stents. Diagnosis is made through an abdominal ultrasound. As with acute cholangitis, the initiation of antibiotics and adequate drainage are critical. Endoscopic drainage through an ERCP is preferred, although it can be technically difficult and requires an experienced endoscopist. If this cannot be accomplished, then percutaneous tube cholecystostomy may be necessary. Cholecystectomy is avoided because of the high risk for tumor dissemination.

Neoadjuvant therapy creates several important issues in the pretransplant management of these patients. The authors administer 5-FU as a continuous infusion because of the improved tolerability compared with bolus administration. Capecitabine (Xeloda) is an oral chemotherapeutic agent that is enzymatically coverted to 5-FU and, thus, has a similar side-effect profile. Chemotherapy side effects are usually mild and do not become significant until near the end of the chemotherapeutic course (ie, during the last week of continuous infusion therapy with 5-FU and during the last few days of each 2-week course of capecitabine). Lethargy and malaise are common. Fortunately, these symptoms typically resolve within 2 weeks of completing neoadjuvant therapy. Significant leukopenia, anemia, and thrombocytopenia can occur and the authors recommend checking a complete blood count (CBC) on a weekly basis to monitor for these because they can require a dose reduction in the chemotherapy. A painful rash most commonly involving the palms and soles (hand-foot syndrome) and stomatitis can develop and frequently requires dose reduction to prevent progression of these side effects. Nausea, vomiting, anorexia, and diarrhea are common gastrointestinal side effects and are usually mild and well controlled with medications and dietary changes. In addition, the authors have observed that chemotherapy will occasionally induce a flare of previously quiescent inflammatory bowel disease. If symptoms during neoadjuvant therapy are suggestive of an inflammatory bowel disease flare, the authors recommend performing a colonoscopy to evaluate for active inflammatory bowel disease and to exclude an infectious cause. Flares of inflammatory bowel disease in this setting typically respond well to routine treatments.

Radiation therapy has several side effects that the clinician should be cognizant of. Patients receiving neoadjuvant therapy are at a significant risk for duodenal ulcer. Therefore, ulcer prophylaxis is important in these patients. The authors routinely administer a proton pump inhibitor daily throughout neoadjuvant therapy and extending for a month after completion of brachytherapy. Radiation therapy can result in the development of radiation gastropathy, which involves multiple gastric vascular ectasias and may present as iron-deficiency anemia and melena. This condition responds well to argon plasma coagulation, although several sessions may be required. Radiation therapy can result in significant impairment of gastric and duodenal motility. This impairment can manifest itself as postprandial nausea and vomiting. Onset can be delayed for weeks after radiation therapy and can extend well into the posttransplant period. Symptoms are particularly common when other exacerbating factors are present, such as narcotics. Symptoms are typically managed by moving to a low-residue diet with frequent meals. Occasionally patients require a liquid diet or even jejunal feeding tubes for a limited period of time.

Involuntary weight loss is a frequent and important issue in patients with CCA. Weight loss likely occurs through multiple mechanisms. Chemotherapy, antibiotics, and elevated bilirubin from impaired biliary drainage can all result in anorexia and dysgeusia that impair adequate oral intake. As in several other cancers, weight loss is also likely mediated through immune system antitumor activity via cytokines, such as tumor necrosis factor. The authors work to treat any correctable causes and to help patients maintain their weight through nutritional counseling, dietary changes, and nutritional supplements.

Posttransplant Management

There are several issues in the management of patients after transplant for CCA that deserve special attention.

Because patients receiving transplantation for CCA have received neoadjuvant radiation therapy, particular attention needs to be paid to late effects of radiation injury. There is an increased incidence of late vascular complications in this patient population compared with patients receiving an OLT for other indications.[58] Because of the frequent hepatic artery thrombosis when the native hepatic artery is used for deceased donor arterial reconstruction, the Mayo Clinic transplant group preferentially performs arterial reconstruction with a donor iliac artery interposition graft to the infrarenal aorta. When an interposition graft is used, the deceased donor arterial complication rate in patients transplanted for CCA is significantly decreased and is similar to patients undergoing OLT for other indications. These patients remain at risk for late portal venous stenosis, which can be detected on follow-up CT. When present, this complication has been successfully treated by transhepatic transportal angioplasty and intraluminal stent insertion.[59]

Living donor liver transplant has been used successfully in this patient population. However, radiation-induced injury to the hilar vessels and the location of the tumor result in significant technical challenges given the short vessels of a living donor allograft. Hepatic artery complications, such as stenosis and thrombosis, occur at a higher rate in patients with CCA receiving a living donor compared with a deceased donor allograft.[59] If detected in time by a Doppler study, then stenting of the artery can often prevent early graft loss or the late sequelae of chronic biliary injury and hepatic abscesses. As with deceased donor recipients, living donor recipients are also at risk for portal venous stenosis.

Impaired gastric motility is common following neoadjuvant therapy and can persist for a long time after transplantation. The postoperative state and narcotic pain medications tend to exacerbate this issue. These patients typically have postprandial nausea and vomiting without evidence of mechanical obstruction. Small frequent meals that are primarily liquid are usually the best tolerated. Occasionally jejunal tube feeding is required for a period to maintain nutrition.

Patients requiring pancreatoduodenectomy are particularly challenging in postoperative management. Potential difficulties arise because of the hostile operative field as a result of the prior radiation therapy. Patients are at high risk for a pancreatic leak or a vascular complication because of the proximity of the pancreatic and vascular anastomosis.

SUMMARY

CCA is a rare malignancy that arises from malignant transformation of the cells that line the biliary tree. The incidence of CCA is increasing globally. Primary sclerosing cholangitis and other conditions with chronic inflammation of the biliary tree are risk factors for the development of CCA. Hilar CCA usually presents with obstructive jaundice. Diagnostic techniques have significantly improved in the past 2 decades, enabling more accurate and less-invasive evaluation. Surgical resection and liver transplantation following neoadjuvant therapy in carefully selected patients are the only curative modalities currently available. Surgical therapy is guided by the pattern of bile duct and vasculature involvement noted on preoperative imaging. Complete tumor extirpation usually involves major hepatic resection and reconstruction of the biliary tree. Liver transplantation following neoadjuvant therapy is effective therapy for patients with unresectable hilar CCA or hilar CCA arising in PSC. Biliary stenting, chemotherapy, radiation therapy, and PDT are palliative therapies for CCA.

REFERENCES

1. Khan SA, Taylor-Robinson SD, Toledano MB, et al. Changing international trends in mortality rates for liver, biliary and pancreatic tumours. J Hepatol 2002;37(6): 806–13.
2. Patel T. Increasing incidence and mortality of primary intrahepatic cholangiocarcinoma in the United States. Hepatology 2001;33(6):1353–7.
3. Patel T. Worldwide trends in mortality from biliary tract malignancies. BMC Cancer 2002;2:10.
4. Shaib YH, Davila JA, McGlynn K, et al. Rising incidence of intrahepatic cholangiocarcinoma in the United States: a true increase? J Hepatol 2004;40(3):472–7.
5. Shaib Y, El-Serag HB. The epidemiology of cholangiocarcinoma. Semin Liver Dis 2004;24(2):115–25.
6. Bergquist A, Ekbom A, Olsson R, et al. Hepatic and extrahepatic malignancies in primary sclerosing cholangitis. J Hepatol 2002;36(3):321–7.

7. Burak K, Angulo P, Pasha TM, et al. Incidence and risk factors for cholangiocarcinoma in primary sclerosing cholangitis. Am J Gastroenterol 2004;99(3):523–6.

8. Broome U, Olsson R, Loof L, et al. Natural history and prognostic factors in 305 Swedish patients with primary sclerosing cholangitis. Gut 1996;38(4):610–5.

9. Rosen CB, Nagorney DM, Wiesner RH, et al. Cholangiocarcinoma complicating primary sclerosing cholangitis. Ann Surg 1991;213(1):21–5.

10. Chalasani N, Baluyut A, Ismail A, et al. Cholangiocarcinoma in patients with primary sclerosing cholangitis: a multicenter case-control study. Hepatology 2000;31(1):7–11.

11. Shin HR, Lee CU, Park HJ, et al. Hepatitis B and C virus, Clonorchis sinensis for the risk of liver cancer: a case-control study in Pusan, Korea. Int J Epidemiol 1996;25(5):933–40.

12. Vatanasapt V, Uttaravichien T, Mairiang EO, et al. Cholangiocarcinoma in northeast Thailand. Lancet 1990;335(8681):116–7.

13. Mecklin JP, Jarvinen HJ, Virolainen M. The association between cholangiocarcinoma and hereditary nonpolyposis colorectal carcinoma. Cancer 1992;69(5): 1112–4.

14. Lee SS, Kim MH, Lee SK, et al. Clinicopathologic review of 58 patients with biliary papillomatosis. Cancer 2004;100(4):783–93.

15. Lipsett PA, Pitt HA, Colombani PM, et al. Choledochal cyst disease. A changing pattern of presentation. Ann Surg 1994;220(5):644–52.

16. Edil BH, Cameron JL, Reddy S, et al. Choledochal cyst disease in children and adults: a 30-year single-institution experience. J Am Coll Surg 2008;206(5): 1000–5 [discussion: 1005–8].

17. El-Serag HB, Engels EA, Landgren O, et al. Risk of hepatobiliary and pancreatic cancers after hepatitis C virus infection: a population-based study of U.S. veterans. Hepatology 2009;49(1):116–23.

18. Nakajima T, Kondo Y, Miyazaki M, et al. A histopathologic study of 102 cases of intrahepatic cholangiocarcinoma: histologic classification and modes of spreading. Hum Pathol 1988;19(10):1228–34.

19. Chen TC, Ng KF, Kuo T. Intrahepatic cholangiocarcinoma with lymphoepithelioma-like component. Mod Pathol 2001;14(5):527–32.

20. Iguchi T, Yamashita N, Aishima S, et al. A comprehensive analysis of immunohistochemical studies in intrahepatic cholangiocarcinoma using the survival tree model. Oncology 2009;76(4):293–300.

21. Lau SK, Prakash S, Geller SA, et al. Comparative immunohistochemical profile of hepatocellular carcinoma, cholangiocarcinoma, and metastatic adenocarcinoma. Hum Pathol 2002;33(12):1175–81.

22. Patsenker E, Wilkens L, Banz V, et al. The alphavbeta6 integrin is a highly specific immunohistochemical marker for cholangiocarcinoma. J Hepatol 2010;52(3): 362–9.

23. Klatskin G. Adenocarcinoma of the hepatic duct at its bifurcation within the porta hepatis. An unusual tumor with distinctive clinical and pathological features. Am J Med 1965;38:241–56.

24. Bismuth H, Corlette MB. Intrahepatic cholangioenteric anastomosis in carcinoma of the hilus of the liver. Surg Gynecol Obstet 1975;140(2):170–8.

25. De Bellis M, Sherman S, Fogel EL, et al. Tissue sampling at ERCP in suspected malignant biliary strictures (part 1). Gastrointest Endosc 2002;56(4):552–61.

26. Baron TH, Harewood GC, Rumalla A, et al. A prospective comparison of digital image analysis and routine cytology for the identification of malignancy in biliary tract strictures. Clin Gastroenterol Hepatol 2004;2(3):214–9.

27. Clary B, Jarnigan W, Pitt H, et al. Hilar cholangiocarcinoma. J Gastrointest Surg 2004;8(3):298–302.
28. Steinberg W. The clinical utility of the CA 19-9 tumor-associated antigen. Am J Gastroenterol 1990;85(4):350–5.
29. Nichols JC, Gores GJ, LaRusso NF, et al. Diagnostic role of serum CA 19-9 for cholangiocarcinoma in patients with primary sclerosing cholangitis. Mayo Clin Proc 1993;68(9):874–9.
30. Okabayashi T, Yamamoto J, Kosuge T, et al. A new staging system for mass-forming intrahepatic cholangiocarcinoma: analysis of preoperative and postoperative variables. Cancer 2001;92(9):2374–83.
31. Jarnagin WR, Fong Y, DeMatteo RP, et al. Staging, resectability, and outcome in 225 patients with hilar cholangiocarcinoma. Ann Surg 2001;234(4):507–17 [discussion: 517–9].
32. Deoliveira ML, Schulick RD, Nimura Y, et al. New staging system and a registry for perihilar cholangiocarcinoma. Hepatology 2011;53(4):1363–71.
33. Valle J, Wasan H, Palmer DH, et al. Cisplatin plus gemcitabine versus gemcitabine for biliary tract cancer. N Engl J Med 2010;362(14):1273–81.
34. Bengala C, Bertolini F, Malavasi N, et al. Sorafenib in patients with advanced biliary tract carcinoma: a phase II trial. Br J Cancer 2010;102(1):68–72.
35. Gruenberger B, Schueller J, Heubrandtner U, et al. Cetuximab, gemcitabine, and oxaliplatin in patients with unresectable advanced or metastatic biliary tract cancer: a phase 2 study. Lancet Oncol 2010;11(12):1142–8.
36. Lubner SJ, Mahoney MR, Kolesar JL, et al. Report of a multicenter phase II trial testing a combination of biweekly bevacizumab and daily erlotinib in patients with unresectable biliary cancer: a phase II consortium study. J Clin Oncol 2010; 28(21):3491–7.
37. Prat F, Chapat O, Ducot B, et al. Predictive factors for survival of patients with inoperable malignant distal biliary strictures: a practical management guideline. Gut 1998;42(1):76–80.
38. Zoepf T, Jakobs R, Arnold JC, et al. Palliation of nonresectable bile duct cancer: improved survival after photodynamic therapy. Am J Gastroenterol 2005;100(11): 2426–30.
39. Kiefer MV, Albert M, McNally M, et al. Chemoembolization of intrahepatic cholangiocarcinoma with cisplatinum, doxorubicin, mitomycin C, Ethiodol, and polyvinyl alcohol: a 2-center study. Cancer 2011;117(7):1498–505.
40. Stieber AC, Marino IR, Iwatsuki S, et al. Cholangiocarcinoma in sclerosing cholangitis. The role of liver transplantation. Int Surg 1989;74(1):1–3.
41. Goere D, Wagholikar GD, Pessaux P, et al. Utility of staging laparoscopy in subsets of biliary cancers: laparoscopy is a powerful diagnostic tool in patients with intrahepatic and gallbladder carcinoma. Surg Endosc 2006;20(5):721–5.
42. Lai ECH, Lau WY. Aggressive surgical resection for hilar cholangiocarcinoma. ANZ J Surg 2005;75(11):981–5.
43. Nagorney DM, Donohue JH, Farnell MB, et al. Outcomes after curative resections of cholangiocarcinoma. Arch Surg 1993;128(8):871–7 [discussion: 870–9].
44. Murakami Y, Uemura K, Sudo T, et al. Prognostic factors after surgical resection for intrahepatic, hilar, and distal cholangiocarcinoma. Ann Surg Oncol 2011; 18(3):651–8.
45. Nakeeb A, Tran KQ, Black MJ, et al. Improved survival in resected biliary malignancies. Surgery 2002;132(4):555–63 [discussion: 563–4].

46. Uenishi T, Hirohashi K, Kubo S, et al. Histologic factors affecting prognosis following hepatectomy for intrahepatic cholangiocarcinoma. World J Surg 2001; 25(7):865–9.
47. Uenishi T, Hirohashi K, Kubo S, et al. Clinicopathological factors predicting outcome after resection of mass-forming intrahepatic cholangiocarcinoma. Br J Surg 2001;88(7):969–74.
48. Rea DJ, Munoz-Juarez M, Farnell MB, et al. Major hepatic resection for hilar cholangiocarcinoma: analysis of 46 patients. Arch Surg 2004;139(5):514–23 [discussion: 523–5].
49. Kelley ST, Bloomston M, Serafini F, et al. Cholangiocarcinoma: advocate an aggressive operative approach with adjuvant chemotherapy. Am Surg 2004; 70(9):743–8 [discussion: 748–9].
50. Pitt HA, Nakeeb A, Abrams RA, et al. Perihilar cholangiocarcinoma. Postoperative radiotherapy does not improve survival. Ann Surg 1995;221(6):788–97 [discussion: 797–8].
51. Iwatsuki S, Todo S, Marsh JW, et al. Treatment of hilar cholangiocarcinoma (Klatskin tumors) with hepatic resection or transplantation. J Am Coll Surg 1998; 187(4):358–64.
52. Jonas S, Kling N, Guckelberger O, et al. Orthotopic liver transplantation after extended bile duct resection as treatment of hilar cholangiocarcinoma. First long-terms results. Transpl Int 1998;11(Suppl 1):S206–8.
53. Shimoda M, Farmer DG, Colquhoun SD, et al. Liver transplantation for cholangiocellular carcinoma: analysis of a single-center experience and review of the literature. Liver Transpl 2001;7(12):1023–33.
54. Heimbach JK, Gores GJ, Haddock MG, et al. Liver transplantation for unresectable perihilar cholangiocarcinoma. Semin Liver Dis 2004;24(2):201–7.
55. Sudan D, DeRoover A, Chinnakotla S, et al. Radiochemotherapy and transplantation allow long-term survival for nonresectable hilar cholangiocarcinoma. Am J Transplant 2002;2(8):774–9.
56. Rea DJ, Heimbach JK, Rosen CB, et al. Liver transplantation with neoadjuvant chemoradiation is more effective than resection for hilar cholangiocarcinoma. Ann Surg 2005;242(3):451–8 [discussion: 458–61].
57. De Palma GD, Galloro G, Siciliano S, et al. Unilateral versus bilateral endoscopic hepatic duct drainage in patients with malignant hilar biliary obstruction: results of a prospective, randomized, and controlled study. Gastrointest Endosc 2001; 53(6):547–53.
58. Mantel HT, Rosen CB, Heimbach JK, et al. Vascular complications after orthotopic liver transplantation after neoadjuvant therapy for hilar cholangiocarcinoma. Liver Transpl 2007;13(10):1372–81.
59. Heimbach JK. Successful liver transplantation for hilar cholangiocarcinoma. Curr Opin Gastroenterol 2008;24(3):384–8.

Liver Transplantation for Hepatocellular Carcinoma: Lessons Learned and Future Directions

David M. Levi, MD[a,b,*], Seigo Nishida, MD, PhD[a,b]

KEYWORDS

- Hepatocellular carcinoma • Liver transplant • Cirrhosis
- Bridge therapy • Downstaging • Recurrence
- Adoptive immunotherapy • Natural killer cells

Whereas hepatocellular carcinoma (HCC) has long been a major cause of cancer-related morbidity and mortality in Asia and Africa,[1] its prominence in the United States is a more recent phenomenon. The incidence of HCC in the United States, which has more than doubled in the past 2 decades,[2] can be attributed to the frequency of hepatitis C infection in the 1960s and 1970s[3] as well as the increasing incidence of nonalcoholic fatty liver disease related to diabetes and obesity.[4]

Hepatic resection may be curative, but most patients with HCC are cirrhotic and would not tolerate major resection. In addition, apparently curative resection is often complicated by tumor recurrence. Liver transplantation removes the cirrhotic liver, the carcinogenic substrate for HCC development, provides the widest possible oncologic margins, and restores normal liver function. The major limitation to its application is the requirement for therapeutic immunosuppression and the finite supply of donor organs.

Initial experience with liver transplantation for HCC in the 1980s and early 1990s was disappointing.[5–7] In retrospect, high recurrence rates and poor survival reported in early series reflected inclusion of many patients with advanced HCC, including those with large tumors, multifocal disease, and major vascular invasion. By the mid 1990s, however, several groups had reported more encouraging results with transplant in

The authors have nothing to disclose.
[a] DeWitt Daughtry Family Department of Surgery, University of Miami Miller School of Medicine, Miami, FL, USA
[b] Miami Transplant Institute, Highland Professional Building, 1801 North West 9th Avenue, Miami, FL 33136, USA
* Corresponding author. Miami Transplant Institute, Highland Professional Building, 1801 North West 9th Avenue, Miami, FL 33136.
E-mail address: dlevi@med.miami.edu

patients with early HCC, specifically those with small, often incidentally discovered tumors.[8,9] In 1996, Mazzaferro and colleagues[10] established the Milan Criteria, defining early disease based on a pretransplant, radiologic assessment of tumor size and number using the tumor-node-metastasis (TNM) classification system (**Table 1**). The Milan Criteria included T1 HCC, one lesion less than 2 cm in diameter, and T2 HCC, one lesion between 2 and 5 cm or up to 3 lesions all being less than 3 cm in diameter. In their series of 48 patients with early HCC, the investigators reported an impressive a 4-year recurrence-free survival rate of 83% and a patient survival rate of 75%.

Since March 2002, the United Network for Organ Sharing (UNOS) has utilized the Model for End-Stage Liver Disease (MELD) system for the allocation of livers in the United States. The MELD formula assigns a chronic liver disease severity score that is highly predictive of short-term mortality for patients awaiting liver transplant. It effectively stratifies cirrhotic patients according to easily obtained, objective measures of liver disease severity, namely serum creatinine, total bilirubin, and international normalized ratio (INR). The intent of the system was to facilitate liver transplantation for patients at highest risk of mortality while not increasing posttransplant mortality.[11]

When the MELD system was implemented the Milan Criteria were incorporated, giving priority to patients with early HCC. The allowance of additional points based on the tumor's imaging characteristics and assessment of stage has facilitated transplantation for cirrhotic patients with unresectable HCC. The MELD system has had a dramatic effect on the allocation of donor organs; the number of patients with HCC transplanted has increased substantially.[12,13] In response, the organ allocation system has been amended periodically. MELD points granted for T2 HCC have been decreased, and extra points for T1 HCC were eliminated when it was recognized that the risk of dropout from the waiting list because of tumor progression was low with smaller tumors.[14]

Experience with liver transplantation for HCC in the MELD era confirms the principal findings of the Milan group, namely that it is effective treatment for early, unresectable

Table 1
United Network for Organ Sharing modified TNM staging classification for primary HCC

T1	One nodule ≤1.9 cm
T2	One nodule 2.0–5.0 cm; 2 or 3 nodules, all <3.0 cm
T3	One nodule >5.0 cm; 2 or 3 nodules, at least one >3.0 cm
T4a	Four or more nodules, any size
T4b	T2, T3, or T4a plus gross intrahepatic portal or hepatic vein involvement
N1	Regional (porta hepatis) nodes, involved
M1	Metastatic disease, including extrahepatic portal or hepatic vein involvement
Stage 1	T1
Stage II	T2
Stage III	T3
Stage IVA1	T4a
Stage IVA2	T4b
Stage IVB	Any N1, any M1

Data from American Liver Tumor Study Group. A randomized prospective multi-institutional trial of orthotopic liver transplantation or partial hepatic resection with or without adjuvant chemotherapy for hepatocellular carcinoma. Investigators booklet and protocol; 1998.

HCC.[15,16] In view of these favorable results, several transplant groups have suggested that the Milan Criteria might be modestly expanded without adversely affecting results. Yao and colleagues[17] proposed the University of California, San Francisco (UCSF) criteria in 2001 based on their experience; patients transplanted for HCC with one tumor up to 6.5 cm or no more than 3 tumors, none greater than 4.5 cm with a total tumor diameter of less than 8 cm, achieved a remarkable 75.2% 5-year patient survival rate. Applying the UCSF criteria retrospectively to a large group of patients transplanted over more than 2 decades, Duffy and colleagues[18] from the University of California, Los Angeles reported similar findings and concluded that expansion of the existing criteria was justified. In the authors' series at the University of Miami, patients whose HCC exceeded the Milan Criteria based on their pretransplant staging achieved a 5-year recurrence-free survival that was not statistically different to that observed for those that met the Milan Criteria, further supporting the idea of modestly expanding the current criteria.[15] The argument advocating expansion of the current criteria is countered by concerns that, because of the scarcity of organs for transplant, even a modest change in organ allocation will deprive some patients without HCC who are in need a of liver transplant.

Important lessons have been learned from the experience with liver transplantation for HCC since the introduction of the MELD system. In a cirrhotic liver, early HCC remains difficult to diagnose and accurately stage using current imaging modalities.[19] Although the pathologic assessment of tumor stage (size and number) is a predictor of HCC recurrence,[15,18] contrast-enhanced multiphase computed tomography (CT) and magnetic resonance (MR) imaging often underestimate the extent of disease.[20] Even when accurately staged as early HCC and transplanted promptly, some patients experience tumor recurrence.

The authors' experience at the University of Miami includes some 300 liver transplants for HCC in the 9 years of the current allocation system. An analysis of the first 244 patients, transplanted between 2002 and 2009,[15] revealed 4 factors that affect recurrence-free survival, corroborating the findings of others. As stated, the crude measure of tumor burden—pathologic stage—is one prognostic factor. In the authors' series, because of the limitations of CT and MR to reliably stage cirrhotic patients with HCC, the radiologically assessed stage has not been an accurate predictor of disease recurrence. Besides the pathologic stage, Kaplan-Meier survival analysis revealed that peak serum α-fetoprotein (AFP) prior to transplant, histologic degree of differentiation, and the presence or absence of lymphovascular invasion all affected recurrence-free survival (**Box 1**). Of these variables, only AFP is routinely available before transplant. Although its performance as a screening test is unsatisfactory,[21] it is a valuable predictor of HCC recurrence and, in some series, patient survival after

---

Box 1
Predictors of HCC recurrence-free survival after liver transplantation

Pathologic stage: tumor size (diameter) and number

Peak serum AFP prior to transplant: 100 ng/mL threshold

Histologic degree of differentiation: mild, moderate, and poor

Lymphovascular invasion: present or absent

Data from Levi DM, Tzakis AG, Martin P, et al. Liver transplantation for hepatocellular carcinoma in the model for end-stage liver disease era. J Am Coll Surg 2010;210:727–34.

transplant.[22,23] In Korea, a scoring system incorporating tumor size, number, and AFP has been proposed for the selection of transplant candidates in the living donor transplantation setting.[24] The authors' data suggest that serum AFP could be integrated with the Milan Criteria to enhance the MELD system's HCC selection criteria for prioritization of patients on the waiting list. The only HCC-related predictors of patient survival were lymphovascular invasion and posttransplant tumor recurrence.

In the series reported from Milan in 1996, 27 of the 48 patients transplanted received some form of locoregional, ablative therapy prior to transplant.[11] The utilization of ablative technologies including radiofrequency ablation, percutaneous ethanol injection, microwave ablation, and irreversible electroporation and/or catheter-based modalities including transarterial chemoembolization (TACE) and radioembolization to preoperatively treat HCC has evolved considerably in recent years. Conceptually, these modalities are used in patients with cirrhosis and HCC who are potential transplant candidates in two ways: (1) in liver transplant candidates with preserved liver function to prevent tumor progression while awaiting transplant, (2) in an attempt to downstage a tumor to within accepted criteria thus rendering the patient a transplant candidate.[25] The strategy of ablation of small tumors, close radiological surveillance, and repeat ablation for recurrence is increasingly being considered definitive therapy for many in well-compensated, asymptomatic cirrhotics with early HCC.[26]

Percutaneous radiofrequency ablation[27] for those awaiting transplant has been advocated, although others have been unable to show a survival benefit for various modalities when used as "bridge therapy."[28,29] Belghiti and colleagues,[30] in their 2008 review, recognized the wide acceptance of bridge therapy in the absence of convincing data supporting its benefit either on waiting list dropout rate or posttransplant outcome. The investigators reasoned that benefit is most likely to be realized by patients expected to experience a prolonged waiting time for transplant. At the authors' transplant center, located in a region where most patients granted additional points for having early HCC are transplanted within 3 months, there was a trend toward a recurrence-free survival benefit in the patients who received pretransplant ablative therapy as a bridge, although this trend did not reach statistical significance.[15]

There is also increasing evidence in support of the concept of downstaging of patients with HCC beyond the Milan Criteria in an attempt to facilitate liver transplantation with acceptable outcomes. Presented in an elegant intention-to-treat analysis, the UCSF group has been able to successfully downstage patients with HCC beyond the Milan Criteria and to proceed with transplantation, with excellent results.[31] In Miami, fewer than 20% of patients transplanted for HCC had disease assessed to be beyond the Milan Criteria, nearly 80% of whom received some form of pretransplant, locoregional therapy in an attempt to downstage their disease. The remaining patients had decompensated liver function and a tumor burden modestly beyond the Milan Criteria, and consequently were transplanted without an attempt at downstaging therapy. This group's outcome was not statistically different from that of the group with disease within the Milan Criteria.[15] It seems that a subset of patients with HCC beyond the Milan Criteria can be downstaged and transplanted, with acceptable outcomes. However, whether the authors' results reflect a true benefit of downstaging therapy or an ability to exclude from transplant patients with unfavorable tumor biology is uncertain.

Ironically, as the treatment options for HCC have expanded and results have improved, the diagnosis and management of HCC in the patient with cirrhosis has become quite complex. An "alphabet soup" of treatment algorithms and practice guidelines have been devised[32–34] to address the problem, including the Barcelona Clinic Liver Cancer (BCLC) algorithm (perhaps the most widely accepted, data-supported model), the Metroticket model, UNOS consensus conference recommendations, and American Association for the Study of Liver Diseases (AASLD) practice guidelines, to name a few. While each has its strengths, none can encompass all the variables and logistic issues that contribute to the treatment decision-making process for individual patients. Michael Abecassis,[35] in his "State of the Art" address on the subject delivered at the AASLD Conference in October 2010, illuminated the limits of these algorithms. Many do not consider important clinical variables such as recipient age, comorbid conditions, liver disease etiology, donor availability, and type. In addition, classic treatment algorithms are inherently inflexible and static, failing to account for clinical changes and responses to therapy over time. Abecassis made a compelling argument for the use of dynamic influence diagrams[36] over limited, decision-tree type algorithms to facilitate the individualization of treatment for the cirrhotic patient with HCC. He advocates carefully designed, randomized, controlled clinical trials to address specific areas where data needed to populate these diagrams are lacking.

At the University of Miami, the authors have formed a multidisciplinary team of clinicians to manage patients with HCC. The group includes hepatology and gastroenterology, transplant surgeons, medical and surgical oncologists, radiologists, interventional radiologists, pathologists, and radiation oncologists. Physicians, nurses, coordinators, residents, and fellows from these services meet weekly to present cases and formulate comprehensive treatment plans. This multidisciplinary approach has been recognized as beneficial for patients with HCC and cirrhosis.[8,37]

Patients with cirrhosis and suspected HCC are considered for liver transplant if a radiologically typical tumor(s) is demonstrated on contrast-enhanced CT or MR imaging, a suspicious tumor is seen that does not meet radiologic criteria but is associated with an AFP level greater than 200 ng/mL, a biopsy of a tumor reveals histologic evidence of HCC, or if no tumor is seen but the AFP level is greater than 500 ng/mL. Noncirrhotic patients and those with resectable tumors are not considered for transplant. All patients deemed suitable candidates for transplant are, after a comprehensive evaluation, placed on the waiting list and prioritized according to the MELD system. The authors are presently not performing living donor transplants in Miami because of the relative availability of deceased donor livers. Although tumor progression resulting in removal of patients from the waiting list occurs, it is not common.

At the authors' institution, the treatment strategy for patients with HCC and cirrhosis is determined primarily by the preoperative stage of the tumor and the degree of hepatic decompensation (**Box 2**).[15] Patients with T1 HCC and well-compensated cirrhosis are treated with resection or ablative therapy, usually radiofrequency ablation or irreversible electroporation. Those with T1 HCC and poor liver function are evaluated for transplant. Patients with cirrhosis and unresectable T2 HCC are evaluated for transplant. However, if a patient's liver function is well preserved with minimal or absent portal hypertension, some T2 HCCs are treated with ablation as definitive therapy over transplant or resection. Patients' comorbid conditions that may increase the risks associated with transplant or concern for issues such as posttransplant hepatitis C recurrence may contribute to this decision. Preoperative treatment, usually transarterial therapy and/or ablation, is utilized as a bridge to transplant in T2 HCC patients selectively, commonly in cases where the time from diagnosis to transplant is expected to be protracted. Patients with T3 HCC and preserved liver function are routinely treated with transarterial therapy in an effort to downstage the HCC to within Milan Criteria. Those with T3 HCC who are successfully downstaged or those with disease nominally beyond the Milan Criteria who are not able to undergo locoregional therapy, due to hepatic decompensation, are considered for transplant. Patients with

---

Box 2
Factors considered when formulating HCC treatment plan

Patient Parameters

  Age

  Comorbid conditions

  Performance status

  Liver disease etiology

Liver Function

  Biological MELD score

  Total bilirubin

  Index complications: ascites, hepatic encephalopathy, and so forth

  Portal hypertension

Tumor Characteristics

  Size (greatest diameter)

  Number

  AFP

  Radiologically measured tumor stage

  Histologic data (if available): differentiation and lymphovascular invasion

Logistic and Nonclinical Variables

  Organ availability

  Psychosocial issues and social support

  Financial constraints and access to care

---

locally advanced HCC, major portal or hepatic vein invasion, or extrahepatic, metastatic disease are not considered for transplant. In the authors' treatment strategy, compensated liver function is characterized by minimal or absent portal hypertension, total bilirubin less than 3 mg/dL, and a MELD score of less than 15.

For the foreseeable future, liver transplantation will remain an effective, potentially curative treatment option in a relatively small number of selected patients with HCC. The main limitations will be those that affect liver transplantation in general, the requirement for immunosuppression, and the scarcity of quality donor livers. Progress will likely come in several areas. It is hoped that improved imaging technologies will allow earlier detection and more accurate staging of HCC. The application of advanced imaging modalities, such as positron emission tomography, may reliably and noninvasively detect the presence of lymphovascular invasion and predict HCC recurrence after transplant.[38,39] The advent of gene expression–based predictors of HCC recurrence[40,41] may eventually supplant the current tumor size-based and number-based MELD system criteria for prioritizing HCC candidates.

Even as results improve, some patients undergoing liver transplant for HCC will develop recurrence of cancer. Posttransplant surveillance protocols for detecting recurrence and effective treatments for those who experience recurrence are needed. One novel approach being applied that may decrease the risk of recurrent HCC after transplant is through adoptive immunotherapy using activated donor natural killer (NK)

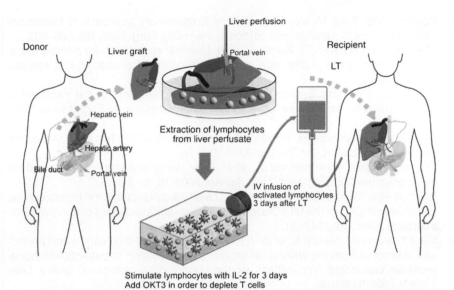

Fig. 1. Outline of adoptive immunotherapy with lymphocytes (natural killer cells) extracted from liver allograft perfusate. IL-2, interleukin-2; IV, intravenous; LT, liver transplantation; OKT-3, muromonab CD-3. (*Data from* Ohira M, Ishiyama K, Tanaka Y, et al. Adoptive immunotherapy with liver allograft-derived lymphocytes induces anti-HCV activity after liver transplantation in humans and humanized mice. J Clin Invest 2009;119:3226–35; with permission; and *Courtesy of* Hideki Ohdan, MD, PhD, Hiroshima University.)

cells. Developed by Ohdan and colleagues[42] at Hiroshima University, interleukin-2–stimulated NK cells extracted from donor liver graft perfusate possess potent anti-HCC cytotoxicity. Their protocol (**Fig. 1**) is used in living donor liver transplantation and has yielded encouraging preliminary results. The authors are replicating this protocol in Miami using deceased donor grafts. The hope is that the adoptive transfer of NK cells will result in less HCC recurrence and will ultimately allow the expansion of the Milan Criteria without negatively affecting recurrence-free survival.

REFERENCES

1. Bosch FX, Ribes J, Diaz M, et al. Primary liver cancer: worldwide incidence and trends. Gastroenterol 2004;127(5 Suppl 1):S5–16.
2. El-Serag HB, Davila JA, Petersen NJ, et al. The continuing increase in the incidence of hepatocellular carcinoma in the United States: an update. Ann Intern Med 2003;139:817–23.
3. El-Serag HB, Mason AC. Risk factors for the rising rates of primary liver cancer in the United States. Arch Intern Med 2000;160(21):3227–30.
4. Bugianesi E. Non-alcoholic steatohepatitis and cancer. Clin Liver Dis 2007;11:191–207.
5. Iwatsuki S, Starzl TE, Sheahan DG, et al. Hepatic resection versus transplantation for hepatocellular carcinoma. Ann Surg 1991;214:221–9.
6. Bismuth H, Chiche L, Adam R, et al. Liver resection versus transplantation for hepatocellular carcinoma in cirrhotic patients. Ann Surg 1993;218:145–51.
7. Ringe B, Wittekind C, Bechstein WO, et al. The role of liver transplantation in hepatobiliary malignancy: a retrospective analysis of 95 patients with particular regard to tumor stage and recurrence. Ann Surg 1989;209:88–98.

8. Schwartz ME, Sung M, Mor E, et al. A multidisciplinary approach to hepatocellular carcinoma in patients with cirrhosis. J Am Coll Surg 1995;180:596–603.

9. McPeake JR, O'Grady JG, Zaman S, et al. Liver transplantation for primary hepatocellular carcinoma: tumor size and number determine outcome. J Hepatol 1993;18:226–34.

10. Mazzaferro V, Regalia E, Doci R, et al. Liver transplantation for the treatment of small hepatocellular carcinomas in patients with cirrhosis. N Engl J Med 1996; 334:693–9.

11. Freeman RB, Wiesner RH, Edwards E, et al. Results of the first year of the new liver allocation plan. Liver Transpl 2004;10:7–15.

12. Sharma P, Balan V, Hernandez JL, et al. Liver transplantation for hepatocellular carcinoma: the MELD impact. Liver Transpl 2004;10:36–41.

13. Ioannou GN, Perkins JD, Carithers RL. Liver transplantation for hepatocellular carcinoma: impact of the MELD allocation system and predictors of survival. Gastroenterol 2008;134:1342–51.

14. Yao FY, Bass NM, Nikolai B, et al. A follow-up analysis of the pattern and predictors of dropout from the waiting list for liver transplantation in patients with hepatocellular carcinoma: implications for the current organ allocation policy. Liver Transpl 2003;9:684–92.

15. Levi DM, Tzakis AG, Martin P, et al. Liver transplantation for hepatocellular carcinoma in the model for end-stage liver disease era. J Am Coll Surg 2010;210:727–34.

16. Thuluvath PJ, Maheshwari A, Thuluvath NP, et al. Survival after liver transplantation for hepatocellular carcinoma in the MELD and pre-MELD eras and the independent impact of the hepatitis C virus. Transplantation 2009;15:754–62.

17. Yao FY, Ferrell L, Bass NM, et al. Liver transplantation for hepatocellular carcinoma: expansion of tumor size limits does not adversely impact survival. Hepatology 2001;33:1394–403.

18. Duffy JP, Vardanian A, Benjamin E, et al. Liver transplantation criteria for hepatocellular carcinoma should be expanded. Ann Surg 2007;246:502–11.

19. Forner A, Vilana R, Ayuso C, et al. Diagnosis of hepatic nodules 20 mm or smaller in cirrhosis: prospective validation of the noninvasive diagnosis criteria for hepatocellular carcinoma. Hepatology 2008;47:97–104.

20. Shah SA, Tan JC, McGilvray ID, et al. Accuracy of staging as a predictor for recurrence after liver transplantation for hepatocellular carcinoma. Transplantation 2006;81:1633–9.

21. Farinati F, Marino D, De Giorgio M, et al. Diagnostic role of alpha-fetoprotein in hepatocellular carcinoma: both or neither? Am J Gastroenterol 2006;101:524–32.

22. Vivarelli M, Cuchetti A, La Barba G, et al. Liver transplantation for hepatocellular carcinoma under calcineurin inhibitors: reassessment of risk factors for tumor recurrence. Ann Surg 2008;248:857–62.

23. Yao FY, Xiao L, Bass NM, et al. Liver transplantation for hepatocellular carcinoma: validation of the UCSF-expanded criteria based on preoperative imaging. Am J Transpl 2007;7:2587–96.

24. Yang SH, Suh K, Lee HW, et al. A revised scoring system utilizing serum alpha-fetoprotein levels to expand candidates for living donor transplantation in hepatocellular carcinoma. Surgery 2007;141:598–609.

25. Schwartz M, Roayaie S, Uva P. Treatment of HCC in patients awaiting liver transplantation. Am J Transplant 2007;7:1875–81.

26. Rossi S, Ravetta V, Rosa L, et al. Repeated radiofrequency ablation for management of patients with small hepatocellular carcinomas: a long-term cohort study. Hepatology 2011;53:136–47.

27. Lu DSK, Yu NC, Raman SS, et al. Percutaneous radiofrequency ablation of hepatocellular carcinoma as a bridge to liver transplantation. Hepatology 2005;41: 1130–7.
28. Porrett PM, Peterman H, Rosen H, et al. Lack of benefit of pre-transplant locoregional hepatic therapy for hepatocellular carcinoma in the current MELD era. Liver Transpl 2006;12:665–73.
29. Lesurtel M, Mullhaupt B, Pestalozzi BC, et al. Transarterial chemoembolization as a bridge to liver transplantation for hepatocellular carcinoma: an evidence based analysis. Am J Transplant 2006;6:2644–50.
30. Belghiti J, Carr BI, Greig PD, et al. Treatment before liver transplantation for HCC. Ann Surg Oncol 2008;15:993–1000.
31. Yao YF, Kerlan RK, Hirose R, et al. Excellent outcome following down-staging of hepatocellular carcinoma prior to liver transplantation: an intention to treat analysis. Hepatology 2008;48:819–27.
32. Forner A, Reig ME, de Lope CR, et al. Current strategy for staging and treatment: BCLC update and future prospects. Semin Liver Dis 2010;30:61–74.
33. Pomfret EA, Washburn K, Wald C, et al. Report of a national conference on liver allocation in patients with hepatocellular carcinoma in the United States. Liver Transpl 2010;16:62–78.
34. Mazzaferro V, Llovet JM, Miceli R, et al. Predicting survival after liver transplantation in patients with hepatocellular carcinoma beyond the Milan Criteria: a retrospective, exploratory analysis. Lancet Oncol 2009;10:35–43.
35. Avilable at: http://74.43.177.57/courses/2010/sal/abecassis/player.html. Accessed August 19, 2011.
36. Van Gerven MAJ, Diez FJ, Taal BG, et al. Selecting treatment strategies with dynamic limited-memory influence diagrams. Artif Intell Med 2007;40:171–86.
37. Chang TT, Sawhney R, Monto A, et al. Implementation of a multidisciplinary treatment team for hepatocellular cancer at a Veterans Affairs Medical Center improves survival. HPB 2008;10:405–11.
38. Kornberg A, Freesmeyer M, Barthel E, et al. ^{18}F-FDG-uptake of hepatocellular carcinoma on PET predicts microvascular tumor invasion in liver transplant patients. Am J Transpl 2009;9:592–600.
39. Lee JW, Paeng JC, Kang KW, et al. Prediction of tumor recurrence by ^{18}F-FDG PET in liver transplantation for hepatocellular carcinoma. J Nucl Med 2009;50: 682–7.
40. Iizuka N, Oka M, Yamada-Okabe H, et al. Oligonucleotide microarray for prediction of early intrahepatic recurrence of hepatocellular carcinoma after curative resection. Lancet 2003;361:923–9.
41. Hoshida Y, Villanueva A, Kobayashi M, et al. Gene expression in fixed tissues and outcome in hepatocellular carcinoma. N Engl J Med 2008;359:1995–2004.
42. Ishiyama K, Ohdan H, Ohira M, et al. Difference in cytotoxicity against hepatocellular carcinoma between liver and periphery natural killer cells in humans. Hepatology 2006;43:362–72.

Alcohol and Substance Use in Liver Transplant Patients

Andrea DiMartini, MD[a],*, Catherine Crone, MD[b],
Mary Amanda Dew, PhD[c,d]

KEYWORDS

• Alcohol use • Substance use • Liver transplant patients

Of the many causes of end-organ damage, excess alcohol and illicit drug use are more likely to result in the need for liver transplantation (LT) than for other types of transplantation. Equally importantly hepatitis C virus (HCV) and alcoholic liver disease (ALD) are the first and second most frequent indications for LT in the United States and Europe, in combination accounting for more than 60% of LTs performed.[1-3] Because hepatologists and gastroenterologists commonly see these patients, a thorough understanding of alcohol and other substance use is important for these patients' care and their preparation for and progress through the LT process.

In this article the epidemiology of substance use and substance disorders in the United States and their association with liver disease are reviewed. Tobacco use is commonly associated with other substance use disorders and its relevance to LT is discussed. Issues of candidacy as it pertains to substance use are also addressed. It is essential to understand the differences in perspectives and listing criteria between LT programs for patients with addiction disorders. The controversial issues such as the use of alcohol while on the waitlist and short sobriety are also addressed. The

---

[a] Consultation Liaison to the Liver Transplant Program, Starzl Transplant Institute, University of Pittsburgh Medical Center, 3811 O'Hara Street, Pittsburgh, PA 15213, USA
[b] Department of Psychiatry at Inova Fairfax Hospital, George Washington University Medical Center, Inova Fairfax Hospital, Virginia Commonwealth University, 3300 Gallows Road, Falls Church, VA 22042, USA
[c] Clinical Epidemiology Program, Research Methods and Biostatistics Core, Advanced Center for Interventions and, Services Research in Late Life Mood Disorders, University of Pittsburgh School of Medicine and Medical Center, 3811 O'Hara Street, Pittsburgh, PA 15213, USA
[d] Quality of Life Research, Artificial Heart Program, Adult Cardiothoracic Transplantation, University of Pittsburgh School of Medicine and Medical Center, 3811 O'Hara Street, Pittsburgh, PA 15213, USA
* Corresponding author.
E-mail address: dimartiniaf@upmc.edu

Clin Liver Dis 15 (2011) 727–751
doi:10.1016/j.cld.2011.08.002
1089-3261/11/$ – see front matter © 2011 Elsevier Inc. All rights reserved.

merits of monitoring of patients both during the waiting period before LT and in the long-term after LT are discussed. The outcomes of these patients after LT including the rates of return to substance use as well as the impact of substance use on morbidity and mortality are examined. The article concludes with a summary of recommendations for clinicians working with these patients and possible future directions for both clinical care and research. The preponderance of the literature is on ALD and LT. Only a small body of literature exits for drug use disorders. When possible data are also presented from Europe and other countries as they pertain to these areas, recognizing that the bulk of the literature is from the United States.

SUBSTANCE USE AND DISORDERS IN GENERAL AND END-STAGE LIVER DISEASE POPULATIONS
Physical Versus Psychiatric Disorders in the End-stage Liver Disease Population

The overlap of the psychiatric disorders (alcohol and substance abuse/dependence disorders) with the physical disorder of end-stage liver disease (ESLD) (specifically end-stage alcoholic and viral liver disease) is extensive but not complete. Consider that the physical and psychiatric disorders are separate categories of disorders (represented by the Venn diagram in **Fig. 1**). Both the physical and psychiatric disorders need to be formally diagnosed; individuals could have either type of disorder or both. For example an individual who injected drugs once or twice decades ago may not meet criteria for a substance use disorder but could have ESLD as a result of HCV contracted from injected drug use. Many individuals meet criteria for an alcohol dependence diagnosis but may never develop liver disease. Conversely some individuals drink modestly and develop end-stage ALD but never meet criteria for an alcohol dependence disorder.[4,5] Exposure alone to alcohol or substances even in substantial quantities does not necessarily result in the development of an addictive disorder. These complexities require a formal psychiatric evaluation to identify the correct psychiatric diagnoses even for individuals who have ESLD caused by alcohol or substance use (see section on assessment). The following statistics aid in the understanding of at risk populations in the United States.

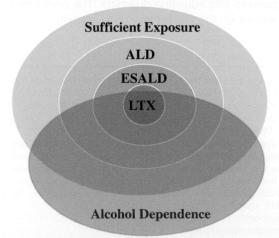

Fig. 1. Psychiatric versus physical diagnoses. (*From* DiMartini A, Weinrieb R, Lane T, et al. Defining the alcoholic liver transplant population: implications for future research. Liver Transplant 2001;7(5):429; with permission.)

Alcohol Use, ALD, and Alcohol Addiction Disorders

The cumulative exposure required to create alcoholic cirrhosis is variable. Although the risk increases with regular consumption of approximately 8 standard drinks/d (80 g) for men and as little as 2 standard drinks/d (20 g) for women, other studies have shown only 20% of men drinking the equivalent of 12 beers daily for 10 years become cirrhotic.[6] This shows the development of cirrhosis can require years of sustained heavy drinking yet some who drink modestly may also develop liver disease.[6]

From a psychiatric diagnostic perspective, large nationwide epidemiologic studies, although not specifying consumption patterns, show that substantial numbers of individuals, more than 15 million adults in 2009, were identified as having an alcohol dependence or abuse disorder.[7] The lifetime prevalence of an alcohol abuse or dependence disorder is nearly 20% with twice as many men as women being affected.[8,9] In the LT population several studies have reported on the psychiatric diagnoses of alcohol use disorders among candidates and recipients. Seventy-five percent to 80% of ALD LT patients meet psychiatric diagnostic criteria for an alcohol dependence disorder, the more severe form of an alcohol use disorder that commonly has a relapsing remitting course.[4,5] The rest are diagnosed with alcohol abuse, the less severe form of alcohol addiction.

HCV, HCV Cirrhosis, and Injected Drug Use

Approximately 3.2 million persons in the United States have chronic HCV infection, with approximately 17,000 acute cases noted in 2007.[10] Of those infected 75% to 85% develop chronic infection, 60% to 70% develop chronic liver disease, 5% to 20% develop cirrhosis over a period of 20 to 30 years, and without transplantation 1% to 5% die from the consequences of chronic infection (eg, liver cancer or cirrhosis).[10]

Although HCV can be contracted through tattoos, sexual contacts, intranasal drug use, and blood transfusions, injection drug use is the most common means of HCV transmission in the United States. Viral hepatitis can be contracted with a single injection. A large national household survey from 2006 to 2008 revealed that an annual average of nearly half a million US adults used a needle to inject illicit drugs during the past year.[11] Recent surveys of injection drug users show one-third of young users (aged 18–30 years) are HCV infected. Older and former drug users typically have higher prevalence of HCV infection (70%–90%), reflecting both the heightened risks with ongoing injected drug use and the spread of HCV infection in the 1970s to 1980s from needle sharing before the risks of blood-borne viruses were well known and public educational initiatives were implemented.[10]

Approximately 3.2 million US adults are identified with a substance dependence or abuse disorder to both alcohol and illicit drugs (not necessarily injected) and 3.9 million to illicit drugs but not alcohol.[7] The lifetime prevalence of illicit drug abuse (not necessarily injected) is approximately 8% of the adult population, whereas drug dependence is 3% and not all users of drugs become dependent on them.[9]

Data about injection drug use and substance use disorders among LT patients have not been systematically gathered. Thus the exact numbers of LT patients who potentially acquired hepatotropic viruses through injection drug use are not known but based on the most current modes of viral transmission and the number of HCV-infected individuals who are being considered for LT the percentage is expected to be large. In a single-center study of patients diagnosed with ALD (n = 112), 52% were also infected with HCV.[12] All who were infected with HCV admitted use of illicit drugs; nearly 50% had injected drugs at some point in their lifetime and all who injected drugs were infected with HCV. In addition, 25% were diagnosed with a lifetime substance use disorder and 36% had lifetime depressive disorders.[12] At another center 60% of waitlisted ALD LT candidates were HCV infected, with 21% having a previous history of injected drug use.[13,14]

Tobacco Use in LT Candidates

Substances of addiction include tobacco products. In recent years an increasing awareness of the potential deleterious effects of tobacco use on post-LT outcomes (see section on outcomes) has created greater focus on identifying the prevalence of tobacco in this population. Although about 20% of the US population uses tobacco and 50% have ever smoked cigarettes, in several studies up to 60% of LT candidates have a lifetime history of using tobacco products and for those with ALD the percentage is as high as 70%.[15–19] Those with previous substance use histories are more likely to be smokers. In 1 study of LT patients comparing ALD with non-ALD patients, the former had on average consumed 10 more pack-years of cigarettes than non-ALD patients.[20] Although chewing tobacco is associated with mouth/throat cancers few studies have examined this exposure rate to tobacco in LT patients.[15] In 1 study of LT candidates the lifetime history of using smokeless tobacco was 8%.[16]

SUBSTANCE USE ASSESSMENT, PSYCHIATRIC DIAGNOSIS, AND TREATMENT PLANNING FOR LT
General Recommendations

Assessment for substance use disorders should be an integral part of LT evaluation. Questions regarding substance use and possible abuse should be raised by each team member who sees a potential candidate, rather than relegating this to those responsible for providing the psychosocial evaluation. Taking this approach helps to emphasize the importance of this issue to potential candidates and also reduces the chance of obtaining inaccurate information. Patients often minimize information about their substance use histories or provide inconsistent information across different interviews. Depending on the transplant team, social workers, nurse specialists, psychologists, or psychiatrists may be responsible for providing the psychosocial assessment of candidates. Addictions specialists may also be asked to evaluate a patient who has a clear or suspected history of a substance use disorder. Most LT programs rely on the input of mental health clinicians for the assessment of ALD candidates.[21] This assessment includes careful evaluation for the presence of substance use disorders and knowledge about its implications for organ transplantation. Even patients not referred for ALD, especially those with HCV, may have significant alcohol use disorders that are missed on referral but would be identified by structured psychiatric interview (12% in 1 study).[22–24]

The approach to assessing and diagnosing substance use disorders among transplant candidates begins with adopting a direct and nonjudgmental stance. Similar to obtaining the history of concurrent medical conditions or psychiatric disorders, patients should be asked about their use of tobacco, alcohol, illicit and prescription drugs. Information about the duration, quantity, and frequency of use of these substances should be obtained. Questions regarding activities to obtain these substances (eg, drug dealing, stealing) and consequences of use (eg, physical withdrawal, legal complications, loss of job, disciplinary actions, relationship problems) should be included. Information on previous attempts to reduce usage, mandated or voluntary participation in addiction rehabilitation or 12-step groups, and reasons for ending use should be obtained. Transplant candidates may have stopped using drugs or alcohol simply because they have become too ill. Obtaining collateral information from family, close friends, other health care professionals, 12-step sponsors, and rehabilitation programs the patient has attended helps to provide a more accurate assessment. The severity of the candidate's substance use disorder needs to be determined because it helps to predict risk for posttransplant relapse and the necessity for more intensive monitoring and treatment before being listed, during listing, and after transplantation (see sections on ongoing monitoring and predictors of relapse after LT).

In addition to alcohol and illicit drugs, given the number of LT candidates who use tobacco products, assessment of tobacco use and treatment of nicotine dependence should be a routine part of LT evaluation and follow-up.[16,18] Whether tobacco use cessation is a condition for LT listing is a decision made by the individual LT programs.

The Use of Written Behavioral Contracts

Some LT teams use written behavioral contracts for patients with substance use disorders.[25,26] Although this is not a legal document, it can provide patients and transplant teams with a list of clear and explicit expectations. For the transplant team, this document allows them to set forth conditions for the potential candidate such as attendance and completion of inpatient/outpatient rehabilitation, participation in 12-step programs, and use of random toxicology screens. For patients, a contract removes any ambiguity about the LT team's expectations. The contract may include such details as the number and frequency of attendance at treatment sessions or 12-step meetings. Meeting these conditions leads to a patient being placed on the waiting list. Failure to comply with terms of the contract, such as detection of a positive toxicology screen or refusal to attend rehabilitation, delays possible listing or if the candidate is on the list could result in their being removed from the waitlist. Campbell and Punch[27] describe the development of such a contract at their LT program, which is signed by the patient and stipulates that they agree to be abstinent from all illicit drugs and alcohol (see Ref.[27] for a copy of the contract).

Timing of Referral for LT and Mental Health Evaluation

The frequent dictum by LT teams of 6 months of abstinence before LT listing is based on evidence that this time frame allows recovery from possible acute alcoholic hepatitis and may render LT unnecessary.[23,28,29] However, a consensus statement jointly drafted by the American Society of Transplant Physicians and the American Association for the Study of Liver Diseases (AASLD) emphasized that 6 months of abstinence alone is not an adequate minimal standard for placement on the LT waiting list. They recommended patients be evaluated by and comply with the recommendations of a substance abuse professional.[30]

Enforcing a minimum of 6 months' abstinence may place patients in jeopardy because they may not be referred until they are in an advanced state of physical deterioration or cognitively compromised by hepatic encephalopathy. In turn, this situation interferes with their ability to fully participate in the evaluation process, which includes education about the risks and benefits of transplantation. Referring physicians should therefore consider early referral for transplant evaluation in keeping with AASLD guidelines.[28] Although patients referred early may still have listing deferred for 6 months, they are provided with more time to adjust to the prospect of transplantation, develop a relationship with the transplant team, and can participate in efforts to address their substance use disorder.

TREATMENT OPTIONS FOR ADDICTION DISORDERS
Addiction Rehabilitation

Therapeutic options for substance use disorders include counseling and medications. Detoxification may be required if a patient is actively using substances. This brief therapy involves medical treatment, typically in an inpatient setting, to manage frank withdrawal symptoms with medications.[31] The emphasis is to stabilize patients so that they are not in imminent danger of serious physical consequences from substance withdrawal, and the therapy involves minimal counseling.[31]

Addiction rehabilitation programs are recommended when patients are no longer experiencing the acute physiologic or psychological effects of substance use or withdrawal.[31] Programs may be inpatient or outpatient, and involve intensive counseling and education. Patients are educated about their addiction as a chronic medical illness and, like other chronic diseases such as diabetes, patients are taught how to manage their illness. This education is vital even for those who have already achieved some period of abstinence, because those patients often do not have the psychological or behavioral skills to stay sober. Patients meet with counselors individually and in groups, and families may participate in some of the sessions. A variety of psychotherapeutic techniques are used and can include cognitive-behavioral, motivational enhancement, 12-step facilitation, or other therapeutic approaches. Most approaches emphasize teaching coping skills and behaviors as well as strategies to avoid/prevent future relapse. Attendance at 12-step groups (eg, Alcoholics Anonymous or Narcotics Anonymous) is often a component of the rehabilitation process. Individual psychotherapy may be an alternative for some patients who are reluctant to participate in group-based rehabilitation programs. However, it is vital that the therapist have specialized training in addiction counseling. For cases of severe substance use, patients may require treatment in a residential facility or halfway house that provide longer treatment and monitoring than standard rehabilitation programs.

Twelve-step programs such as Alcoholics Anonymous and Narcotics Anonymous consist of peer-led support groups that can assist patients in achieving abstinence and eventual sobriety. Patients may attend these groups without being part of a formal rehabilitation program. Groups are available for general as well as specific populations (eg, women, gay, or professionals). The twelve-step approach encourages patients to develop responsibility and self-efficacy during their recovery, discourages use of denial, and affords greater understanding about the emotions, behaviors, and actions that promote substance use.[32] In addition, these groups provide patients with a stable support system that fosters abstinence/sobriety. To optimize potential gains from participation in 12-step programs, patients should be advised to obtain a sponsor (someone who can provide additional support and emergency assistance if needed), establish a home group, work the steps, and participate in service activities (eg, serve as speaker or sponsor, help with meeting set-up). Often if patients are using 12-step groups as their only form of rehabilitation they are encouraged to attend several times a week for maximal benefit. These groups are free and can be especially useful for patients without mental health insurance. Some transplant programs require formal documentation of meeting attendance.

Although standard addiction therapies are applicable to any patient with an addiction disorder there is evidence that treatment could be tailored more specifically to the needs of transplant patients. Weinrieb and colleagues[13] discovered that ALD LT candidates were different from other types of patients with alcohol dependence in that they did not perceive a need for addiction treatment especially after accruing some abstinence before referral for LT evaluation. In addition, LT patients were preoccupied with transplant management, were less likely to endorse alcohol cravings, and showed little motivation for alcoholism treatments.[13,14] They were also reluctant to take naltrexone, a medication approved for the treatment of alcoholism, because of a small albeit potential risk for hepatotoxicity.[14] Based on these findings Weinrieb decided to investigate a trial of motivational enhancement therapy (MET) as the psychological intervention designed to encourage motivation toward treatment and treatment goals. Their results suggest that MET used during the pre-LT phase can reduce the amount and frequency of alcohol consumption compared with treatment as usual.[33] Another pilot study examined the use of a 3-session motivational-style network-based brief intervention integrated into the LT evaluation process.[34] The intervention provided support and guidance to the patients and their LT support person and focused on relapse prevention and healthy behaviors after LT. Patients also signed an abstinence contract at the completion of the sessions. Georgiou and colleagues[34] found the intervention was feasible and acceptable, but small numbers and nonrandomized design prevented an estimation of efficacy.

Medications for the Treatment of Substance Use Disorders

Medications for the treatment of substance use disorders are primarily used as adjuncts to counseling and are most effective when used in this manner. Among those available, medications for alcohol, opiate, and tobacco use disorders are the most well established. Psychiatrists or addiction medicine specialists should be consulted for the use of these medications, especially for patients with liver disease, because dosages and dosing often require adjustment. In addition some medications may add to symptoms of mental slowing or sedation.

For the management of alcohol use disorders, acamprosate has shown modest effects in reducing relapse and lengthening abstinence periods.[35] It is a synthetic glutamate receptor antagonist the action of which is unclear.[36] Side effects include diarrhea, nausea, vomiting, and abdominal pain, with rare cases of cardiomyopathy, cardiac failure, and renal failure. Acamprosate is renally excreted and not hepatically metabolized. In the presence of moderate renal impairment (creatinine clearance of 30–50 mL/min), acamprosate dosing should be reduced by half, and it should be avoided altogether if creatinine clearance is 30 mL/min or less.[37] Naltrexone, which is discussed later for opiate use disorders, may also be used for alcohol use disorders and has similar efficacy to acamprosate.[35]

Disulfiram is a well-established option for alcohol use disorders that works by negative reinforcement. Intake of alcohol while on disulfiram leads to accumulation of acetaldehyde and the resulting disulfiram-ethanol reaction (ie, sweating, facial flushing, tachycardia, dyspnea, headache, nausea, vomiting, dizziness).[36] However, serious cardiovascular effects (ie, chest pain, tachyarrhythmias, hypertension, hypotension, and hemodynamic instability) have also been described,[38] which may be hazardous in patients with liver disease. Clinical trials have shown the effectiveness of disulfiram in the maintenance of abstinence, with superiority to naltrexone and acamprosate.[39,40] There is a rare risk of hepatotoxicity at normal doses, which can range from asymptomatic increase of liver function tests to fulminant hepatitis requiring transplantation.[40,41] Disulfiram is contraindicated in the presence of severe coronary disease and requires caution in those with hepatic dysfunction or cirrhosis.[40] A metabolite of disulfiram is a CYP3A4 inhibitor, thus it may interfere with the metabolism of other medications including cyclosporine and tacrolimus.[41]

Naltrexone is a μ-opioid antagonist that has been used for relapse prevention for both opioid and alcohol use disorders. Several studies have shown its ability to reduce relapse to heavy drinking, which is believed to be related to its ability to counteract the reward/reinforcing effects of alcohol.[42,43] However, naltrexone does not seem to enhance abstinence. Poor adherence with oral naltrexone led to the development of a monthly depot injection.[36] A recent Cochrane review[44] indicated that naltrexone had effects comparable with placebo for opioid use disorders. Common side effects include sedation, headache, nausea, dizziness, and abdominal pain. Naltrexone may cause hepatotoxicity when used in high doses ($\geq$300 mg/d), and its use is contraindicated in the presence of severe liver disease. Low doses have been found helpful in relief of pruritus caused by liver disease, but acute worsening of hepatic function may rarely occur even at therapeutic dosages.[37] As a μ-opioid antagonist naltrexone blocks the effects of opioid analgesics, therefore its use for patients on opioid pain medications is contraindicated (eg, in the early postoperative period). One study that offered naltrexone to post-LT patients found few patients willing to take it because of concerns over potential hepatotoxicity.[13,14]

Buprenorphine is a partial μ-opioid receptor agonist that also has partial κ-opioid antagonist properties. Prescribed for the treatment of opioid use disorders, it relieves withdrawal symptoms and cravings for 24 hours or longer.[45] Compared with methadone, buprenorphine is safer in overdose and may be used for either maintenance therapy or detoxification. Its combination with naloxone discourages intravenous misuse because it produces withdrawal symptoms.[45] Nausea, dizziness, and somnolence are common side effects, and cases of serious hepatotoxicity have been reported even at therapeutic doses.[46,47] There is reduced risk of QT prolongation compared with methadone.[48] A multisite study sponsored by the National Institute on Drug Abuse is under way to clarify risk of buprenorphine-induced hepatotoxicity.[49] Dose adjustment is advised in the presence of hepatic disease, although specific recommendations are lacking. Buprenorphine should not be used perioperatively because it may cause withdrawal in patients receiving opioid pain medications.[37]

Medications for Smoking Cessation

Because tobacco use increases the risk of hepatic artery thrombosis, malignancies, and all-cause mortality (see section on tobacco-related outcomes), LT programs have become more concerned about nicotine use.[50] Nicotine replacement therapies (NRTs) are readily available in a variety of forms (eg, transdermal patch, gum, lozenges, nasal spray), with most not requiring a prescription. NRTs reduce the pleasurable effects of smoking and reduce both the severity of cravings and withdrawal symptoms.[51] Replacement therapies double the odds of patients achieving long-term abstinence compared with placebo.[52,53] Common side effects include insomnia, headaches, abnormal dreams, dizziness, palpitations, nausea, and other gastrointestinal disturbances.[54]

Bupropion is an antidepressant that is also effective for smoking cessation. Although the exact mechanism is unknown, bupropion is a dopamine and norepinephrine reuptake inhibitor that also has nicotine acetylcholine receptor antagonist properties (ie, blocks the reinforcing effects of nicotine).[51] Bupropion increases 2-fold the likelihood of a patient achieving abstinence.[52] Initial dosing and dose adjustments should be reduced in patients with advanced liver disease.[55,56] Headache, insomnia, nausea, diarrhea, and anxiety are common side effects. Its use has been implicated in the onset of seizures, with an incidence of 0.1% to 0.4%, with those predisposed to seizures (eg, history of alcohol withdrawal seizures, head trauma at highest risk).[54] In 2009, a black box warning was included when an association between bupropion SR for smoking cessation and neuropsychiatric symptoms including suicidal ideation/behavior was noted.[54] However, large postmarketing studies and a Cochrane review failed to establish a risk of suicidality.[57,58]

Varenicline is a long-acting partial agonist of the nicotine acetylcholine receptor that lessens craving and withdrawal symptoms and also reduces the reinforcing effects of smoking by competitively inhibiting nicotine binding.[52] Recent meta-analyses have shown that varenicline is more effective than bupropion and pharmacologically unassisted approaches in assisting patients in reaching sustained abstinence.[59] Varenicline does not undergo significant hepatic metabolism, with 90% excreted unchanged in the urine. Caution and dose reduction are required when varenicline is used in patients with severe renal impairment.[60] Side effects include nausea, insomnia, abnormal dreams, dizziness, and headache.[36] In 2008, a black box warning was added regarding potential neuropsychiatric symptoms (eg, agitation, suicidal ideation, attempted and completed suicide) but a clear cause-and-effect relationship has not been established.[52,54,61]

ONGOING MONITORING: VERIFYING ABSTINENCE AND PARTICIPATION IN SUBSTANCE USE TREATMENT
Pretransplant Monitoring

While patients are on the waiting list, transplant teams should monitor those with substance use disorders to determine whether they are maintaining abstinence or struggling with relapse. For those attending a rehabilitation program or individual counseling, regular updates from the addictions program provides teams with a measure of the patient's progress in treatment. In some cases, physical deterioration or hepatic encephalopathy interfered with a patient's ability to complete a specific period of abstinence or formal treatment of a substance use disorder. By monitoring the patient's rehabilitation efforts during the waiting period, the team can make an informed decision about whether to proceed with transplantation despite these shortcomings. Patients may also be requested to complete substance use treatment after transplantation.

Random toxicology screens using blood or urine samples that include all substances of interest should also be used for monitoring. Patients are notified about the need to provide a sample of blood or urine and given a limited time in which they may do this. Because some substances (eg, alcohol, cocaine) are only detectable for a short period, failure to provide a sample within a specified time limit is considered equivalent to a positive sample. Positive screen results should be confirmed by gas chromatography and mass spectroscopy because of the risk of false-positive results, especially if a patient denies use.[62] Carbohydrate-deficient transferrin is a marker of heavier sustained alcohol use, but can be increased (falsely suggesting alcohol use) simply because of liver disease.[63] Haller and colleagues[64] suggest because of strong incentives to obscure continued substance use that hair toxicology analyses should be considered for patients seeking transplantation. Hair analysis provides a longer window of ascertainment (90 days) and can identify alcohol and other drug use. In these investigators' study of transplant candidates, hair analysis indicated twice as many cases of use as other tests (self-report, breathalyzer, and urine).[64] Based on the detection window for hair analyses, 2 negative tests help confirm 6 months of continuous abstinence.[64]

Monitoring After Transplantation

Monitoring should also continue after LT. Every routine posttransplant appointment should include questions about any substance use and education about the risks and dangers of use. It is useful for LT teams to develop an approach that continues to foster abstinence and encourages the patient's continued awareness about vulnerability to relapse. A direct, nonjudgmental, supportive approach is recommended to promote disclosure of problems and the desire to seek appropriate addiction treatment.[24] In 1 study of post-LT ALD recipients comparing multiple methods of alcohol use identification (both interviewing and toxicologic screening), patients were found to be open to discussing their use with a transplant team member. Although blood alcohol levels did identify a few cases of covert drinking, patient interviews in the LT clinic were most likely to identify use.[65] Collateral information from primary social supports should also be sought. Random toxicology screens are helpful, especially when relapse is suspected and the patient denies substance abuse. Patients who have relapsed need to be offered assistance in reentering substance use treatment and may benefit from seeing a mental health professional to determine the type of addiction treatment needed and whether a comorbid psychiatric disorder is contributing to relapse.

COMPLEX AND CONTROVERSIAL SUBSTANCE USE ISSUES IN LT CANDIDACY
Access to LT and Beliefs of General Public, Other Nontransplant Physicians, and LT Programs

Although ALD remains the second most common indication for LT, a larger percentage of patients, by some estimates up to 95% of those with end-stage ALD, are not being referred for evaluation, even when AASLD guidelines for referral are satisfied.[66,67] Although some of these potential candidates may still be using alcohol,[66] for those who are abstinent the low rate of referral is attributed to perceptions of ALD as a self-induced disease, low support for transplantation of patients with ALD by physicians and public, unawareness of this therapeutic option, or concerns over possible return to alcohol use after transplantation or nonadherence to long-term post-LT medical requirements, socioeconomic, and possibly racial barriers.[66–73] Although earlier views that patients with ALD are less deserving of transplantation because of self-induced disease, or that they should have sought help to prevent the development of ALD,[74] are no longer widely held in the medical community, surveys of physicians and the general public show they consistently assigned a lower priority for LT to patients with ALD.[75–77] At the level of the transplant programs a more favorable view of patients with ALD is held, especially amongst transplant psychiatrists and psychologists who would prefer to allow a patient to address listing requirements such as achieving sobriety and alcohol rehabilitation rather than reject them unequivocally.[78] Nevertheless, negative beliefs about candidates with ALD may still prevent some potential candidates from being referred to transplant programs when addictions issues could be successfully addressed in preparation for LT. A recent study at a large Veterans Affairs center[66] highlights this issue: compared with other causes of cirrhosis, patients with ALD were significantly less likely to be informed that transplantation was a treatment option and were less likely to be referred for evaluation.

Ethical Perspectives

The United Network for Organ Sharing (UNOS) Ethics Committee and US and UK consensus panels hold the view that a person's past behavior (including alcohol consumption) should not be considered as an exclusion criterion for LT and that equal respect and concern be given to all patients in need of an organ (principle of justice).[30,79,80] In 1 ethicist's view "if we grant the claim that alcoholics are morally responsible for their liver diseases, using moral responsibility as an allocation criterion would undermine the physician-patient relationship necessary for the practice of medicine with its current commitments."[81] Nevertheless, these consensus groups recognize that donated organs are a limited resource and thus recommend identifying the best potential recipients in whom the probability of a good outcome must be highly emphasized to achieve the maximum benefit for all transplants (principle of medical usefulness).[79,82] However, "medical professionals, while honoring the moral obligations to extend life and relieve suffering, must also recognize the limitations of transplantation in meeting these ends."[79]

LT Programs Differ in Listing Criteria

There are no national guidelines for candidacy requirements either in the United States or Europe. Each LT team must decide how to consider complex cases (eg, when the length of sobriety is short, addiction rehabilitation has not been performed, or adequate social support is lacking), optimally with input from mental health or addiction specialists. In an older survey of transplant psychiatrists and psychologists at 14 academic programs, the consensus opinion was to observe, refer for alcohol addictions counseling, and reconsider rather than refuse outright when such issues existed for a potential candidate.[78] However, in that survey there was great variability, with some centers being willing to consider recently drinking individuals and other centers recommending they be turned down outright.[78] A UK consensus panel also acknowledged that equity for patients with ALD might be considered improbable because there exists no nationwide standardized approach for selection, and individuals turned down at 1 UK program because of their alcohol history might be accepted at another.[82] A US consensus panel determined that there should be no absolute contraindication to LT listing in ALD.[30] However, relative contraindications to LT listing included alcohol use by a patient with alcohol abuse or dependence or illicit substance use by a patient with a diagnosis of substance abuse within the past 6 months. Such patients may be referred to regional review boards for consideration if the individual is still deemed to be a good candidate after assessment by the LT team and a substance abuse professional.[30]

As noted earlier, a minimal criterion of 6 months' abstinence for patients with ALD is widely held by programs both in the United States and Europe.[30] However, consensus panels emphasize that 6 months' abstinence alone is not sufficient for placement on the LT list but that patients must be evaluated by a substance abuse professional and must comply with the recommendations of the substance abuse professional.[21,30] In addition consensus panels have recognized that criteria regarding abstinence from alcohol and assessment by a substance abuse professional also apply to other illicit substances.[30,82]

However, a threshold of specifically 6 months' abstinence has limited prognostic value in determining those who remain abstinent, especially abstinence achieved in the context of deteriorating health and lengthy hospital stays.[23,82] It is well known that short sobriety, especially if measured in months, predicts future relapse (see section on predictors of alcohol use after LT). Drawing from large cohorts of alcohol-dependent individuals (general population not LT patients) followed longitudinally for years, 60% to 80% relapse rates are common.[83,84] In 1 such cohort of alcohol-dependent individuals followed 8 to 12 years after an index hospitalization for alcohol treatment, although at least 59% were able to achieve 6 months' sobriety at some point, 95% also relapsed to alcohol dependence and 50% of those who continued to have serious alcohol problems to the end of the 8-year to 12-year follow-up had also at some point achieved 6 months' sobriety.[83] Analogous to cancer remission, stable sobriety is measured in years, and after 5 years of abstinence from alcohol dependence future relapse could be considered unlikely.[83,84]

Alcohol Use on the Waitlist

Three studies have identified up to 25% of waitlisted candidates with ALD using alcohol.[85–87] In 1 study women and those with short sobriety (>6 months but <12 months) were more likely to drink on the waitlist.[86] The prevailing view is that these patients should be removed from the list but allowed to reenter the evaluation process after completing addiction treatment as directed by the mental health or addictions professional of the transplant program.[21,30,88] A 1997 survey of LT program responses to alcohol use on the waitlist ranged from 15% of programs permanently delisting such a patient to a few programs that did not remove the individual but required them to receive counseling.[21] There are no mandated regulations regarding removing a person from the UNOS waitlist or decisions about relisting. These decisions are left to the clinical expertise and individual decisions of the LT programs.[30] Ultimately, these patients need closer monitoring and likely more intensive treatment.

Considerations in advanced liver disease when patients have short sobriety
Patients who first come to the LT evaluation with advanced disease and short sobriety create significant controversy for most LT teams. The extent of recovery and potential for acute decompensation are often difficult to predict, and such patients require close monitoring to ensure that the timing of transplantation is appropriate.[80] There are few data on patients with very short sobriety (eg, <6 months) and whether they benefit from LT.[89] In addition, the potential role of LT in managing patients with severe alcoholic hepatitis remains unsettled.[82] A large study of 340 patients with severe alcoholic hepatitis (Maddrey discrimination function $\geq$32) treated with corticosteroids found only 67% were alive at 6 months,[90] highlighting the limited time frame to work with such patients, including meeting psychosocial and addiction rehabilitation listing requirements. In a study of 74 patients with severe alcoholic cirrhosis (Child-Pugh grade C who were mostly emergency admissions), Vedlt and colleagues[73] found 26% died during the initial hospitalization, but for those who survived hospitalization abstinence was the strongest predictor of survival. Their results indicate if liver improvement is to occur it begins within 3 months and few abstinent patients died within 6 months. These investigators suggested rather than waiting the full 6 months, to consider LT in those patients when a Child-Pugh score of C persists after 3 months of abstinence.[73] This strategy allows patients to be waitlisted sooner and potentially transplanted before dying of acute decompensation. To accomplish this goal, a social and psychological evaluation was recommended at the initial hospitalization with proven patient compliance with directives.[73]

Methadone-maintained LT Candidates

Methadone maintenance therapy (MMT) is a source of confusion and misgiving for much of the public as well as the medical community, but is the most effective treatment of opioid use disorders.[91] Methadone is a μ-opioid agonist that suppresses withdrawal symptoms and blocks the euphoric effects of opioids such as heroin and morphine. Numerous long-term follow-up studies have shown that MMT reduces relapse to opioid use disorders and its associated risks (eg, injection-related health problems, criminal behavior). Patients are able to remain on stable doses of 80 to 120 mg/d of methadone long-term without misuse.[36] Dose adjustment may be necessary in renal or hepatic failure.[37] Higher doses may be required after LT when hepatic metabolic activities are normalized: in 1 study an average post-LT dose increase from baseline was 60%.[92] MMT is available only through licensed treatment centers, which also provide counseling and toxicology monitoring for relapse. Despite little clinical experience with patients receiving MMT, surveys indicate that only one-quarter to one-half of US LT centers are willing to accept a candidate on MMT and many would only do so if the patient tapered off methadone.[93,94] This situation is because of a lack of understanding of MMT as a treatment of opioid use disorders, rather than an alternative addiction.[95] Discontinuation of methadone potentially places patients at high risk for relapse, and relapse could make them ineligible for LT.[91,95] Several studies have reported similar survival outcomes for small cohorts of MMT compared with non-MMT LT recipients[96,97] with isolated opioid use that did not affect outcomes.[96] Two studies have suggested perhaps slightly higher perioperative morbidity and longer hospital stays for these patients[92,97] and in 1 study a higher percentage of severe recurrent HCV infections,[92] but all studies supported the consideration of patients on MMT for LT if supported by psychosocial assessment.

Third-party Payer Contributions

Although the transplant teams may decide to list a patient for LT, in the United States third-party payers (eg, a health insurance carrier) may require their own specific period of abstinence, introduce their own addiction treatment requirements or monitoring of abstinence or treatment compliance, or deny insurance coverage for LT.[21] Some insurers have refused reimbursement pending smoking cessation.[98]

POSTTRANSPLANT OUTCOMES
General Outcomes for ALD and HCV

The outcome and survival after LT for ALD (without comorbid HCV) in general is comparable with or better than that of patients transplanted for other types of liver disease.[2,99,100] The cumulative experience from multiple transplant centers in the United States and Europe show that the 1-year and 5-year actuarial survival rates after LT are similar for patients with and without ALD.[1,3] The overall 1-year and 5-year survival rates of patients with ALD were 82% and 68%, respectively, in the UNOS database, and 85% and 73%, respectively, in the European Liver Transplant Registry.[1,3,89] Some experts regard ALD as an excellent indication for LT based on patient/graft survival and functional outcomes.[89]

Compared with the positive survival outcomes for those with ALD, it has been well established that patients transplanted for HCV consistently have markedly lower long-term patient and graft survival rates compared with patients transplanted for other liver diseases. Recurrent HCV is an inevitable post-LT outcome and the incidence of cirrhosis by 5 years after LT can be as high as 30%.[101] Compared with the referent of primary biliary cirrhosis (PBC) the risk of graft loss to recurrence HCV is 11 times higher.[99] An analyses of a decade of UNOS data found HCV recurrence to be the cause of graft failure in 55.2% to 61.3% of failures.[102] One study investigating the combination of HCV and ALD on post-LT outcomes found those with HCV alone had the poorest post-LT survival, followed by those with both ALD and HCV, and those with ALD alone having the best survival.[103]

Quality of Life and Other Psychosocial Aspects

In an earlier study, data from 139 patients transplanted for ALD and a control group of 486 non-ALD recipients were analyzed from the National Institute of Diabetes and Digestive Diseases-Liver Transplant Registry (a 7-year prospective study of LT recipients from 3 LT programs).[104] Wiesner and colleagues[104] found that the quality of life of

ALD recipients (including perceptions of health, well-being, affective distress, and psychological symptoms) was slightly worse for the ALD group before LT and also diminished slightly after LT, with a significant difference between groups emerging by 3 years after LT. However, by 1 year after LT the percentages of patients who were not able to work or who improved in their ability to work were similar in both groups. In a single-center study of 47 ALD LT recipients quality of life was assessed using the Nottingham Health Profile (NHP) and the Short Form-36 (SF-36) Health Survey, and scores were found to be similar between the subgroup of patients with harmful drinking and those with none or mild alcohol relapse.[105] Overall, NHP and SF-36 health dimension scores were similar to community controls.[105]

RELAPSE RATES AND RELATED OUTCOMES
Use of Alcohol After LT for ALD

After initial estimates of 20% to 40% 2-year to 5-year relapse rates[21,27,65] seem to compare favorably with the 2-year alcohol relapse rates of 60% to 80% after conventional treatment of alcohol dependence (nontransplant patients) and up to 95% 5-year relapse rates noted in many conventional treatment studies.[83] Lower rates of heavy or pathologic drinking have been reported in US, UK, and European cohorts of ALD recipients, with only 10% to 20% reaching this consumption pattern.[60,88,99,106,107] Although many reports emphasize that the onset of drinking is more common in the first 2 years after LT,[108] onset of first use or heavy patterns of use can begin years later,[60,107,109] highlighting the chronic nature of alcohol addiction and the need for long-term monitoring.[60,107] That the overall rates are substantially lower in ALD LT recipients compared with the general population of individuals with alcohol dependence may be because of the selection process for LT, careful monitoring by the LT team after transplant, and the life-altering experience of LT.[4,80,83,110]

A critical issue in establishing accurate alcohol use rates involves the definition of alcohol relapse. In most studies alcohol relapse has been defined as any alcohol at all including only a single drink, whereas from an addiction perspective this may be considered a slip. Definitions of heavier use vary across studies, with investigators setting different thresholds of alcohol use with respect to the parameters of quantity, frequency, and duration of use. To overcome these methodological limitations a recent meta-analysis included 50 studies of ALD recipients, including studies from North America and Europe.[109] This analysis found that relapse to any alcohol use was 5.6% of patients per year of observation, and 2.5% of patients per year for relapse to heavy use.[109] The European studies had a significantly higher average rate (6.7% of patients per year) than North American studies (4.4%). European studies also found significantly higher rates of relapse to heavy alcohol use (3.2% vs 1.2% of patients per year).[109]

Beyond rates of return to alcohol use, specific patterns of alcohol consumption can emerge both during the early recovery period and years later. In 1 study when the consumption of alcohol was prospectively surveyed 2 early-onset patterns (1 moderate use and 1 heavy use) were identified, as well as a sustained pattern of low-level use that evolved into a heavy use pattern 3 years after LT (Fig. 2).[60] In this study the moderate use pattern (defined as nearly 4 standard drinks/wk) and heavy use patterns (defined as 2 or more standard drinks/d) accounted for 20% of the cohort.[60]

Illicit Drug Use After LT

Few studies have examined the use of drugs in LT recipients and often studies have examined substance use in ALD recipients only. For example, 1 single-center study

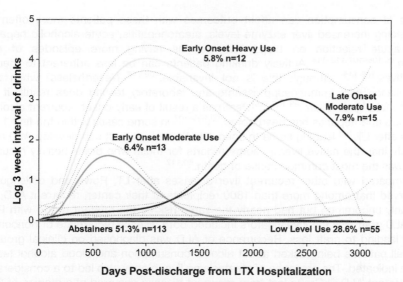

Fig. 2. Specific alcohol use trajectories from the point of transplant. (*From* DiMartini A, Dew MA, Day N, et al. Trajectories of alcohol consumption following liver transplantation. Am J Transplant 2010;10(10):2308–12; with permission.)

of ALD recipients with a median follow-up of 41 months found 17.2% had documented drug use after LT (mostly marijuana).[111] Drug abuse before transplantation was the only independent predictor of drug abuse after transplantation.[111] A recent meta-analysis[109] that included 4 studies reporting on return to illicit drug use in LT recipients who were identified as having used illicit drugs before transplantation found the rate of return to any use was very low (1.9% of patients per year). In that meta-analysis, Dew and colleagues[109] also found the rate of illicit drug relapse was significantly lower in LT recipient studies than in studies of other types of organ recipients.

Tobacco Use After LT

Various rates of tobacco use have been identified in single-center studies. A recent single-center cross-sectional telephone survey of recipients found 15% smoked, with most smoking less than 1 pack per day.[16] Higher smoking rates are observed among cohorts of ALD recipients of up to 40% to 50% within the first 2 years after LT.[15,19] However, these rates underestimate the rates among previous smokers, which can be as high as 60% to 70%.[15,19] In a recent meta-analysis of substance use after transplantation for patients with alcohol or substance use histories, a post-LT smoking rate of 10% of patients per year of observation was determined.[109]

Outcomes Related to Alcohol Use After LT for ALD

Although the definition of alcohol relapse varies widely between studies, to examine the specific contribution of alcohol use to outcomes, a threshold of exposure that includes both quantity and frequency should be used and a rationale for choosing defined levels of exposure should be proposed. Several studies have investigated outcomes using specific quantity/frequency definitions for moderate to heavy use of alcohol (defined variously as approximately 4 or more standard drinks/wk or 4 or more standard drinks/d or more than 21 units/wk for men and 14 units/wk for women or periods of 3.5 or more units a day). These studies found that moderate to heavy levels of consumption can affect outcomes with these patients more often experiencing increased liver enzyme levels, steatohepatitis, acute alcoholic hepatitis, and acute rejection on biopsy as well as having more episodes of graft failure.[60,105–107,112–114] Actively drinking patients can be less adherent to medical directives,[106,115] although this is not invariable.[109,116] Nevertheless, when poor compliance with immunosuppressants and laboratory testing does result, it can lead to fatal graft failure.[99,106,115] Death as a result of early-onset recurrent alcoholic cirrhosis and hepatitis has been noted,[60,105–107] in some cases within the first 1 to 2 years after LT,[105] leading some to speculate that a liver graft can develop ALD more quickly than the native liver. In some reports for those who drank heavily recurrent ALD was the most common cause of death.[60,117]

Compared with other recurrent liver diseases after LT, Rowe and colleagues[99] observed that among more than 1800 recipients at their center, recurrent ALD was not only uncommon but had nearly the same risk as the referent group with PBC. For ALD graft loss the investigators included both disease recurrence or noncompliance leading to graft loss. Recurrence of ALD was diagnosed on clinical grounds, with all patients being asked about alcohol consumption and blood alcohol testing when indicated. The presence of steatosis on liver biopsy also led to a consideration of recurrent ALD.[99] Grafts lost from recurrent disease occurred at a median of 2543 days (nearly 7 years) for ALD, 2833 days for PBC, 1429 days for HCV, and 581 days for hepatocellular carcinoma. Graft loss to recurrent disease was only 3.2% for ALD compared with 1.3% for PBC and 14.3% for HCV. The cumulative risk for graft loss for ALD by 10 years was approximately equivalent to PBC (about 2%). No difference was seen when comparing the rate of graft loss from all causes after 90 postoperative days between ALD and PBC (hazard ratio [HR] 1.4; 95% confidence interval 0.9–2.0).[99] These investigators acknowledged that, although a significant proportion (up to 50%) of patients return to drinking alcohol, the return to harmful drinking at their center was less common, with less than 10% of patients returning to drinking more than 21 units per week.[99] This number is similar to the rates of harmful drinking reported at many centers, suggesting that comparatively ALD recurrence could be expected to be low.

Tobacco-related Outcomes

Cancer

Oropharyngeal cancer, lung cancer, and digestive tract cancers are important causes of death after LT,[115,117] with the rate of upper airway malignances significantly higher in ALD compared with non-ALD recipients.[20,115,118] The higher prevalences of oropharyngeal and lung cancers are likely related to the higher percentage of tobacco users in the ALD group.[60,115] Of the de novo malignancies that developed in a cohort of ALD recipients, 89% were upper aerodigestive malignancies; these cancers were significantly associated with male gender and smoking but not with post-LT alcohol use.[119] These investigators concluded the significant decline in survival after 10 years was largely because of aerodigestive malignancies, which was a greater cause of morbidity and mortality than recurrent alcohol liver disease.[119] In 1 study the cumulative rate of malignancies at 10 years was 12.7% in active smokers versus 2.1% of nonsmokers ($P = .02$), although smoking did not have an effect on cardiovascular disease.[19] Not uncommonly lung cancers are identified at an advanced stage when prognosis is poor. In 1 study of LT recipients the mean survival after tumor diagnosis was 5.4 months.[118] Even all other nonskin malignancies seem to be higher in ALD recipients, who have a higher probability of developing such malignancies by 10 years (18% for ALD compared with recipients transplanted for most other types of liver diseases, which were only 10%).[120] Multivariate analysis showed that older age, a history of smoking (HR = 1.6, P = .046), and ALD (HR = 2.1, P = .01) were associated with development of solid malignancies after LT.[120]

Vascular Complications

In a study of LT recipients (not limited to patients with ALD) Pungpapong and colleagues[18] observed that patients with a history of cigarette smoking had a higher incidence of vascular complications than nonsmokers (17.8% vs 8%) and a higher incidence of arterial complications (hepatic artery stenosis or thrombosis) (13.5% vs 4.8%). These investigators also found having quit cigarette smoking 2 years before LT reduced vascular complications by 58.6% and reduced arterial complications by 77.6%.[18] The calculated absolute risk reduction was 15.9%, and therefore the number of the patients needed to quit cigarette smoking 2 years before LT to prevent 1 arterial complication after LT was 7 patients.[18] Post-LT active smokers also have poorer 5-year and 10-year survival than nonsmokers (68% and 54% vs 83%, and 77%, respectively) (P = .04).[121] Smoking independently predicted death (HR 2.23, P = .03) and active smokers showed increased cardiovascular-specific mortality (P = .01) and sepsis-specific mortality (P = .02).[121]

PREDICTORS OF ALCOHOL USE AFTER LT

One of the strongest and most consistent predictors of alcohol use after LT for ALD is shorter length of sobriety. Whether measured as a specific cut point, such as 6 months, or as a continuous variable, length of sobriety predicts future alcohol use. This finding is most likely because many ALD recipients have alcohol dependence, which is a relapsing remitting disorder. In addition, as pointed out earlier (see section on LT programs differ in listing criteria), stable sobriety is measured in years, not by months as is common before LT. Thus attempts to identify a specific threshold of months of pre-LT sobriety that predicts future abstinence have been unsuccessful; it has been shown only that longer sobriety predicts less risk for future use.[108]

In a recent review of the literature on predictors of relapse to alcohol use after LT for ALD, McCallum and Masterton[122] concluded that it was difficult to firmly establish predictors because most studies were retrospective in design, using single-center, small cohorts. Factors of the psychosocial history that were more consistently reported in predicting better outcomes (ie, less risk of post-LT alcohol use) were social stability, no close relatives with an alcohol problem, older age, no repeated alcohol treatment failures, good compliance with medical care, no current polydrug misuse, and no coexisting severe mental disorder.[122] Other studies have shown in addition to length of abstinence that a diagnosis of alcohol dependence, family history of alcoholism,[107,108] number of alcohol withdrawal experiences,[107] rehabilitation or failed rehabilitation attempts,[88,108] poor social support,[67,117] and a history of other substance use[88,108] predict return to alcohol use after LT. In the meta-analysis by Dew and colleagues[109] risk factors for any alcohol use included poorer social support, family alcohol history, and pre-LT abstinence of 6 months or less, which showed small but significant associations with alcohol use (r = 0.17–0.21). A study that examined psychological stresses in the 3-month period after transplant found those ALD recipients who were more stressed and reported worse health compared with 1 year earlier, had more pain, less vitality, felt less confident they would receive another liver if they needed it, and regretted undergoing LT were more likely to relapse to an early-onset moderate to heavy pattern of alcohol use.[60]

FUTURE DIRECTIONS
Clinical Initiatives

Although alcoholic recipients can experience significant alcohol-related morbidity and mortality after LT, the relatively good outcomes and apparent minimal impact of such occurrences can be explained by the infrequency of heavy alcohol use after LT and the amount and duration of alcohol exposure required to produce an adverse effect on graft, health, and survival. However, although ALD recipients have good physical health outcomes overall, from a clinical perspective, measures to improve the identification and treatment of substance use and modifiable risk factors could further improve outcomes. Improvement would be more likely if all programs provided regular and ongoing monitoring of addiction and behavioral health issues both before and after LT. However, such monitoring is not routine. These initiatives are especially needed for patients with previous substance use disorders. For substance use disorders (alcohol and illicit drugs) this strategy requires implementing consistent and regular screening and monitoring programs for candidates, waitlisted patients, and recipients. In parallel a process for mental health evaluation and treatment is necessary to address any identified substance use. Because many programs have mental health clinicians who perform the initial transplant evaluation, these professionals may be available for follow-up appointments and treatment if needed. These arrangements are especially needed when recipients are only partially able to complete pre-LT addiction rehabilitation or are recommended to receive post-LT treatment. Monitoring for the long-term, not just perioperatively, is also needed as discussed earlier because substance-use issues can emerge years after stable abstinence. Investigations of post-LT ALD recipients support the use of high-frequency regularly scheduled visits with the patient and family as, among other things, an effective monitoring tool.[27] In addition, monitoring and providing treatment of stress during the early postoperative period may help prevent early relapse. The first year may be an especially important time frame to target because of the initial high rates of relapse during this period.

Greater efforts are required to identify post-LT tobacco use and assist with treatment of tobacco cessation. This strategy is especially critical because tobacco-related deaths seem to exceed alcohol and other substance use-related deaths in LT recipients. One investigator[119] reported at their center, to screen for tobacco-related cancers, these patients undergo an upper digestive endoscopy with lugol coloration, a clinical pharyngolaryngeal examination (because otorhinolaryngology screening is insufficient), and a chest radiography, in the case of persistent smoking. Studies of lung cancer screening have not been performed in LT recipients, yet in the general population screening is beneficial for early detection when individualized based on age and years of smoking.[123]

Research Initiatives

Most of the research investigating relapse rates and outcomes has focused on alcohol use, and little is known about relapse rates to other substances, especially among those with drug use histories (with or without HCV infection). Prospective studies that longitudinally monitor illicit drug use are needed, perhaps including a comparison group to examine outcomes. An additional area of particular importance is the examination of outcomes of methadone-maintained patients. From the small and single-center studies to date, there is little evidence that these patients shorten their lives after LT, or damage their health or their graft through drug relapse. Correcting misconceptions about methadone as a valid treatment and greater evidence of comparable outcomes may allow more centers to consider these patients as possible LT candidates. Patients with acute alcoholic hepatitis are not considered for LT, typically because they have very short sobriety, often drinking up until hospitalization. However, given that those with severe acute alcoholic hepatitis who do not respond to treatment have a 50% mortality in 2 months, 1 suggestion has been to conduct pilot studies on a small cohort of patients to determine whether transplantation improves survival in patients with severe alcoholic hepatitis.[124]

We conclude that despite nearly 3 decades of experience with patients with alcohol and more recently other substance use disorders in LT, there is still much work that needs to be done and many questions that are unanswered. We believe such clinical and research initiatives can improve our clinical care and patient and graft outcomes, advance our knowledge and understanding of these specific patient populations, and address disparities in access to transplantation.

REFERENCES

1. European Liver Transplant Registry. Data on recipients. Available at: http://www. eltr.org/. Accessed March 21, 2011.
2. Lucey MR, Schaubel DE, Guidinger MK, et al. Effect of alcoholic liver disease and hepatitis C infection on waiting list and posttransplant mortality and transplant survival benefit. Hepatology 2009;50:400–6.
3. 2009 Annual Report of the U.S. Organ Procurement and Transplantation Network and the Scientific Registry of Transplant Recipients: Transplant Data 1996–2008. Health Resources and Services Administration, Healthcare Systems Bureau, Division of Transplantation, Rockville, MD. Available at: http://optn. transplant.hrsa.gov/ar2009/. Accessed August 18, 2011.
4. Beresford TP. Psychiatric assessment of alcoholic candidates for liver transplantation. In: Lucey MR, Merion RM, Beresford TP, editors. Liver transplantation and the alcoholic patient: medical, surgical, and psychosocial issues. Cambridge (United Kingdom): Cambridge University Press; 1994. p. 29–49.
5. DiMartini A, Beresford T. Alcoholism and liver transplantation. Curr Opin Organ Transplant 1999;4:117–81.
6. Diehl AM. Alcoholic liver disease. Liver transplantation and surgery 1997;3(3): 206–11.
7. The Substance Abuse and Mental Health Services Administration (SAMHSA), agency of the U.S. Department of Health and Human Services (HHS), 2009 annual report. Available at: http://oas.samhsa.gov/NSDUHlatest.htm. Accessed August 18, 2011.
8. Grant BF. Prevalence and correlates of alcohol use and DSM-IV alcohol dependence in the United States: results of the National Longitudinal Alcohol Epidemiologic Survey. J Stud Alcohol 1997;58(5):464–73.
9. Kessler RC, Berglund P, Demler O, et al. Lifetime prevalence and age-of-onset distributions of DSM-IV disorders in the National Comorbidity Survey Replication. Arch Gen Psychiatry 2005;62:593–602.
10. Centers for Disease Control Prevention. Hepatitis C FAQs for health professionals. Available at: http://www.cdc.gov/hepatitis/HCV/HCVfaq.htm#section1. Accessed March 21, 2011.
11. National Survey on Drug Use and Health Report. 2009. The NSDUH Report is published periodically by the Office of Applied Studies, Substance Abuse and Mental Health Services Administration (SAMHSA). Available at: http://oas. samhsa.gov. Accessed March 22, 2011.

12. DiMartini A, Dew MA, Javed L, et al. The pretransplant psychiatric and medical comorbidity of alcoholic liver disease patients who received liver transplant. Psychosomatics 2004;45(6):517–23.
13. Weinrieb RM, Van Horn DH, McLellan AT, et al. Drinking behavior and motivation for treatment among alcohol dependent liver transplant candidates. J Addict Dis 2001a;20(2):105–19.
14. Weinrieb RM, Van Horn DH, McLellan AT, et al. Alcoholism treatment after liver transplantation: lessons learned from a clinical trial that failed. Psychosomatics 2001;42(2):111–5.
15. DiMartini A, Javed L, Russell S, et al. Tobacco use following liver transplantation for alcoholic liver disease: an underestimated problem. Liver Transpl 2005; 11(6):679–83.
16. Ehlers SL, Rodrigue JR, Widows MR, et al. Tobacco use before and after liver transplantation: a single center survey and implications for clinical practice and research. Liver Transpl 2004;10:412–7.
17. Ethics Committee, United Network for Organ Sharing. General principles for allocating human organs and tissues. Transplant Proc 1992;24:2227–35.
18. Pungpapong S, Manzarbeitia C, Ortiz J, et al. Cigarette smoking is associated with an increased incidence of vascular complications after liver transplantation. Liver Transpl 2002;8:582–7.
19. van der Heide F, Dijkstra G, Porte RJ, et al. Smoking behavior in liver transplant recipients. Liver Transpl 2009;15(6):648–55.
20. Duvoux C, Delacroix I, Richardet J, et al. Increased incidence of oropharyngeal squamous cell carcinomas after liver transplantation for alcoholic cirrhosis. Transplantation 1999;67:418–21.
21. Everhart JE, Beresford TP. Liver transplantation for alcoholic liver disease: a survey of transplantation programs in the United States. Liver Transpl Surg 1997;3:220–6.
22. Day E, Best D, Sweeting R, et al. Detecting lifetime alcohol problems in individuals referred for liver transplantation for nonalcoholic liver failure. Liver Transpl 2008;14(11):1609–13.
23. Neuberger J, Schulz KH, Day C, et al. Transplantation for alcoholic liver disease. J Hepatol 2002;36:130–7.
24. Weinrieb RM, Lucey MR. Treatment of addictive behaviors in liver transplant patients. Liver Transpl 2007;13:S79–82.
25. Cupples SA, Steslow B. Use of behavioral contingency contracting with heart transplant candidates. Prog Transplant 2001;11:137–44.
26. Nelson MK, Presberg BA, Olbrisch ME, et al. Behavioral contingency contracting to reduce substance abuse and other high-risk health behaviors in organ transplant patients. J Transpl Coord 1995;5:35–40.
27. Campbell DA, Punch JD. Monitoring for alcohol use relapse after liver transplantation for alcoholic liver disease. Liver Transpl Surg 1997;3(3):300–3.
28. Murray KL, Carithers RF. AASLD practice guidelines: evaluation of the patient for liver transplantation. Hepatology 2005;41(6).
29. O'Shea RS, Dasarathy S, McCullough AJ, the Practice Guideline Committee of the American Association for the Study of Liver Diseases and the Practice Parameters Committee of the American College of Gastroenterology. AASLD practice guidelines alcoholic liver disease. Hepatology 2010;51(1):307–28.
30. Lucey MR, Brown KA, Everson GE, et al. Minimal criteria for placement of adults on the liver transplant waiting list: a report of a national conference organized by the American Society of Transplant Physicians and the American Association for the Study of Liver Diseases. Liver Transpl Surg 1997;3(6):628–37.

31. McLellan AT. Evolution in addiction treatment concepts and methods. In: Galanter M, Kleber HD, editors. The American Psychiatric Publishing textbook of substance abuse treatment. 4th edition. Washington, DC: American Psychiatric Publishing Inc.; 2008. p. 93–108.

32. Tonigan JS. Alcoholics anonymous outcomes and benefits, in recent developments in alcoholism. In: Galanter M, Kaskutas LA, editors. Research on alcoholics anonymous and spirituality in addiction recovery, vol. 18. New York: Springer; p. 357–72.

33. Weinrieb RM, Van Horn D, Lynch KG, et al. A randomized, controlled study of treatment for alcohol dependence in patients awaiting liver transplantation. Liver Transpl 2011;17:539–47.

34. Georgiou G, Webb K, Griggs K, et al. First report of a psychosocial intervention for patients with alcohol related liver disease undergoing liver transplantation. Liver Transpl 2003;9(7):772–5.

35. Rosner S, Hackl-Herrwerth A, Leucht S, et al. Acamprosate for alcohol dependence. Cochrane Database Syst Rev 2010;9:CD004332.

36. Ross S, Peselow E. Pharmacotherapy of addictive disorders. Clin Neuropharmacol 2009;32:277–89.

37. DiMartini AF, Crone CC, Fireman M. Organ transplantation. In: Ferrando SJ, Levenson JL, Owen JA, editors. Clinical manual of psychopharmacology in the medically ill. Washington, DC: American Psychiatric Publishing; 2010c. p. 469–99.

38. Chick J. Safety issues concerning the use of disulfiram in treating alcohol dependence. Drug Saf 1999;20(5):427–35.

39. Berglund M. A better widget? Three lessons learned for improving addiction treatment from a meta-analytical study. Addiction 2005;11:742–50.

40. Krampe H, Ehrenreich H. Supervised disulfuram as adjunct to psychotherapy in alcoholism treatment. Curr Pharm Des 2010;16:2076–90.

41. Beresford TP, Martin B. The evidence for drug treatment of alcohol dependence in liver transplant patients. Curr Opin Organ Transplant 2007;12:176–81.

42. Garbutt JC. Efficacy and tolerability of naltrexone in the management of alcohol dependence. Curr Pharm Des 2010;16:2091–7.

43. Garbutt JC, Kranzler HR, O'Malley SS, et al. Efficacy and tolerability of long-acting injectable naltrexone for alcohol dependence. JAMA 2005;293:1617–25.

44. Minozzi S, Amato L, Vecchi S, et al. Oral naltrexone maintenance treatment for opioid dependence. Cochrane Database Syst Rev 2011;4.

45. Kahan M, Srivastava A, Ordean A, et al. Buprenorphine: new treatment of opioid addiction in primary care. Can Fam Physician 2011;57:281–9.

46. Herve S, Riachi G, Noblet C, et al. Acute hepatitis due to buprenorphine administration. Eur J Gastroenterol Hepatol 2004;16:1033–7.

47. Zuin M, Giogini A, Selmi C, et al. Acute liver and renal failure during treatment with buprenorphine at therapeutic dose. Dig Liver Dis 2009;41:e8–10.

48. Wedam EF, Bigelow GE, Johnson RE, et al. QT-interval effects of methadone, levomethadyl, and buprenorphine in a randomized trial. Arch Intern Med 2007;167:2469–75.

49. Bogenschutz MP, Abbott PJ, Kushner R, et al. Effects of buprenorphine and hepatitis C on liver enzymes in adolescents and young adults. J Addict Med 2010;4:211–6.

50. Bright RP. Denial of hepatic transplantation on the basis of smoking: is it ethical? Curr Opin Organ Transplant 2010;15:249–53.

51. Herman AI, Sofuoglu M. Comparison of available treatments for tobacco addiction. Curr Psychiatry Rep 2010;12:433–40.

52. McNeil JJ, Piccenna L, Ioannides-Demos LL. Smoking cessation: recent advances. Cardiovasc Drugs Ther 2010;24:359–67.

53. Moss A, Siegler M. Should alcoholics compete equally for liver transplantation? JAMA 1991;265:1296–8.

54. Hays JT, Ebbert JO. Adverse effects and tolerability of medications for the treatment of tobacco use and dependence. Drugs 2010;70:2357–72.

55. Crone CC, Marcangelo M, Lackamp J, et al. Gastrointestinal disorders. In: Ferrando SJ, Levenson JL, Owen JA, editors. Clinical manual of psychopharmacology in the medically ill. Washington, DC: American Psychiatric Publishing Inc.; 2010. p. 103–48.

56. Cuadrado A, Fabrega E, Casafont F, et al. Alcohol recidivism impairs long-term patient survival after orthotopic liver transplantation for alcoholic liver disease. Liver Transpl 2005;11:420–6.

57. Boshier A, Wilton LV, Shakir SA. Evaluation of the safety of bupropion (Zyban) for smoking cessation from experience gained in general practices in England in 2000. Eur J Clin Pharmacol 2003;59:767–73.

58. Hughes JR, Stead LF, Lancaster T. Antidepressants for smoking cessation. Cochrane Database Syst Rev 2007;1:CD000031.

59. Cahill K, Stead LF, Lancaster T. Nicotine receptor partial agonists for smoking cessation. Cochrane Database Syst Rev 2011;2:CD006103.

60. DiMartini A, Dew MA, Day N, et al. Trajectories of alcohol consumption following liver transplantation. Am J Transplant 2010;10(10):2305–12.

61. Purvis TL, Nelson LA, Mambourg SE. Varenicline use in patients with mental illness: an update of the evidence. Expert Opin Drug Saf 2010;9:471–82.

62. Warner EA, Sharma N. Laboratory diagnosis. In: Ries RK, Fiellin DA, Miller SC, et al, editors. Principles of addiction medicine. 4th edition. Philadelphia: Lippincott Williams & Wilkins; 2009. p. 295–304.

63. DiMartini A, Day N, Lane T, et al. Carbohydrate deficient transferrin in abstaining patients with end-stage liver disease. Alcohol Clin Exp Res 2001;25(12): 1729–33.

64. Haller DH, Acosta MC, Lewis D, et al. Hair analysis versus conventional methods of drug testing in substance abusers seeking organ transplantation. Am J Transplant 2010;10:1305–11.

65. DiMartini A, Day N, Dew M, et al. Alcohol use following liver transplantation: a comparison of follow-up methods. Psychosomatics 2001;42:55–62.

66. Julapalli VR, Kramer JR, El-Serag HB. Evaluation for liver transplantation: adherence to AASLD referral guidelines in a large veterans affairs center. Liver Transpl 2005;11:1370–8.

67. Kotlyar DS, Burke A, Campbell MS, et al. Critical review of candidacy for orthotopic liver transplantation in alcoholic liver disease. Am J Gastroenterol 2008; 103:734–43.

68. Bryce CL, Angus DC, Arnold RM, et al. Sociodemographic differences in early access to liver transplantation services. Am J Transplant 2009;9:2092–101.

69. Cahill K, Stead LF, Lancaster T. Nicotine receptor partial agonists for smoking cessation. Cochrane Database Syst Rev 2010;2:CD006103.

70. Douglas D. Should everyone have equal access to organ transplantation? An argument in favor. Arch Intern Med 2003;163(16):1883–5.

71. Dumortier J, Guillaud O, Adham M, et al. Negative impact of de novo malignancies rather than alcohol relapse on survival after liver transplantation for alcoholic cirrhosis: a retrospective analysis of 305 patients in a single center. Am J Gastroenterol 2007;102:1032–41.

72. Neuberger J. Public and professional attitudes to transplanting alcoholic patients. Liver Transpl 2007;13(11 Suppl 2):S65–8.
73. Veldt BJ, Lainé F, Guillygomarc'h A, et al. Indication of liver transplantation in severe alcoholic liver cirrhosis: quantitative evaluation and optimal timing. J Hepatol 2002;36:93–8.
74. Moss AH, Siegler M. Should alcoholics compete equally for liver transplantation? JAMA 1991;265(10):1295–8.
75. Ubel P, Jepson C, Baron J, et al. Allocation of transplantable organs: do people want to punish patients for causing their illness? Liver Transpl 2001;7(7):600–7.
76. Neuberger J, Adams D, MacMaster P, et al. Assessing priorities for allocation of donor liver grafts: survey of public and clinicians. BMJ 1998;317:172–5.
77. McMaster P. Transplantation for alcoholic liver disease in an era of organ shortage. Lancet 2000;355:424–5.
78. Snyder SL, Drooker M, Strain J. A survey estimate of academic liver transplant teams' selection practices for alcohol-dependent applicants. Psychosomatics 1996;37:432–7.
79. OPTN/UNOS Ethics Committee general considerations in assessment for transplant candidacy. Available at: http://optn.transplant.hrsa.gov/resources/bioethics. asp?index=10. Accessed March 30, 2011.
80. Webb K, Shepherd L, Day E, et al. Transplantation for alcoholic liver disease: report of a consensus meeting. Liver Transplant 2006;12:301–5.
81. Ho D. When good organs go to bad people. Bioethics 2008;22(2):77–83.
82. Webb K, Shepherd L, Day E, et al. Transplantation for alcoholic liver disease: report of a consensus meeting. Liver Transpl 2006;12:301–5.
83. Vaillant GE. The natural history of alcoholism and its relationship to liver transplantation. Liver Transpl Surg 1997;3:304–10.
84. Vaillant GE. A 60-year follow-up of alcoholic men. Addiction 2003;98:1043–51.
85. Iasi MS, Vieira A, Anez CI, et al. Recurrence of alcohol ingestion in liver transplantation candidates. Transplant Proc 2003;35(3):1123–4.
86. Vieira A, Rolim EG, De Capua A Jr, et al. Relapse of alcohol consumption in liver transplant candidates. Risk factor analysis. Arq Gastroenterol 2007;44(3):205–9.
87. Weinrieb R, Van Horn D, Lucey M, et al. Interpreting the significance of drinking by alcohol dependent liver transplant patients: fostering candor is the key to recovery. Liver Transpl 2000;6(6):769–76.
88. Beresford TP. Predictive factors for alcoholic relapse in the selection of alcohol-dependent persons for hepatic transplant. Liver Transpl Surg 1997;3(3):280–91.
89. Lim JK, Keefe EB. Liver transplantation for alcoholic liver disease: current concepts and length of sobriety. Liver Transpl 2004;10:S31–8.
90. Louvet A, Texier F, Dharancy S, et al. A prognostic model predicting the death at 6 months of patients with severe alcoholic hepatitis. Hepatology 2004;40:274A.
91. Stotts AL, Dodrill CL, Kosten TR. Opioid dependence treatment: options in pharmacotherapy. Expert Opin Pharmacother 2009;10(11):1727–40.
92. Weinrieb RM, Barnett R, Lynch KG, et al. A matched comparison study of medical and psychiatric complications and anesthesia and analgesia requirements in methadone-maintained liver transplant recipients. Liver Transpl 2004; 10(1):97–106.
93. Koch M, Banys P. Liver transplantation and opioid dependence. JAMA 2001; 285:1056–8.
94. Kroeker KI, Basin VG, Shaw-Stiffel T, et al. Adult liver transplant survey: policies towards eligibility criteria in Canada and the United States 2007. Liver Int 2008; 28:1250–5.

95. Jiao M, Greanya ED, Haque M, et al. Methadone maintenance therapy in liver transplantation. Prog Transplant 2010;20:209–15.

96. Liu LU, Schiano TD, Lau N, et al. Survival and risk of recidivism in methadone-dependent patients undergoing liver transplantation. Am J Transplant 2003;3: 1273–7.

97. Kanchana TP, Kaul V, Manzarbeitia C, et al. Liver transplantation for patients on methadone maintenance. Liver Transplant 2002;8(9):778–82.

98. Lee DS, Mathur AK, Acker WB, et al. Effects of smoking on survival for patients with end-stage liver disease. J Am Coll Surg 2009;208(6):1077–84.

99. Rowe IA, Webb K, Gunson BK, et al. The impact of disease recurrence on graft survival following liver transplantation: a single centre experience. Transpl Int 2008;21:459–65.

100. Belle SH, Beringer KC, Deter KM. Liver transplantation for alcoholic liver disease in the United States 1988 to 1995. Liver Transpl Surg 1997;3:212–9.

101. Berenguer M, Ferrell L, Watson J, et al. HCV-related fibrosis progression following liver transplantation: increase in recent years. J Hepatol 2000;32:673–84.

102. Futagawa Y, Terasaki PI, Waki K, et al. No improvement in long-term liver transplant graft survival in the last decade: an analysis of the UNOS data. Am J Transplant 2006;6:1398–406.

103. Aguilera V, Berenguer M, Rubín A, et al. Cirrhosis of mixed etiology (hepatitis C virus and alcohol): posttransplantation outcome–comparison with hepatitis C virus-related cirrhosis and alcoholic-related cirrhosis. Liver Transpl 2009;15:79–87.

104. Wiesner RH, Lombardero M, Lake JR, et al. Liver transplantation for end-stage alcoholic liver disease: an assessment of outcomes. Liver Transpl Surg 1997; 3(3):231–9.

105. Pereira SP, Howard LM, Muiesan P, et al. Quality of life after liver transplantation for alcoholic liver disease. Liver Transpl 2000;6:762–8.

106. Pageaux GP, Bismuth M, Perney P, et al. Alcohol relapse after liver transplantation for alcoholic liver disease: does it matter? J Hepatol 2003;38(5):629–34.

107. Perney P, Bismuth M, Sigaud H, et al. Are preoperative patterns of alcohol consumption predictive of relapse after liver transplantation for alcoholic liver disease? Transpl Int 2005;18:1292–7.

108. DiMartini A, Day N, Dew MA, et al. Alcohol consumption patterns and predictors of use following liver transplantation for alcoholic liver disease. Liver Transpl 2006;12:813–20.

109. Dew MA, DiMartini AF, Steel J, et al. Meta-analysis of risk for relapse to substance use after transplantation of the liver or other solid organs. Liver Transpl 2008;14(2):159–72.

110. Starzl TE, Van Thiel D, Tzakis A, et al. Liver transplant for alcoholic liver disease. JAMA 1988;260:2542–4.

111. Gedaly R, McHugh PP, Johnston TD, et al. Predictors of relapse to alcohol and illicit drugs after liver transplantation for alcoholic liver disease. Transplantation 2008;86(8):1090–5.

112. Bellamy CO, DiMartini A, Ruppert K, et al. Liver transplantation for alcoholic cirrhosis: long term follow-up and impact of disease recurrence. Transplantation 2001;72(4):619–26.

113. Belle SH, Beringer KC, Detre KM. Liver transplantation for alcoholic liver disease in the United States: 1988 to 1995. Liver Transpl Surg 1997;3:212–9.

114. Benich JJ. Opioid dependence. Prim Care Clin Office Pract 2011;38:59–70.

115. Jain A, DiMartini A, Kashyap R, et al. Long-term follow-up after liver transplantation for alcoholic liver disease under tacrolimus. Transplantation 2000;70:1335–42.

116. Berlakovich GA, Langer F, Freundorfer E, et al. General compliance after liver transplantation for alcoholic cirrhosis. Transpl Int 2000;13(2):129–35.
117. Pfitzmann R, Schwenzer J, Rayes N, et al. Long-term survival and predictors of relapse after orthotopic liver transplantation for alcoholic liver disease. Liver Transpl 2007;13:197–205.
118. Jimenez C, Manrique A, Marques E, et al. Incidence and risk factors for the development of lung tumors after liver transplantation. Transpl Int 2007;20:57–63.
119. Dumortier J, Guillaud O, Adham M, et al. Negative impact of De Novo malignancies rather than alcohol relapse on survival after liver transplantation for alcoholic cirrhosis: A retrospective analysis of 305 patients in a single center. Am J Gastroenterol 2007;102:1032–41.
120. Watt KDS, Pedersen RA, Kremers WK, et al. Long-term probability of and mortality from de novo malignancy after liver transplantation. Gastroenterology 2009;137(6):2010–7.
121. Leithead JA, Ferguson JW, Hayes PC. Smoking-related morbidity and mortality following liver transplantation. Liver Transpl 2008;14(8):1159–64.
122. McCallum S, Masterton G. Liver transplantation for alcoholic liver disease: a systematic review of psychosocial selection criteria. Alcohol Alcohol 2006; 41(4):358–63.
123. International Early Lung Cancer Action Program Investigators. Computed tomographic screening for lung cancer: individualising the benefit of the screening. Eur Respir J 2007;30(5):843–7.
124. Mathurin P. Is alcoholic hepatitis an indication for transplantation? Current management and outcomes. Liver Transpl 2005;11:S21–4.

Current Status of Liver Transplantation for Hepatitis B Virus

Corinne Buchanan, MSN, ACNP-BC[a], Tram T. Tran, MD[b],*

KEYWORDS

- Hepatitis B virus • Liver transplant
- Hepatitis B immune globulin • Antiviral
- HBcAb positivity • Genotype

There are at least 800,000 to 1,400,000 individuals in the United States chronically infected with hepatitis B virus (HBV) with 3000 deaths annually.[1] Since the mid 1990s, there has been a substantial decrease in the incidence of acute HBV infection in the United States, due to widespread administration of the hepatitis B vaccine.[2] In 2008, the estimated number of acute HBV infections in the United States was 38,000, which significantly decreased from the estimated 73,000 new cases in 2003.[1] Despite improvements in the treatment of HBV, however, it is still associated with significant morbidity and mortality. Before the introduction of antivirals and immunoprophylaxis with hepatitis B immune globulin (HBIg), hepatitis B was considered a relative if not absolute contraindication to liver transplant, due to frequent recurrence of the virus post transplant with poor survival rates. Today, hepatitis B remains the most common etiology for liver transplant in Asia, and still leads to 5% to 10% of all liver transplants in the United States.[3]

BEFORE LIVER TRANSPLANT

Viral Load

Persistently high levels of HBV replication are implicated in long-term risk of cirrhosis, decompensation, hepatocellular carcinoma, and liver-related mortality.[4] In chronic hepatitis B (CHB) patients with active replication, 15% to 20% will progress to cirrhosis within 5 years.[5] Furthermore, patients who are viremic at the time of transplantation have a higher rate of recurrence after transplantation.[6] Viral replication in a cirrhotic patient can result in acute HBV exacerbation and clinical decompensation;

[a] Center for Liver Transplantation, Cedars-Sinai Medical Center, Los Angeles, CA, USA
[b] Center for Liver Transplantation, Cedars Sinai Medical Center, Geffen UCLA School of Medicine, 8635 West 3rd Street, Suite 590W, Los Angeles, CA 90048, USA
* Corresponding author. Center for Liver Transplantation, Cedars Sinai Medical Center, Geffen UCLA School of Medicine, 8635 West 3rd Street, Suite 590W, Los Angeles, CA 90048.
E-mail address: TranT@cshs.org

Clin Liver Dis 15 (2011) 753–764
doi:10.1016/j.cld.2011.08.011
1089-3261/11/$ – see front matter © 2011 Published by Elsevier Inc.

liver.theclinics.com

therefore, timely and appropriate treatment of HBV is crucial. However, specific difficulties exist in the treatment of decompensated patients. For example, adefovir (ADV) and tenofovir (TDF) may have some increased risk of nephrotoxicity, especially in critically ill patients with existing comorbidities. Nucleos(t)ide analogues require dose adjustment if renal function is impaired, and carry warnings about lactic acidosis.

Goals of antiviral therapy in the pretransplant patient include reduction of viral load to low or nondetectable serum HBV DNA levels. This reduction helps both to stabilize the disease, thereby delaying or possibly preventing the need for transplantation, and to decrease the risk of recurrent hepatitis B after transplantation. Recurrent HBV infection previously occurred in 70% to 90% of patients who are hepatitis B surface antigen (HBsAg) positive at the time of transplantation without immunoprophylaxis. Patients with high serum HBV DNA levels and hepatitis B e antigen (HBeAg) positivity had the highest rate of posttransplant recurrence, with a corresponding decrease in patient and graft survival.[7,8] With sustained viral suppression by oral therapy, reversal of hepatic fibrosis and overt decompensation can be seen in patients with end-stage liver disease,[2] which has led to a decrease in liver transplants for hepatitis B.[2]

Interferon

Interferon (IFN) is an antiviral medication that frankly decompensated cirrhotic patients have difficulty tolerating.[9,10] It may, however, be beneficial in the treatment of carefully selected compensated cirrhotic patients.[11] Multiple studies have shown that interferon is effective in achieving loss of HBeAg as well as undetectable levels of HBV DNA.[3] The use of interferon prior to transplant is now uncommon, as it may increase the risk of decompensation due to an immune flare, and aggravate thrombocytopenia and neutropenia. In an era with well-tolerated oral therapies, IFN use in the cirrhotic patient is currently not recommended.

Lamivudine

Although newer, more potent nucleos(t)ide agents are now available and are considered first-line therapies, initial studies supported the safety and efficacy of lamivudine (LAM) for the pretransplant patient. LAM was approved for use in HBV in 1998, and can be employed in both compensated and decompensated cirrhotic patients. LAM improves liver function and decreases the occurrence of hepatocellular carcinoma.[4,12–14] It also reduces fibrosis and the need for liver transplantation.[4,15–20] Dienstag and colleagues[15] observed that 70% of cirrhotic patients treated with long-term lamivudine therapy had a diminution in their fibrosis score to noncirrhotic levels.

The benefit of LAM therapy on hepatocellular function can take up to 3 to 6 months, and even with clinical improvement hepatocellular carcinoma can still occur.[21] Longer-term treatment with LAM in patients with HBV results in a 15% to 20% incidence of resistance[3] leading to cross-resistance to newer antivirals, most notably entecavir (ETV).

Adefovir

Adefovir (ADV) was approved for the treatment of HBV in 2002. Though ADV does have a lower rate of resistance compared with LAM it is a less potent antiviral, with reports of response as low as 25% to 50%.[3,22] ADV has also been implicated in nephrotoxicity, which makes it not ideal as first-line therapy in liver transplant patients.[23] Nevertheless, ADV was considered a relatively safe and effective second-line therapy for wait-listed patients with chronic hepatitis B,[22,24,25] being well tolerated for extended periods of time (48–52 weeks) in decompensated cirrhotic patients.[21,26,27] In a study that examined patients with decompensated cirrhosis, 81% had undetectable HBV DNA and 90% had improved Child-Pugh Score after 48 weeks of treatment with ADV. There is also the risk of development of mutations, though less so with LAM. Adefovir-associated mutations include rtN236T and rtA181V. ADV has been shown to be effective in inhibiting replication of wild-type HBV and YMDD mutants.[22,27,28] Thus, it has been advocated for use as rescue therapy for LAM in both the pretransplant and posttransplant setting. Reports have indicated that in patients with LAM resistance, low-dose ADV yielded greater than 80% viral remission and that development of ADV resistance was not seen.[27–29] However, its use has now been superseded by newer antivirals.

Entecavir

ETV is a newer antiviral agent (approved in 2005), highly potent and successful in the treatment of chronic HBV infection.[3,30,31] ETV has a low intrinsic rate of viral resistance—in patients who are treatment naïve, there is a 1.2% resistance rate at 5 years of therapy.[32] There is, however, a relationship between LAM and ETV resistance, as 9% of patients who are LAM resistant become resistant to ETV within 2 years of initiating ETV use.[29] Although there are not many data available comparing ETV with older antivirals, the data that exist are promising and support the use of ETV as a first-line agent for transplant patients. ETV is well tolerated, with adverse effects similar to those of LAM or placebo. ETV should still be dose adjusted in the setting of renal insufficiency. There are ongoing studies examining its safety and efficacy in decompensated cirrhotic patients.[21] A recent study by Lange and colleagues[33] examined 16 patients with chronic HBV and cirrhosis who were started on therapy with ETV. Five of these patients, with Model for End-stage Liver Disease (MELD) scores of at least 20, developed lactic acidosis, which subsided once ETV was discontinued. The relationship to ETV therapy is still not clear. Of note, none of the patients with MELD scores of less than 18 developed lactic acidosis, which led to the hypothesis that persons with impaired liver function had a higher risk of contracting lactic acidosis. These observations await confirmation.

Tenofovir

TDF is the newest antiviral, approved for use in hepatitis B in 2008, and has a robust clinical profile in human immunodeficiency virus (HIV) infection. It is considered potent, with no resistance mutations in HBV therapy identified to date. One concern in the transplant population is the risk of nephrotoxicity observed in previous HIV studies.[9] TDF is effective in patients who are resistant to LAM and have viral breakthrough with ADV rescue therapy.[9] When compared with ADV over a 48-week trial period, TDF has been shown to decrease alanine aminotransferase levels more than ADV.[10] Another benefit of TDF is that it has been found to be effective and safe for patients who are dually infected with HBV and HIV.[10]

Genotype

There are at least 10 hepatitis B genotypes. Multiple studies have concluded that specific genotypes can predict clinical outcome. In addition, various genotypes have not only been associated with geographic region, but a recent study by Chu and colleagues[34] noted that genotype is also associated with mode of transmission. Genotype A was found to be more common among persons infected with hepatitis B from sexual or parenteral transmission. Genotypes B and C were prevalent in those who were infected via vertical (mother-to-child) transmission.[34]

Patients with genotype B have a lower likelihood of hepatic decompensation than those with genotype C.[34] These patients also have less likelihood of progression to cirrhosis and hepatocellular carcinoma as well as earlier HBeAg seroconversion.[21] However, genotype B patients tend to have higher risk of hepatitis flares.[35] Genotype C has been associated with higher rates of hepatitis B recurrence after transplant, due to lamivudine resistance.[35] Rates of hepatocellular carcinoma are also higher with genotype C.[36] In terms of graft survival following transplant, 3-year rates were similar between genotypes B and C.[35] Genotype D has been associated with increased mortality, graft loss, and disease recurrence.[37,38] A small study from Australia found that genotype D was associated with a more severe recurrence of disease.[39] This genotype has also been linked to an increased incidence of fulminant hepatic failure.[40]

In 2008, Gaglio and colleagues[36] reported on 123 patients from the National Institutes of Health HBV-OLT study group (a retrospective-prospective observational study that enrolled patients 13 years of age and older who were HBsAg-positive, and either were on the liver transplant waiting list or had been transplanted within the past 12 months). The investigators observed differences in pretransplant and posttransplant outcomes and indications for transplant related to HBV genotype. Hepatocellular carcinoma was the indication for transplant in 49% of patients with genotype C, 25% of those with genotype D, 23% of those with genotype A, and 13% of those with genotype B. Thirteen percent of patients with genotype D were listed for transplant for acute liver failure (ALF), followed by 12% and 2% for genotypes A and C, respectively. No patient with genotype B was listed for ALF. Genotypes A (69%) and C (47%) were associated with HBeAg positivity. Precore variants were most commonly found in genotypes B and D. Genotype D was associated with the highest wait-list mortality rate. Although statistical significance was not achieved, patients with genotype C had a trend toward lower posttransplant survival compared with those with genotype non-C (4-year survival of 67% vs 89%).

The most commonly occurring natural variants of HBV include the precore mutation ($G_{1896}A$), which stops HBeAg production, and the core promoter mutation ($A_{1762}T$, $G_{1764}A$), which downregulates HBeAg production.[41–44] A study by Chu and colleagues[45] that enrolled 694 patients from 17 liver centers in the United States over a 1-year period found a relationship between the core promoter variant and development of cirrhosis. Hepatic decompensation was found more commonly in patients with the core promoter variant with or without with the precore variant. The precore variant was found in patients with genotypes D and B, whereas the core promoter variant was seen more often in patients with genotype C.

AFTER LIVER TRANSPLANT

In patients undergoing liver transplant for CHB, posttransplant immunosuppression can increase or induce viral replication. Without antiviral prophylaxis, the rate of HBV recurrence following transplantation is 80%.[6,46] With the widespread use of HBIg and oral antiviral therapy, outcomes of HBV patients after transplantation have vastly improved.[47] Using nucleos(t)ide analogues pretransplantation and posttransplantation in conjunction with HBIg postoperatively, the 3-year posttransplant recurrence rate for HBV has dropped to 7.9%.[36] IFN is not currently used for treatment of hepatitis B after transplantation, given the risk of graft rejection (**Table 1**).[48–51] Patients transplanted for HBV currently have the highest graft survival among all adult diseases.[7]

Bzowej and colleagues[52] recently reported on liver transplantation outcomes among Caucasians, Asian Americans, and African Americans with HBV. This study retrospectively examined 274 patients from 15 transplant centers within the United States. Five-year survival was greatest in African Americans, followed by Caucasians and Asian Americans (94%, 89%, and 85%, respectively). The only independent

Table 1
Considerations for hepatitis B treatment

	Noncirrhotic/Compensated Cirrhotic	Decompensated Cirrhotic	Posttransplant	Safety Profile	Resistance Profile
IFN	Only in noncirrhotics and selected compensated cirrhotics	Not recommended	Not recommended	Significant	None
LAM	✓	✓	✓	Negligible	20% resistance year 1 70% resistance year 5
ADV	✓	✓	✓	Possible renal toxicity	29% resistance year 5
ETV	✓	✓	✓	Reported lactic acidosis in high MELD score	1.2% resistance year 5
TDF	✓	✓	✓	Possible renal toxicity	None reported

Abbreviations: ADV, adefovir; ETV, entecavir; IFN, interferon; LAM, lamivudine; MELD, model for end-stage liver disease; TDF, tenofovir.

risk factor for mortality was recurrence of hepatocellular carcinoma; race was not a statistically significant predictor ($P = .93$). Caucasians had the highest rate of HBV recurrence (19%) in comparison with Asian Americans (7%) and African Americans (6%). On Cox regression analysis only HBeAg status at listing was significantly associated with HBV recurrence; race showed a trend toward significance ($P = .057$). The investigators concluded that Caucasians, Asian Americans, and African Americans with hepatitis B can be managed similarly in the transplant setting and have similar outcomes after transplantation, in contrast to an earlier era in which Asian Americans had inferior outcomes due to disease recurrence.

Hepatitis B Immune Globulin

HBIg has been a mainstay of posttransplant prophylaxis of recurrent hepatitis B since the early 1990s. prior to the use of HBIg, HBV had a recurrence rate of 80% to 100% and a 2-year mortality of 50% following transplantation.[46,53] With the combination of HBIg and LAM, posttransplant HBV recurrence is as low as 0% to 11%.[47,54–58]

The most commonly accepted strategy for posttransplant prophylaxis of hepatitis B recurrence is now the combination of lifelong HBIg plus an oral antiviral agent (LAM).[10] However, the lifelong use of HBIg has limitations, chiefly high cost, supply, parenteral administration, and need for frequent laboratory monitoring.[59] In general, most transplant centers administer high doses of HBIg (10,000 IU) during the anhepatic phase of transplantation followed by daily intravenous (IV) dosing for the first week post transplant.[3] Subsequent treatment regimens vary from center to center. Some centers have attempted to transition long-term IV HBIg administration to the intramuscular (IM) route in an effort to reduce the cost associated with IV infusions. Saab and colleagues[60] reported the annual cost of LAM plus IV HBIg as $181,130 compared with $13,500 for LAM plus IM HBIg. Still, the cost of lifetime IM HBIg administration remains substantial. Some investigators have described discontinuation of HBIg after a certain period of time after liver transplant, continuing with oral antiviral medications only. In one study, 61 patients transplanted for HBV were converted from HBIg plus one nucleoside agent to dual combination therapy with one nucleoside and one nucleotide analogue 12 months after transplant. HBV recurrence occurred in 2 patients (3.3%), a rate similar to that achieved with continued HBIg plus LAM.[59]

Lamivudine

A study of 206 patients transplanted for HBV showed 2-year survival of 85% for those who received HBIg only versus 94% who received combination therapy with LAM and HBIg. The 2-year recurrence rate for the two groups was 42%, compared with 8% for those receiving HBIg alone or HBIg plus LAM, respectively.[7]

Long-term LAM monotherapy has recently been examined as a potential option for posttransplant prophylaxis. A retrospective study at the University of Michigan looked at 21 patients transplanted for hepatitis B; HBIg was discontinued at a median of 26 months after transplant and the patients, 19 of whom were on LAM monotherapy, were continued on nucleoside analogue therapy. Of these only one patient, who was noncompliant with oral medication, developed recurrent HBV.[53] Other reports have indicated that in patients with HBV DNA levels less than 100,000 copies/mL before transplantation, recurrence rates were similar in patients receiving long-term LAM monotherapy after completing a 1-month course of HBIg and LAM in comparison with patients receiving long-term combination HBIg/LAM treatment.[47,61–64] LAM resistance is of particular concern in patients who are immunosuppressed; in some studies resistance was detected in 45% of immunosuppressed patients within the first year of treatment following liver transplantation.[3]

Adefovir

ADV has been another option for liver transplant recipients.[22,65,66] In carefully selected patients, no significant renal toxicity was noted.[22] Some transplant centers have reported that the combination of ADV in addition to LAM/HBIg combination therapy post transplant is beneficial in highly viremic patients.[67] In patients who are known to have LAM-resistant HBV, ADV has been shown to be a good option for posttransplant antiviral therapy.[25,65] Following recurrence of HBV after transplant, one study showed 34% of patients had undetectable viral loads 48 weeks after initiating treatment with ADV.[66]

Combination of Lamivudine and Adefovir

The combination of nucleoside and nucleotide analogues has proved to be effective, owing to the lack of cross-resistance. LAM plus ADV has been shown to be useful in patients with the YMDD mutation.[22] Due to the lack of documented viral breakthrough and cost efficacy, it is now proposed that LAM and ADV combination therapy be used following the first year after transplantation.[60,68] In a small study by Angus and colleagues,[68] recurrence rates were found to be similar when comparing ADV/LAM with the standard HBIg/LAM initiated as early as 6 months after transplant. The University of Minnesota suggests using combination LAM/ADV beginning at 1 week after transplant with discontinuation of HBIg. In the 32 patients studied with mean follow-up of 2 years, only one patient was found to have recurrence.[8]

Hepatitis B Core Antibody–Positive Donor Livers

Hepatitis B core antibody (HBcAb)-positive donor livers have been used for many years in HBsAg-positive recipients. With the increasing number of patients on liver transplant lists, the use of extended criteria donors (eg, HBcAb-positive donors) has increased. The frequency of HBcAb-positive donor availability has also increased with older donors being used. In 1988, 2.5% of liver transplant donors were older than 50 years and 0.05% were older than 65 years; in 2010, the percentages had increased to 34% and 9%, respectively.[69] Transmission of HBV to recipients varies depending on recipient HBcAb status: in HBcAb-negative recipients, the transmission rate was shown to be 33% to 87.5% compared with 0% to 13% for HBcAb-positive recipients in the absence of prophylaxis.[70–75]

HBIg and antiviral therapy to prevent hepatitis B reactivation after HBcAb-positive liver donation has become the standard of care in most centers. However, it is not clear whether HBIg or antiviral therapy needs to be given to all recipients of HBcAb-positive organs. Studies examining HBcAb-negative and HBsAb-negative recipients receiving HBcAb-positive organs have shown excellent protection with use of HBIg plus LAM. Holt and colleagues[76] reported 100% (n = 12) prevention of seroconversion to HBsAg positivity with the use of HBIg and LAM. Uemoto and colleagues[77] examined HBsAg-negative recipients who received HBcAb-positive livers and reported that with no immunoprophylaxis, 15 of 16 patients had seroconversion to HBsAg positivity. In this study, 3 patients received HBIg and remained HBsAg-negative, and with undetectable HBV DNA levels. Dodson and colleagues[78] studied 41 transplants using HBcAb-positive organs in which 7 of the recipients were HBsAb-positive. These patients were screened 6 months after transplantation, and all were negative for HBV without receiving HBIg or antiviral therapy. Thus, it may be suggested that whereas HBsAb-negative recipients require prophylaxis, HBsAb-positive recipients may not, although this requires additional confirmation (**Table 2**).[79] It must be noted that the rate of anti-HBs seroprotection with HBV vaccination is lower in patients with liver disease and cirrhosis, so many recipients, despite vaccination, may remain anti-HBs negative.

Table 2
Recipient and donor status recommendations for prophylaxis

Recipient Status	Donor Status	Prophylaxis
HBsAg positive Anti-HBs negative Anti-HBc +	Any	Recommended
HBsAg positive Anti-HBs negative Anti-HBc +	HBsAg positive Anti-HBs negative Anti-HBc +	Recommended
HBsAg negative Anti-HBs +/− Anti-HBc +/−	HBsAg negative Anti-HBs +/− Anti-HBc +	Recommended
HBsAg negative Anti-HBs +/− Anti-HBc +/−	HBsAg negative Anti-HBs +/− Anti-HBc −	Not recommended

SUMMARY

Progress in the management of hepatitis B in liver transplant has been remarkable over the past 2 decades, from the initiation of HBIg and antivirals in the posttransplant setting to genotype being used as a potential prognostic factor, and widespread use of HBcAb-positive donors with prophylaxis. The use of HBIg and antiviral agents has changed the posttransplant survival and prognosis in this population. With the newer oral antivirals with their better resistance profile and increased potency, it is anticipated that fewer and fewer patients will require liver transplantation for decompensated CHB alone. Further studies are needed regarding the optimal posttransplant immunoprophylaxis regimen that will keep recurrence rates low, yet will cost less and be less burdensome for the patients who require HBIg.

REFERENCES

1. CDC-Viral hepatitis statistics & surveillance. Available at: www.cdc.gov/heptatitis/statistics/index.htm. Accessed 13, February 2011.
2. Kim WR, Terrault NA, Pedersen RA, et al. Trends in waiting list registration for liver transplantation for viral hepatitis in the United States. Gastroenterology 2009;137: 1680–6.
3. Jiang L, Jiang L, Cheng N, et al. Current prophylactic strategies against hepatitis B virus recurrence after liver transplantation. World J Gastroenterol 2009;15:2489–99.
4. Gane EJ. The roadmap concept: using early on-treatment virologic responses to optimize long-term outcomes for patients with chronic hepatitis B. Hepatol Int 2008;2:304–7.
5. Liaw Y, Sung JJ, Chow WC, et al. Lamivudine for patients with chronic hepatitis B and advanced liver disease. N Engl J Med 2004;351:1521–31.
6. Samuel D, Roque-Afonso AM. New sensitive tools for hepatitis B virus (HBV) detection in liver transplantation: what will be their impact on the prophylaxis of HBV infection. Liver Transpl 2007;13:1084–7.
7. Steinmuller T, Seehofer D, Rayes N, et al. Increasing applicability of liver transplantation for patients with hepatitis B-related liver disease. Hepatology 2002; 35:1528–35.
8. Lake JR. Do we really need long-term hepatitis B hyperimmune globulin? What are the alternatives? Liver Transpl 2008;14:S23–6.

9. van Bommel F, Zollner B, Sarrazin C, et al. Tenofovir for patients with lamivudine-resistant hepatitis B virus (HBV) infection and high HBV DNA level during adefovir therapy. Hepatology 2006;44:318–25.

10. Peters MG, Anderson J, Lynch P, et al. Randomized control study of tenofovir and adefovir in chronic hepatitis B virus and HIV infection: ACTG A5127. Hepatology 2006;44:1110–6.

11. Janssen HL, van Zonneveld M, Schalm SW. Hepatitis B. N Engl J Med 2004; 350(26):2719–20.

12. Lok AS, Lai C, Leung N, et al. Long-term safety of lamivudine treatment in patients with chronic hepatitis B. Gastroenterology 2003;125:1714–22.

13. Fontana RJ. Management of patients with decompensated HBV cirrhosis. Semin Liver Dis 2003;23:89–100.

14. Perrillo RP, Wright T, Rakela J, et al. A multi-center United States-Canadian trial to assess lamivudine monotherapy before and after liver transplantation for chronic hepatitis B. Hepatology 2001;33:424–32.

15. Dienstag JL, Goldin RD, Heathcote J, et al. Histological outcome during long-term lamivudine therapy. Gastroenterology 2003;124:105–17.

16. Goodman Z, Dhillon AP, Wu PC, et al. Lamivudine treatment reduced progression to cirrhosis in patients with chronic hepatitis B. J Hepatol 1999;30(Suppl 1):59.

17. Villeneuve J, Condreay LD, Willems B, et al. Lamivudine treatment for decompensated cirrhosis resulting from chronic hepatitis B. Hepatology 2000;31:207–10.

18. Yao FY, Bass NM. Lamivudine treatment in patients with severely decompensated cirrhosis due to replicating hepatitis B infection. J Hepatol 2000;33:301–7.

19. Kapoor D, Guptan RC, Wakil S, et al. Beneficial effects of lamivudine in hepatitis B virus related decompensated cirrhosis. J Hepatol 2000;33:308–12.

20. Yao FY, Terrault NA, Freise C, et al. Lamivudine treatment is beneficial in patients with severely decompensated cirrhosis and actively replicating hepatitis B infection awaiting liver transplantation: a comparative study using matched, untreated cohort. Hepatology 2001;34:411–6.

21. Lok AS, McMahon BJ. Chronic hepatitis B: update 2009. Hepatology 2009;50: 1–36.

22. Lo CM, Liu CL, Lau GK, et al. Liver transplantation for chronic hepatitis B with lamivudine-resistant YMDD mutant using add-on adefovir dipivoxil plus lamivudine. Liver Transpl 2005;11:807–13.

23. Lok A, Tan J. Antiviral therapy for pre- and post-liver transplantation patients with hepatitis B. Liver Transpl 2007;13:323–6.

24. Marcellin P, Chang TT, Lim SG, et al. Long-term efficacy and safety of adefovir dipivoxil for the treatment of hepatitis B e antigen-positive chronic hepatitis B. Hepatology 2008;48:750–8.

25. Schiff E, Lai C, Hadziyannis S, et al. Adefovir dipivoxil for wait-listed and post-liver transplantation patients with lamivudine-resistant hepatitis B: final long-term results. Liver Transpl 2007;13:349–60.

26. Schiff ER, Neuhaus P, Tillmann H, et al. Safety and efficacy of adefovir dipivoxil for the treatment of lamivudine-resistant HBV in patients post liver transplantation. Hepatology 2001;34:446A.

27. Lampertico P, Vigano M, Manenti E, et al. Low resistance to adefovir combined with lamivudine: a 3-year study of 145 lamivudine-resistant hepatitis B patients. Gastroenterology 2007;133:1445–51.

28. Perrillo R, Hann H, Mutimer D, et al. Adefovir dipivoxil added to ongoing lamivudine in chronic hepatitis B with YMDD mutant hepatitis B virus. Gastroenterology 2004;126:81–90.

29. Rapti I, Dimou E, Mitsoula P, et al. Adding-on versus switching-to adefovir therapy in lamivudine-resistant HBeAg-negative chronic hepatitis B. Hepatology 2007;45: 307–13.
30. Kamar N, Milioto O, Alric L, et al. Entecavir therapy for adefovir-resistant hepatitis B virus infection in kidney and liver allograft recipients. Transplantation 2008;86:611–4.
31. Gish RG, Lok AS, Chang TT, et al. Entecavir therapy for up to 96 weeks in patients with HBeAg-positive chronic hepatitis B. Gastroenterology 2007;133:1437–44.
32. Tenney DJ, Rose RE, Baldick C, et al. Long-term monitoring shows hepatitis B virus resistance to entecavir in nucleoside-naïve patients is rare through 5 years of therapy. Hepatology 2009;49:1503–14.
33. Lange CM, Hofmann WP, Wunder K, et al. Severe lactic acidosis during treatment of chronic hepatitis B with entecavir in patients with impaired liver function. Hepatology 2009;50(6):2000–9.
34. Chu CJ, Keefe EB, Han SH, et al. Hepatitis B virus genotypes in the United States: results of a nationwide study. Gastroenterology 2003;125:444–51.
35. Lo CM, Cheung CK, Lau GK, et al. Significance of hepatitis B virus genotype in liver transplantation for chronic hepatitis B. Am J Transplant 2005;5:1893–900.
36. Gaglio P, Singh S, Degertekin B, et al. Impact of the hepatitis B genotype on pre- and post-liver transplantation outcomes. Liver Transpl 2008;14:1420–7.
37. Devarbhavi HC, Cohen AJ, Patel R, et al. Preliminary results: outcome of liver transplantation for hepatitis B virus varies by hepatitis B virus genotype. Liver Transpl 2002;8:550–5.
38. Girlanda R, Mohsen AH, Smith H, et al. Hepatitis B virus genotype A and D and clinical outcomes of liver transplantation for HBV-related disease. Liver Transpl 2004;10:58–64.
39. McMillan JS, Bowden DS, Angus PW, et al. Mutations in the hepatitis B virus pre-core/core gene and core promoter in patients with severe recurrent disease following liver transplantation. Hepatology 1996;24:1371–8.
40. Gish RG, McCashland T. Hepatitis B in liver transplant recipients. Liver Transpl 2006;12:S54–64.
41. Carman WF, Jacyna MR, Hadziyannis S, et al. Mutation preventing formation of hepatitis B e antigen in patients with chronic hepatitis B infection. Lancet 1989; 2:588–91.
42. Akahane Y, Yamanaka T, Suzuki H, et al. Chronic active hepatitis and active hepatitis B virus DNA and antibody against e antigen in the serum. Disturbed synthesis and secretion of e antigen from hepatocytes due to a point mutation in the precore region. Gastroenterology 1990;99:1113–9.
43. Brunetto MR, Giarin M, Oliveri F, et al. Wild-type and e antigen-minus hepatitis B viruses and course of chronic hepatitis. Proc Natl Acad Sci U S A 1991;88: 4186–90.
44. Buckwold VE, Xu Z, Chen M, et al. Effects of a naturally occurring mutation in the hepatitis B virus basal core promoter on precore gene expression and viral replication. J Virol 1996;70:5845–51.
45. Chu AJ, Keefe EB, Han SH, et al. Prevalence of HBV precore/core promoter variants in the United States. Hepatology 2003;38(3):619–28.
46. O'Grady JG, Smith HM, Davies SE, et al. Hepatitis B virus reinfection after orthotopic liver transplantation. Serological and clinical implications. J Hepatol 1992; 14:104–11.
47. Buti M, Mas A, Prieto M, et al. Adherence to lamivudine after an early withdrawal of hepatitis B immune globulin plays an important role in the long-term prevention of hepatitis B virus recurrence. Transplantation 2007;84:650–4.

48. Baid-Agrawal S, Pascual M, Moradpour D, et al. Hepatitis C virus infection in haemodialysis and kidney transplant patients. Rev Med Virol 2007;18:97–115.
49. Durlik M, Gaciong Z, Rowinska D, et al. Long-term results of treatment of hepatitis B, C and D with interferon-alpha in renal allograft recipients. Transpl Int 1998;11: S135–9.
50. Rostaing L, Modesto A, Baron E, et al. Acute renal failure in kidney transplant patients treated with interferon alpha 2b for chronic hepatitis C. Nephron 1996; 74:512–6.
51. Walter T, Dumortier J, Guillaud O, et al. Rejection under alpha interferon therapy in liver transplant recipients. Am J Transplant 2007;7:177–84.
52. Bzowej N, Han S, Degertekin B, et al. Liver transplantation outcomes among Caucasians, Asian Americans, and African Americans with hepatitis B. Liver Transpl 2009;15:1010–20.
53. Wong SN, Chu C, Wai C, et al. Low risk of hepatitis B virus recurrence after withdrawal of long-term hepatitis B immunoglobulin in patients receiving maintenance nucleos(t)ide analog therapy. Liver Transpl 2007;13:374–81.
54. Dan YY, Wai CT, Yeoh KG, et al. Prophylactic strategies for hepatitis B patients undergoing liver transplant: a cost effective analysis. Liver Transpl 2006;12: 736–46.
55. Dumortier J, Chevallier P, Scoazec JY, et al. Combined lamivudine and hepatitis B immunoglobulin for the prevention of hepatitis B recurrence after liver transplantation: long term results. Am J Transplant 2003;3:999–1002.
56. Han SH, Ofman J, Holt C, et al. An efficacy and cost-effectiveness analysis of combination hepatitis B immune globulin and lamivudine to prevent recurrent hepatitis B after orthotopic liver transplantation compared with hepatitis B immune globulin monotherapy. Liver Transpl 2000;6:741–8.
57. Han SH, Martin P, Edelstein M, et al. Conversion from intravenous to intramuscular hepatitis B immune globulin in combination with lamivudine is safe and cost-effective in patients receiving long-term prophylaxis to prevent hepatitis B recurrence after liver transplantation. Liver Transpl 2003;9:182–7.
58. Markowitz JS, Martin P, Conrad AJ, et al. Prophylaxis against hepatitis B recurrence following liver transplantation using combination lamivudine and hepatitis B immune globulin. Hepatology 1998;28(2):585–9.
59. Saab S, Desai S, Tsaoi D, et al. Posttransplantation hepatitis B prophylaxis with combination oral nucleoside and nucleotide analog therapy. Am J Transplant 2011;11:511–7.
60. Saab S, Ham MY, Stone MA, et al. Decision analysis model for hepatitis B prophylaxis one year after liver transplantation. Liver Transpl 2009;15:413–20.
61. Neff GW, O'Brien CB, Nery J, et al. Outcomes in liver transplant recipients with hepatitis B virus: resistance and recurrence patterns from a large transplant center over the last decade. Liver Transpl 2004;10:1372–8.
62. Naoumov NV, Ross Lopes A, Burra P, et al. Randomized trial of lamivudine versus hepatitis B immunoglobulin for long-term prophylaxis of hepatitis B recurrence after liver transplantation. J Hepatol 2001;34:888–94.
63. Buti M, Mas A, Prieto M, et al. A randomized study comparing lamivudine monotherapy after a short course of hepatitis B immune globulin (HBIg) and lamivudine with long-term lamivudine plus HBIg in the prevention of hepatitis B virus recurrence after liver transplantation. J Hepatol 2003;38:811–7.
64. Dodson SF, De Vera ME, Bonham CA, et al. Lamivudine after hepatitis B immune globulin is effective in preventing hepatitis B recurrence after liver transplantation. Liver Transpl 2000;6:434–9.

65. Barcena R, Del Campo S, Moraleda T, et al. Study on the efficacy and safety of adefovir dipivoxil treatment in post-liver transplant patients with hepatitis B virus infection and lamivudine-resistant hepatitis B virus. Transplant Proc 2005;37: 3960–2.

66. Schiff ER, Lai C, Hadziyannis S, et al. Adefovir dipivoxil therapy for lamivudine-resistant hepatitis B in pre- and post-liver transplantation patients. Hepatology 2003;38:1419–27.

67. Marzano A, Lampertico P, Mazzaferro V, et al. Prophylaxis of hepatitis B virus recurrence after liver transplantation in carriers of lamivudine-resistant mutants. Liver Transpl 2005;11:532–8.

68. Angus PW, Patterson SJ, Strasser SI, et al. A randomized study of adefovir dipivoxil in place of HBIG in combination with lamivudine as post-liver transplant hepatitis B prophylaxis. Hepatology 2008;48:1460–6.

69. United Network for Organ Sharing. Available at: http://www.unos.org. Accessed June 6, 2011.

70. Chotiyaputta W, Pelletier SJ, Fontana RJ, et al. Long-term efficacy of nucleoside monotherapy in preventing HBV infection in HBsAg-negative recipients of anti-HBc-positive donor livers. Hepatol Int 2010;4:707–15.

71. Burton JR, Shaw-Stiffel TA. Use of hepatitis B core antibody-positive donors in recipients without evidence of hepatitis B infection: a survey of current practices in the United States. Liver Transpl 2003;9:837–42.

72. Munoz SJ. Use of hepatitis B core antibody-positive donors for liver transplantation. Liver Transpl 2002;8:S82–7.

73. Prieto M, Gomez MD, Berenguer M, et al. De novo hepatitis B core antibody-positive donors in an area with high prevalence of anti-HBc positivity in the donor population. Liver Transpl 2001;7:51–8.

74. Perrillo R. Hepatitis B virus prevention strategies for antibody to hepatitis B core antigen-positive liver donation: a survey of North American, European, and Asian-Pacific transplant programs. Liver Transpl 2009;15:223–32.

75. Manzarbeitia C, Reich DJ, Ortiz JA, et al. Safe use of livers from donors with positive hepatitis B core antibody. Liver Transpl 2002;8:556–61.

76. Holt D, Thomas R, Van Thiel D, et al. Use of hepatitis B core antibody-positive donors in orthotopic liver transplantation. Arch Surg 2002;137:572–5.

77. Uemoto S, Sugiyama K, Marusawa H, et al. Transmission of hepatitis B virus from hepatitis B core antibody-positive donors in living related liver transplants. Transplantation 1998;65:494–9.

78. Dodson SF, Issa S, Araya V, et al. Infectivity of hepatic allografts with antibodies to hepatitis B virus. Transplantation 1997;64:1582–4.

79. Nery JR, Nery-Avila C, Reddy KR, et al. Use of liver grafts from donors positive for antihepatitis B-core antibody (Anti-HBc) in the era of prophylaxis with hepatitis-B immunoglobulin and lamivudine. Transplantation 2003;75:1179–86.

Management of Pulmonary Complications in Pretransplant Patients

Michael J. Krowka, MD[a,b,*]

KEYWORDS

- Hepatic hydrothorax • Hepatopulmonary syndrome
- Portopulmonary hypertension • Overnight oximetry

OVERVIEW

Selected pulmonary complications of liver disease pose additional concerns when liver transplantation (LT) is being considered. How should one screen for certain complications? Will these complications affect the indication, priority, or intraoperative risk for LT? Will these complications affect outcome and/or resolve with successful LT? This brief review focuses on the management of the major pulmonary clinical problems for which these questions are frequently posed (**Box 1**).

CHRONIC OBSTRUCTIVE LUNG DISEASE

Patients with advanced liver disease have well-known abnormalities in pulmonary function testing.[1,2] Lung volumes are commonly decreased by ascites, hepatomegaly, basal atelectasis, or pleural effusions. Screening studies of patients with chronic liver disease have demonstrated arterial blood gas abnormalities in as many as 45%. However, little is known about the prevalence and impact of chronic obstructive pulmonary disease (COPD), with its associated degrees of expiratory airflow obstruction, in patients with advanced liver disease considered for LT. In 1991, Hourani and colleagues[1] published a study of 116 consecutive patients admitted for evaluation for LT and found that only 3% had obstruction by spirometry (defined as forced expiratory volume in 1 second divided by the forced vital capacity [FEV_1/FVC] less than 2 standard deviations below the predicted value). Krowka and colleagues[2]

[a] Division of Pulmonary and Critical Care, Mayo Clinic, Rochester, MN 55905, USA
[b] Division of Gastroenterology and Hepatology, Mayo Clinic, Rochester, MN 55905, USA
* Division of Pulmonary and Critical Care, Mayo Clinic, Rochester, MN 55905.
E-mail address: krowka@mayo.edu

Clin Liver Dis 15 (2011) 765–777
doi:10.1016/j.cld.2011.08.012
1089-3261/11/$ – see front matter © 2011 Elsevier Inc. All rights reserved.

> **Box 1**
> **Major pulmonary issues prior to liver transplantation**
>
> Chronic obstructive pulmonary disease
>
> α1-Antitrypsin deficiency
>
> Hepatic hydrothorax
>
> Hepatopulmonary syndrome
>
> Portopulmonary hypertension
>
> Sleep-disordered breathing

studied 95 patients who underwent LT who had preoperative and postoperative pulmonary function testing. Although 75% of these patients had either primary biliary cirrhosis or primary sclerosing cholangitis, these investigators found that 17% had an FEV_1/FVC percentage ratio of less than 75%, which did not affect or change after LT.

Smoking is an important risk factor for COPD and is common in candidates for LT; however, the risk factors for and outcomes of COPD in this population have received little attention. A recent prospective cohort study of 373 patients who were evaluated for LT at 7 academic centers in the United States has provided necessary insight.[3] COPD was characterized by expiratory airflow obstruction (prebronchodilator FEV_1/FVC <0.70). Sixty-seven patients (18%) had COPD, and 224 (60%) had a history of smoking. Eighty percent of patients with airflow obstruction did not previously carry a diagnosis of COPD, and 27% were still actively smoking. Patients with COPD had higher right ventricular systolic pressure (RVSP) by transthoracic echocardiography compared with patients without COPD. This finding may be explained by ventilation-perfusion mismatch with local hypoxic vasoconstriction/remodeling, as well as parenchymal destruction with loss of capillary beds. These echo findings are of unknown clinical significance.

The degree of COPD (as measured by FEV_1) per se has not been reported to be a contraindication to LT, although patients with severe COPD (FEV_1 <1.00 L) are at higher risk for hypoxemia, $PaCO_2$ retention, and prolonged mechanical ventilation post LT.

Of importance, smoking (with or without COPD) has been linked to immediate posttransplant liver engraftment problems, specifically hepatic artery thrombosis.[4,5] This correlation is perhaps the most important reason for consultation on smoking cessation prior to LT.[6] Absolute smoking cessation may intuitively decrease the increased risk of respiratory tract cancers observed post LT.[7] At present, every liver candidate at the Mayo Clinic undergoes complete pulmonary function testing as part of the routine preoperative evaluation; smokers are offered nicotine dependence center counseling and may be denied LT consideration if smoking is not stopped.

α1-ANTITRYPSIN DEFICIENCY

Abnormal α_1-antitrypsin (AAT) genetics and the development of either hepatic cirrhosis or panacinar emphysema (or both concomitantly) are well-documented relationships associated with selected AAT mutant alleles ("S" or "Z" alleles; "M" being normal).[8] The AAT protein is the main inhibitor of intrapulmonary neutrophil elastase.[9] Severe circulating deficiency of AAT is clearly associated with severe, early-onset emphysema (FEV_1 <50% predicted).[9] Although it is a rare form of COPD (accounting for about 2% of all COPD diagnosed), AAT mutations (Z and S alleles) are not uncommon (~15%) in the LT population.[8] The hepatic manifestations in ZZ and SZ patients (cirrhosis and perhaps hepatocellular carcinoma) are presumably caused by abnormal folding, polymer formation, and accumulation of abnormal AAT protein synthesized within by the mutated genes within hepatocytes. LT is the only current treatment for the advanced hepatic manifestations of severe AAT deficiency.[8]

If significant COPD due to AAT deficiency is documented before LT, current guidelines suggest a benefit from weekly or biweekly infusion of replacement AAT protein from pooled human plasma.[9] Specifically, those individuals with predicted FEV_1 between 35% and 65% or those with accelerated decline in FEV_1 are thought to derive the best benefit.[10] The goal of such therapy is reduce or minimize the deterioration of lung function and offset the pulmonary damage caused by unopposed intrapulmonary neutrophil elastase. Therefore, assessment of pulmonary function testing in ZZ and SZ LT candidates is imperative. There is no role for augmentation therapy to treatment the hepatic aspects of ZZ or SZ liver disease.[10]

LT is considered by many authorities to be equivalent to the "ultimate gene therapy" in that the severe circulating AAT deficiency and consequences of portal hypertension are totally corrected by replacing the affected liver by a normal allograft.[8] As a caveat, pre-LT evaluation of any patient with the Z or S allele considered for living donor LT should be cautiously considered. The siblings of such individuals may harbor a worse genotype than the potential recipient. For example, a potential LT candidate with MZ genotype could have an asymptomatic, potential ZZ sibling wishing to be a donor. Successful transplant would result in the recipient having a severe deficiency in circulating AAT protein.

HEPATIC HYDROTHORAX

Although not an indication for LT per se, the accumulation of pleural fluid caused by the formation of ascitic fluid, termed hepatic hydrothorax (HH), poses several challenges because of the symptoms that result from fluid-induced lung atelectasis, hypoxemia due to impaired ventilation-perfusion matching, and potential pleural space infection.[11] Diagnostic thoracentesis should be conducted on all patients with liver disease who have pleural fluid accumulations ($\sim$6% of all liver transplant candidates) with fever, chest pain, or a diagnosis of hepatocellular carcinoma.[11] Classic management emphasizes sodium restriction (<90 mg/d), aggressive diuresis (maximum combination of spironolactone 400 mg/d plus furosemide 160/mg/d to control the formation of ascitic fluid), and repetitive therapeutic thoracenteses (no more than 2 L per tap, every 2 weeks) to alleviate dyspnea.[11] As these measures fail to control the accumulation of pleural fluid, HH is considered to be refractory, and more invasive procedures can be attempted. Specifically, continual chest tube drainage, video-assisted thoracoscopy with pleurodesis, and transjugular intrahepatic portosystemic shunts (TIPS) have been used with varying degrees of success and morbidity.[12] TIPS for refractory HH is the best studied and should be considered as a bridge to LT as opposed to a definitive treatment for HH.[11] LT is the ultimate intervention to resolve refractory HH. In the largest series reported to date, Xiol and colleagues[13] described 28 patients with HH; 16 of 28 were considered refractory HH. Compared with 56 matched controls, there was no significant difference in post-LT mechanical ventilation, transfusion requirements, or long-term survival.

HEPATOPULMONARY SYNDROME

In the setting of portal hypertension (with or without cirrhosis) in adults and children, pulmonary vascular dilatation frequently develops, as documented by contrast-enhanced echocardiography.[14] Such dilatations are usually diffuse microscopic abnormalities and are not seen on routine chest radiographs or chest computed to-mography scanning. These vascular abnormalities may lead to ventilation-perfusion mismatch (excess perfusion for given ventilation), oxygen diffusion-perfusion limita-tion (due the size of the dilatations), and anatomic right to left shunts (new vessels that abut or even bypass normal alveoli). Of importance, such abnormalities can lead to arterial hypoxemia that can be severe and extremely debilitating.[15] The clinical triad of (1) portal hypertension, (2) hypoxemia, and (3) pulmonary vascular dilatations defines the concept of hepatopulmonary syndrome (HPS), with most, but not all cases associated with cirrhosis of any cause.[14] Specific diagnostic criteria suggested by the European Respiratory Society/European Association for Study of the Liver Task Force are shown in **Box 2**.[15] HPS occurs in up to 30% of LT candidates, with no specific relationship to the cause or severity of liver disease as measured by the Model for End-Stage Liver Disease (MELD) score.[15] The very existence of HPS in association with advanced liver disease portends a poorer prognosis.[16]

Screening for the hypoxemia of HPS can be accomplished by finger-pulse oxime-try.[17] Hemoglobin saturation of less than 92% in the sitting position should trigger further arterial blood gas (ABG) measurements, keeping in mind oxygenation may worsen with the standing position (orthodeoxia), with exercise and during sleep.[15] Although PaO_2 measured from a radial artery sample is the frequent ABG determina-tion reported, arterial oxygenation determined by the alveolar-arterial gradient is more accurate, because it takes into account age, altitude effects (barometric pressure, assumed alveolar oxygen levels, patterns of breathing, and $PaCO_2$), all of which ulti-mately effect PaO_2.[15] It is well documented that up to 30% of HPS patients may have other reasons for hypoxemia that include HH, interstitial lung disease, and COPD due to smoking.[18] In such cases the use of lung perfusion scanning (see later discussion) can usually characterize the degree of hypoxemia due to HPS, because all other conditions mentioned will not cause pulmonary vascular dilatation and result in brain uptake of radiolabeled macroaggregated albumin (^{99m}Tc MAA).[19]

Box 2
Diagnostic criteria for hepatopulmonary syndrome (HPS) and portopulmonary hypertension (POPH)

HPS

1. Portal hypertension (clinical diagnosis)

2. Arterial hypoxemia

    a. Alveolar-oxygen gradient >15 mm Hg (>20 if >64 years of age); or

    b. PaO_2 <80 mm Hg (room air/sitting position)

3. Pulmonary vascular dilatation

    a. Positive contrast-enhanced echocardiography; or

    b. Abnormal brain uptake ($\geq$6%) after ^{99m}Tc macroaggregated albumin lung perfusion scan

POPH

1. Portal hypertension (clinical diagnosis)

2. Right heart catheterization criteria:

    a. Mean pulmonary artery pressure (MPAP) >25 mm Hg

    b. Pulmonary artery occlusion pressure (PAOP) <15 mm Hg

    c. Pulmonary vascular resistance (PVR) >240 dynes/s/cm^5

The definitive diagnosis of pulmonary vascular dilatations can be made using either contrast-enhanced transthoracic echocardiography (qualitative) or ^{99m}Tc MAA lung perfusion scanning with brain uptake imaging (quantitative) (**Fig. 1**).[15] Contrast-enhanced echocardiography is more sensitive than lung perfusion scanning and, importantly, precedes the development of hypoxemia.[20,21] In situations where trans-thoracic contrast-enhanced echocardiography remains equivocal for the observation of abnormal opacification in the left atrium following peripheral administration of agitated saline, a transesophageal echocardiography study can easily discern the existence of intracardiac pathways of microbubbles entering the left atrium versus the passage of microbubbles into the left atrium from the pulmonary veins.[22] Pulmonary angiography is not necessary in most cases, but should be considered if severe hypoxemia (PaO$_2$ <50 mm Hg) breathing room air and poor response to 100% inspired oxygen (PaO$_2$ <300 mm Hg) exists.[15] The goal of angiography is to document discrete arteriovenous communications (usually >5 mm in diameter) that could be embolized.

Supplemental oxygen administration (up to 5 L/min) via nasal cannula usually improves the degree of hypoxemia due to HPS. There are no proven pharmacologic treatment options for HPS to improve hypoxemia.[15] TIPS has resulted in minimal effects on arterial oxygenation, and is generally not employed or advised to treat HPS.[15] Stenting of the inferior vena cava has been reported to resolve the hypoxemia of HPS.[23] Inhaled prostacyclin as a means to alter ventilation-perfusion within the lung, thus improving hypoxemia due to HPS, has been reported.[24]

Once considered as an absolute contraindication for LT, HPS is now considered an indication for LT in appropriate circumstances, due to the extensive documentation for complete resolution of HPS with successful LT with 5-year survivals of 70%.[25,26]

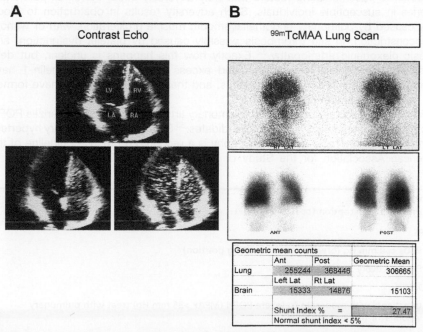

Fig. 1. Imaging methods to detect pulmonary vascular dilations. (*A*) Contrast-enhanced transthoracic echocardiography. (*B*) ^{99m}Tc macroaggregated albumin lung scan with brain uptake.

Current practice guidelines in the United States suggest that all patients considered for LT should have arterial blood gases measured in the sitting position at rest.[27] Higher priority (MELD exception) for LT can be granted in the United States if the PaO_2 is less than 60 mm Hg, in attempts to improve post-LT survival and reduce morbidity associated with severe arterial hypoxemia (**Box 3**).[27,28] The severity of pre-LT hypoxemia correlates directly with the length of time needed for HPS resolution post LT.[29] No intraoperative deaths have been reported when HPS patients have undergone LT.[25] Once PaO_2 is less than 60 mm Hg, supplemental inspired oxygen to main SaO_2 greater than 90% and reassessment of PaO_2 every 3 months is advised.[28] Although screening pulse oximetry for hypoxemia is important in the LT candidate, once SaO_2 is less than 94% it is necessary to obtain an ABG reading to accurately assess oxygenation with the PaO_2 determination, because the implications for MELD exception are based on PaO_2.

PORTOPULMONARY HYPERTENSION

Pulmonary artery hypertension that occurs as a consequence of portal hypertension is termed portopulmonary hypertension (POPH).[14] Intraoperative death and immediate posttransplant mortality are feared clinical events when transplantation is attempted in the setting of untreated, moderate to severe pulmonary artery hypertension.[30,31] Specific pulmonary vasodilator medications appear to be effective in reducing pulmonary artery pressures, improving right ventricular function, and improving survival.[32] Thus, screening for and accurately diagnosing POPH prior to LT has become a standard of care.[33]

The pulmonary vascular bed, downstream from the dysfunctional liver, is exposed to potential vasomediating factors that may adversely affect the small pulmonary arteries in susceptible individuals. Such adversity results in obstruction to blood flow caused by pulmonary endothelial/smooth muscle proliferation, with or without vasoconstriction, in situ thrombosis possibly caused by platelet dysfunction, and classic plexogenic arteriopathy.[32] Exactly how this happens is unclear, but deficiencies in endothelial prostacyclin and excess in circulating endothelin-1 have been well documented in POPH patients, and these two observations have formed the basis for treatment options.[32]

Pulmonary vascular obstruction to pulmonary arterial flow that characterizes POPH occurs in approximately 5% of all LT candidates.[33] Screening for pulmonary hypertension using transthoracic echocardiography is a recognized practice guideline of the American Association for the Study of Liver Diseases (AASLD).[27] The goal is to

---

Box 3
Current MELD exception for HPS and POPH

HPS

- PaO_2 <60 mm Hg (breathing room; sitting position)
- Reassess every 3 months

POPH

- In patients with moderate to severe POPH (MPAP >35 mm Hg) treat with pulmonary vasodilator therapy to attain:
  - MPAP <35 mm Hg and PVR <400 dynes/s/cm⁵; or
  - Normal PVR <240 dynes/s/cm⁵. Reassess every 3 months

determine the RVSP and qualitatively describe right ventricular size and function. Right heart catheterization (RHC) should be accomplished when threshold abnormalities are noted. An RVSP greater than 50 mm Hg (normal <30 mm Hg) is an indication for RHC in the Mayo Clinic management algorithm to evaluate pulmonary hypertension suspected by echocardiography. Using Mayo Clinic screening criteria, approximately 10% of all LT candidates will need RHC to confirm or rule out POPH. Specific diagnostic criteria for POPH were put forth by the 2004 European/US Study Group, based on RHC, and are summarized in **Box 2**.

Poor cardiac output and Child C severity of liver disease in the setting of POPH portends a poor prognosis,[34] yet the therapeutic role for prostacyclins, oral endothelin antagonists, and oral phosphodiesterase inhibition is compelling.[35] The hemodynamic goal of any such therapy is to reduce both MPAP and PVR and improve right ventricular function. Treatment is generally initiated when MPAP is greater than 35 mm Hg and PVR is greater than 240 dynes/s/cm^5. Once hemodynamic improvement with pulmonary vasomodulating therapy has been attained in POPH, MELD exception may be granted to allow earlier LT (see **Box 3**).[36] The management goal is to allow LT within a presumed hemodynamic and time window that will halt or possibly reverse right ventricular dysfunction caused by POPH.[37] Which POPH medication approach is optimal has yet to be determined. Uncontrolled studies are summarized in **Table 1**.[38–49] The Mayo Clinic algorithm for evaluating and treating POPH patients who are otherwise LT candidates is shown in **Fig. 2**. Finally, it should be noted that there are potential adverse effects on right ventricular function in using β-blockers, TIPS, and calcium-channel blockers in the setting of POPH.[32]

The outcome of POPH when LT is attempted continues to be problematic and unpredictable.[25] Therefore, POPH is not considered an indication for LT as is the case for HPS, and pre-LT management approaches in POPH need controlled study. Mortality during and after the transplant procedure has been a significant clinical problem when pre-LT MPAP is greater than 35 mm Hg (14% intraoperative death; 22% during the transplant hospitalization in the largest multicenter series to date

Table 1		
Effective medications used to treat portopulmonary hypertension[a]		
Medication	**Route/Dose**	**References**
Prostacyclin		
Epoprostenol[a]	Intravenous (24/7)	43–47
Treprostinil[a]	Intravenous (24/7)/Subcutaneous (24/7)	48
Iloprost	Inhaled (6–9 times per day)	38
Endothelin Receptor Antagonists		
Bosentan		
(ET$_A$ and ET$_B$)	Oral (62.5 or 125 mg twice a day)	38
Ambrisentan		
(ET$_A$ only)	Oral (5 or 10 mg twice a day)	39
Phosphodiesterase Inhibitor		
Sildenafil	Oral (20–100 mg 3 times a day)	40–42
Tyrosine Kinase Inhibitor		
Imatinib	200 mg bid (400 mg per day)	49

[a] Via permanent central line; dose titrated and usually ranges up to 25 ng/kg/min for epoprostenol; usually 2 to 3 times that for treprostinil (up to 75 ng/kg/min).

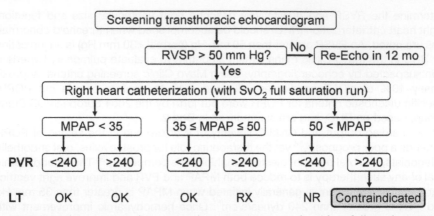

Fig. 2. Portopulmonary pre–liver transplant management algorithm followed at Mayo Clinic based on screening echocardiography and right heart catheterization results. Contraindicated, high risk of intraoperative event at graft reperfusion—case cancelled; LT, liver transplant procedure; MPAP, mean pulmonary artery pressure (normal <25 mm Hg); NR, this hemodynamic pattern never reported in literature to date; OK, risk to proceed with liver transplant is minimal; PVR, pulmonary vascular resistance (normal <240 dyne/s/cm^5 (or 3 Wood units); RVSP, right ventricular systolic pressure estimated by transthoracic echocardiography; RX, vasomodulating treatment advised before liver transplant (prostacyclin ± ambrisentan).

[n = 36]); however, only 1 of 13 patients who died received pre-LT prostacyclin therapy.[50] A 70% 5-year survival (n = 9) was reported from the Mayo Clinic when prostacyclin medications were used pre-LT to improve pulmonary hemodynamics months prior to operation.[35]

SLEEP-DISORDERED BREATHING

The frequency of abnormal overnight oximetry (ovox) in LT candidates is remarkably high, ranging from 20% to 30% depending on the parameter measured and the associated liver disease.[51,52] Abnormalities may be attributable to obstructive sleep apnea, frequent SaO_2 desaturations due to encephalopathy, ascites, and effects of narcotics and/or sedatives. Patients with HPS or POPH are particularly of concern, and overnight oximetry monitoring should be done when those diagnoses are made, because of the further worsening of hypoxemia and strain on the right ventricle that may occur. These abnormal ovox measures correlate poorly with questionnaire measures of sleep complaints, and are frequently confused with the concerns of fatigue that occur in association with hepatic disorders both before and after LT.[53] Using finger-pulse ovox for continued recording as an outpatient, one can easily (and inexpensively) assess for the amount of sleep time spent with hemoglobin saturation (SaO_2) under 90%, frequency of SaO_2 greater than 4%, or ovox SaO_2 patterns that might suggest sleep-disordered breathing (**Fig. 3**). Formal sleep consultation followed by overnight polysomnography can uncover clinically significant sleep issues amenable to therapies that should be known and treated before liver transplant.

PRE-LT PULMONARY EVALUATION

The measurement of arterial oxygenation and transthoracic echocardiography to detect the earliest clinical manifestations of HPS and POPH, respectively, are

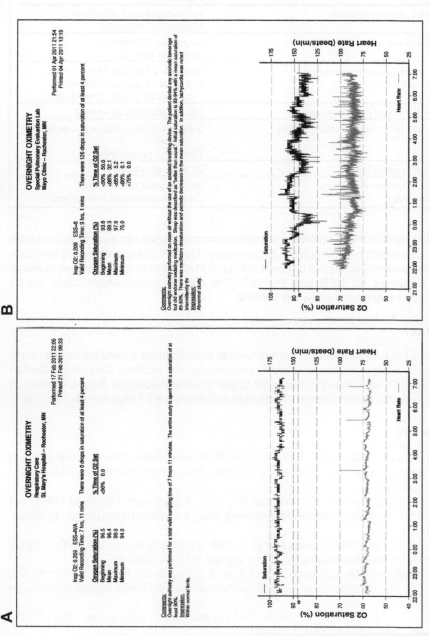

Fig. 3. Overnight finger-pulse oximetry (ovox) tracings measuring saturation of hemoglobin by oxygen (SaO$_2$) and pulse rate. (A) Normal tracing with minimal variation in and no drops of SaO$_2$ below 90%. (B) Markedly abnormal ovox with frequent SaO$_2$ variations greater than 4% (126 episodes; normal <35 for given total sleep time) and significant time (>50%) spent with SaO$_2$ less than 90%.

Table 2
Pre–liver transplant pulmonary evaluation at the Mayo Clinic

Tests	Reason
Standard chest radiograph	Infiltrates/pleural effusions? Masses/cardiomegaly?
Arterial blood gas	Degree of hypoxemia? Acid-base balance?
Contrast-enhanced transthoracic echocardiography	Pulmonary vascular dilatation? Pulmonary hypertension (right ventricular systolic pressure)?
Overnight finger pulse oximetry	Desaturations/sleep apnea?
Complete pulmonary function testing	Smokers/chronic obstructive pulmonary disease Restrictive lung disease?
α1-Antitrypsin genotype	ZZ or SZ genotypes?
Limited physician pulmonary consultation	Review/order further tests Clear for anesthesia and surgery

essential. Both of these screening studies are accomplished because of the potential for MELD exception. A European/US Consensus Conference sponsored by the European Respiratory Society will convene during 2011–2012 to update previous management guidelines for HPS and POPH.[54] The current overall Mayo Clinic pre-LT pulmonary evaluation is shown in **Table 2**.

SUMMARY

The pre-LT pulmonary management of hepatic complications should follow algorithms defined by each institution that are in accordance with evolving Consensus Conference, AASLD, and United network for Organ Sharing guidelines. Post-LT follow-up will be essential in defining the effectiveness of these pre-LT algorithms over time.

REFERENCES

1. Hourani JM, Bellamy PE, Tashkin DP Jr. Pulmonary dysfunction in advanced liver disease: frequent occurrence of an abnormal diffusing capacity. Am J Med 1991; 90:693–700.
2. Krowka MJ, Diskeson ER, Wiesner RH, et al. A prospective study of pulmonary function and gas exchange following liver transplantation. Chest 1992;102: 1161–6.
3. Rybak D, Fallon MB, Krowka MJ, et al. Risk factors and impact of COPD in candidates for liver transplantation. Liver Transpl 2008;14:1357–65.
4. Pungapong S, Manzabeitia C, Ortiz J, et al. Cigarette smoking is associated with an increased incidence of vascular complications after liver transplantation. Liver Transpl 2002;8:582–7.
5. Levy GA, Marsden PA. Cigarette smoking-association with hepatic artery thrombosis. Liver Transpl 2002;8:588–90.
6. Leithead JA, Ferguson JW, Hayes PC. Smoking-related morbidity and mortality following liver transplantation. Liver Transpl 2008;14:1159–64.
7. Jimenez C, Marques L, Manrique A, et al. Incidence and risk factors in the development of lung tumors after liver transplantation. Transplant Proc 2005;39:3970–2.

8. Fairbanks KD, Tavill AS. Liver disease in alpha-1 antitrypsin deficiency. Am J Gastroenterol 2008;103:2136–41.

9. Kelly E, Green CM, Carroll TP, et al. Alpha-1 antitrypsin deficiency. Respir Med 2010;124:763–72.

10. Sandhaus RA. Alpha-1 antitrypsin deficiency: whom to test; whom to treat. Semin Respir Crit Care Med 2010;31:343–8.

11. Roussos A, Philippou N, Mantzaris GJ, et al. Hepatic hydrothorax: pathophysiology, diagnosis and management. J Gastroenterol Hepatol 2007;22:1388–93.

12. Liu LU, Haddadin HA, Bodian CA, et al. Outcome analysis of cirrhotic patients undergoing chest tube placement. Chest 2004;126:142–8.

13. Xiol X, Tremosa G, Castellote J, et al. Liver transplantation in patients with hepatic hydrothorax. Transpl Int 2005;18:672–5.

14. Krowka MJ. Hepatopulmonary syndrome and portopulmonary hypertension: distinctions and dilemmas. Hepatology 1997;25:1282–4.

15. Rodriguez-Roisin R, Krowka MJ. Hepatopulmonary syndrome: a liver induced lung vascular disorder. N Engl J Med 2008;358:2378–87.

16. Schenck P, Schoniger-Hekele M, Fuhrmann V, et al. Prognostic significance of the hepatopulmonary syndrome in patients with cirrhosis. Gastroenterology 2003; 125:1042–52.

17. Kochar R, Tanikella R, Fallon MB. Serial pulse oximetry in hepatopulmonary syndrome. Dig Dis 2011;56(6):1862–8.

18. Martinez G, Barbera JA, Navassa M, et al. Hepatopulmonary syndrome associated with cardiorespiratory disease. J Hepatol 1999;30:882–9.

19. Abrams GC, Jaffe CC, Hoffer PB, et al. Diagnostic utility of contrast echocardiography and lung perfusion scan in patients with hepatopulmonary syndrome. Gastroenterology 1995;109:1283–8.

20. Kim BJ, Lee SC, Parl SW, et al. Characteristics and prevalence of intrapulmonary shunt detected by contrast echocardiography with harmonic analysis in liver transplant candidates. Am J Cardiol 2004;94:525–8.

21. Lenci I, Alvior A, Manzia TM, et al. Saline contrast echocardiography in patients with hepatopulmonary syndrome awaiting liver transplantation. J Am Soc Echocardiogr 2009;22:89–94.

22. Aller R, Moya AR, Moriera V, et al. Diagnosis of hepatopulmonary syndrome with contrast transesophageal echocardiography: advantages over transthoracic echocardiography. Dig Dis Sci 1999;44:1243–8.

23. O'Leary JG, Rees CR, Klintmalm GB, et al. Inferior vena cava stent resolves hepatopulmonary syndrome in an adult with a spontaneous inferior vena cava portal vein shunt. Liver Transpl 2009;15:1897–900.

24. Krug S, Seyfarth HJ, Hagendorff A, et al. Inhaled iloprost for hepatopulmonary syndrome: improvement in hypoxemia. Eur J Gastroenterol Hepatol 2007;19:1140–3.

25. Krowka MJ. Hepatopulmonary syndrome and portopulmonary hypertension: implications for liver transplantation. Clin Chest Med 2005;26:587–97.

26. Swanson KL, Wiesner RH, Kowka MJ. Hepatopulmonary syndrome: impact of liver transplantation. Hepatology 2005;41:1122–9.

27. Murray KF, Carithers RJ Jr. AASLD practice guidelines: evaluation of the patient for liver transplantation. Hepatology 2005;41:1407–32.

28. Fallon MB, Mulligan DC, Gish RG, et al. Model for end-stage liver disease (MELD) exception for hepatopulmonary syndrome. Liver Transpl 2006;12:S105–7.

29. Taille C, Cadranel J, Belloocq A, et al. Liver transplantation for hepatopulmonary syndrome: a ten-year experience in Paris France. Transplantation 2003;75: 1482–9.

30. Ramsay MA, Simpson BR, Nguyen AT, et al. Severe pulmonary hypertension in liver transplant candidates. Liver Transpl Surg 1997;3:494–500.
31. Krowka MJ, Plevak DJ, Findlay JHY, et al. Pulmonary hemodynamics and perioperative cardiopulmonary mortality in patients with portopulmonary hypertension undergoing liver transplantation. Liver Transpl 2000;6:443–50.
32. Stauber RE, Olschewski H. Portopulmonary hypertension: short review. Eur J Gastroenterol Hepatol 2010;22:385–90.
33. Krowka MJ, Swanson KL, Frantz RP, et al. Portopulmonary hypertension: results from a 10-year screening algorithm. Hepatology 2006;44:1502–10.
34. Le Pavec J, Souza R, Herve P, et al. Portopulmonary hypertension: survival and prognostic factors. Am J Respir Crit Care Med 2008;178:637–43.
35. Swanson KL, Wiesner RH, Nyberg SL, et al. Survival in portopulmonary hypertension: Mayo Clinic experience categorized by treatment subgroups. Am J Transplant 2008;8:2445–53.
36. Krowka MJ, Fallon MB, Mulligan DC, et al. MELD exception for portopulmonary hypertension. Liver Transpl 2006;12:S114–6.
37. Krowka MJ. Pulmonary hypertension, (high) risk of orthotopic liver transplantation and some lessons from "primary pulmonary hypertension". Liver Transpl 2002;8:389–90.
38. Hoeper MM, Seyfarth HJ, Hoeffken G, et al. Experience with inhaled iloprost and bosentan in portopulmonary hypertension. Eur Respir J 2007;30:1096–102.
39. Cartin-Ceba R, Swanson KL, Iyer V, et al. Safety and efficacy of ambrisentan or the treatment of portopulmonary hypertension. Chest 2011;139:109–14.
40. Reichenberger F, Voswinckel R, Steveling E, et al. Sildenafil treatment of portopulmonary hypertension. Eur Respir J 2006;28:563–7.
41. Hemmes AR, Robbins IM. Sildenafil monotherapy in POPH can facilitate liver transplantation. Liver Transpl 2009;15:15–9.
42. Gough MS, White RJ. Sildenafil therapy with improved hemodynamics in liver transplantation candidates. Liver Transpl 2009;15:30–6.
43. Krowka MJ, Frantz RP, McGoon MD, et al. Improvement if pulmonary hemodynamics during intravenous epoprostenol (prostacyclin): a study of 15 patients with moderate to severe portopulmonary hypertension. Hepatology 1999;30:641–8.
44. Sussman N, Kaza V, Barshes N, et al. Successful liver transplantation following medical management of portopulmonary hypertension. Am J Transplant 2006;6:2177–82.
45. Ashfaq M, Chinnakotla S, Rogers L, et al. The impact of POPH on survival following liver transplantation. Am J Transplant 2007;7:1258–64.
46. Fix OK, Bass NM, DeMarco T, et al. Long-term follow-up of portopulmonary hypertension: effect of treatment with epoprostenol. Liver Transpl 2007;13:875–85.
47. Sakai T, Planinsic RM, Mathier MA, et al. Initial experience using continuous intravenous treprostinil to manage pulmonary artery hypertension in patients with end-stage liver disease. Transpl Int 2009;22:554–61.
48. Melgosa MT, Ricci GL, Garcia-Pagan JC, et al. Acute and long-term effects of inhaled ilioprost in portopulmonary hypertension. Liver Transpl 2010;16:348–56.
49. Tapper EB, Knowles D, Heffron T, et al. Portopulmonary hypertension: imatinib as a novel treatment and the Emory experience with this condition. Transplant Proc 2009;41(5):1969–71.
50. Krowka MJ, Mandell SM, Ramsay MA, et al. Hepatopulmonary syndrome and portopulmonary hypertension: a report of the multicenter liver transplant database. Liver Transpl 2004;10:174–82.

51. Palma DT, Philips GM, Arguedas MR, et al. Oxygen desaturation during sleep in hepatopulmonary syndrome. Hepatology 2008;47:1253–8.
52. Okcay A, Krowka MJ, Caples S, et al. Prevalence and clinical predictors of abnormal overnight oximetry in patients awaiting liver transplantation [abstract]. Hepatology 2009;50:588.
53. van den Ginneke BT, van der Berg-Emon RJG, van der Windt A, et al. Persistent fatigue in liver transplant recipients: a two-year follow-up study. Clin Transplant 2010;24:E10–6.
54. Rodriguez-Roisin R, Krowka MJ, Fallon MB, et al. Pulmonary-hepatic vascular disorders. Eur Respir J 2004;24:861–80.

Care of the Liver Transplant Candidate

Hui-Hui Tan, MBBS, MRCP(UK)[a],*, Paul Martin, MD, FRCP, FRCPI[b]

> **KEYWORDS**
> - Chronic liver disease • Cirrhosis • Decompensation
> - Surveillance • Prophylaxis • Acute liver failure

Access to liver transplantation (LT) has dramatically altered the management of advanced liver disease, changing the role of the physician from merely managing its complications to proactively assessing potential recipients for this life-saving intervention. LT is indicated when the probability of survival after transplantation exceeds that without or for the relief of intractable symptoms (eg, pruritus, recurrent cholangitis). To rationalize prioritization of waitlist candidates, several disease models have been used to predict survival. In 2002, the Model for End-stage Liver Disease (MELD) model was adopted by United Network for Organ Sharing (UNOS) as the basis for deceased donor liver allocation for adult patients and is currently the most widely used. This model calculates prognosis based on the patient's serum bilirubin, creatinine, and the international normalized ratio (INR) to predict 3-month survival.[1,2] The application and advantages of the MELD model are discussed in greater detail in the article by Kim elsewhere in this issue.

Improved surgical techniques, immunosuppression, and perioperative management allow sicker patients, who previously may have been precluded as candidates, to be transplanted. The supply of donor organs has not matched the increase in demand. Hence, transplant candidates on the waiting list for a protracted period of time are at risk of additional complications from their liver disease. Screening, prophylaxis (where applicable) and the management of complications of end-stage liver disease have become of paramount importance to maximize the likelihood of successful LT.

THE TRANSPLANT CANDIDATE WITH CHRONIC LIVER DISEASE

Patients with early, compensated cirrhosis have good survival rates with low risk of decompensation in the absence of an index complication such as variceal hemorrhage or the development of hepatocellular carcinoma (HCC).[3] However, once an

Disclosures: Dr Paul Martin is consultant/investigator for Gilead and Bristol-Myers Squibb.
[a] Department of Gastroenterology & Hepatology, Singapore General Hospital, Outram Road, Singapore 169608
[b] Division of Hepatology, Department of Medicine, University of Miami, 1500 NW 12th Avenue, Suite 1101, Miami, FL 33136, USA
* Corresponding author.
E-mail address: tan.hui.hui@sgh.com.sg

index complication occurs, the survival rate decreases to less than 50% at 5 years. Ideally, the cause of the liver disease should be treated (eg, abstinence in alcoholic cirrhosis, antivirals in chronic viral hepatitis). However, in many patients currently available therapies may be ineffective. Even with successful therapy (eg, for hepatitis C virus [HCV]), complications such as HCC remain a threat if cirrhosis is already present. Surveillance for varices and HCC, prophylaxis against spontaneous bacterial peritonitis (SBP), and early diagnosis of hepatic encephalopathy (HE) can identify potentially life-threatening complications, reduce the need for or length of hospitalization, and potentially improve survival pending LT (**Table 1**).

Antiviral Therapy for Chronic Viral Hepatitis

HCV

End-stage chronic HCV infection remains a frequent indication for LT.[4] About 40% of liver transplants in the United States are performed in patients with HCV, and the number of transplant candidates with this indication is likely to increase over the next decade.[5,6]

Because pretransplant viral load is a predictor of HCV recurrence in the post-LT graft,[7] HCV treatment is a consideration before LT. Viral clearance may improve liver status and may prevent further disease progression.[8,9] Furthermore, the response to HCV treatment after transplantation is suboptimal because transplant complications (eg, rejection, sepsis, renal dysfunction) and the development of adverse effects from antivirals often result in suboptimal treatment doses or treatment interruption.[10,11] Achieving a sustained virologic response (SVR) (ie, sustained aviremia 6 months after treatment cessation) before LT is highly predictive of a low risk of recurrent HCV infection. As with the noncirrhotic patient, the lack of early virological response (ie, ≥ 2 log decline in viral load by week 12 of treatment) predicts poor treatment response and treatment may be ceased because the pre-LT patient is unlikely to achieve an SVR.[12] SVR rates are known to be reduced in patients with HCV with cirrhosis.[13,14]

The use of direct-acting antiviral agents needs to be carefully studied in LT candidates and recipients before any recommendations about their use in these settings can be made.

The management of HCV in the pre-LT and post-LT patient is discussed in greater detail in the article by Firpi elsewhere in this issue.

Hepatitis B virus

Achieving viral suppression before LT reduces the risk of recurrent disease in the graft. Viral suppression also has the advantage of reducing HCC risk and may improve liver function, sometimes to the point of enabling the patient to be removed from the transplant waiting list.[15–18] Hepatitis B virus (HBV) as an indication for LT in the United States is decreasing, probably as a result of the introduction of effective oral antivirals.[19] Oral therapy (Entecavir, Tenofovir or combination nucleoside-nucleotide analogues) are preferred over the interferons, because the latter are associated with the risk of decompensation in patients with cirrhosis. The current status of LT for HBV is discussed in greater detail in the article by Tran elsewhere in this issue.

Variceal Screening and Management

Varices are present in up to 40% of well-compensated cirrhotic patients with cirrhosis and 60% of patients with overt hepatic decompensation.[20–22] Of these patients, 20% to 30% develop variceal bleeding. Variceal bleeding is a seminal event in the natural history of cirrhosis and is often the first evidence of hepatic decompensation. Mortality used to be high (>50% mortality at 1 year),[23,24] but has improved over the recent

Table 1 Complications of chronic liver disease	
Complication	**Screening/Surveillance/Prophylaxis Recommendations**
Esophageal varices	Screening is recommended for all cirrhotic patients and LT candidates Primary prophylaxis No varices: repeat endoscopic surveillance in 2–3 years; no prophylaxis required Small varices: repeat endoscopic surveillance in 1–2 years; prophylaxis with nonselective β-blocker in CTP class B to C cirrhosis or in varices with red signs Large varices: repeat endoscopic surveillance in 6–12 months; prophylaxis with nonselective β-blocker or EVL Secondary prophylaxis Endoscopy within 12 h of index bleed, then 3-weekly to 4-weekly until EVL eradication, then 6-monthly surveillance endoscopy thereafter; prophylaxis with nonselective β-blocker Consider salvage TIPS for patients who failed first-line prophylaxis or in HVPG nonresponders or at high risk for treatment failure (Child class C or Child class B with active bleeding at endoscopy) Consider tissue sclerosant (eg, histoacryl) for gastric varices
HCC	Screening is recommended for all LT candidates with • cirrhosis, or • high-risk HBV infection (see text), or • current or previous HCC Screening is recommended with liver sonogram or advanced imaging (multi phasic CT or MRI) ± AFP levels
Ascites	No screening/prophylaxis recommendations
SBP	Primary prophylaxis • Recommended for all patients with acute gastrointestinal bleeding Secondary prophylaxis • Recommended in all patients with previous episode of SBP or patients with low ascitic fluid protein <1.5 g/dL and serum creatinine ≥1.2 mg/dL, blood urea nitrogen ≥25 mg/dL, serum sodium levels ≤130 mmol/L, or CTP score ≥9 points with serum bilirubin >3 mg/dL: • oral norfloxacin 400 mg/d, or • oral ciprofloxacin 750 mg/wk, or • oral cotrimoxazole 1 tablet/d
Hepatorenal syndrome	Monitoring of renal function is recommended for patients on diuretics Primary prophylaxis In patients with SBP: IV albumin 1.5 g/kg on day 1 and 1 g/kg on day 3 In patients with alcoholic hepatitis: by mouth pentoxifylline 400 mg 3 times a day In patients undergoing large-volume paracentesis: IV albumin 6–8 g/L of ascitic fluid removed
HE	No screening/primary prophylaxis recommendations Secondary prophylaxis Lactulose or lactitol Rifaximin
Osteoporosis/ osteopenia	Screening of bone mineral density is recommended for all LT candidates at time of evaluation and 2-yearly thereafter
Vaccination	Active immunization is recommended against hepatitis A, hepatitis B, neumococcus, influenza

Abbreviations: AFP, alpha-fetoprotein; CT, computed tomography; CTP, Child-Turcotte-Pugh; EVL, endoscopic variceal ligation; HVPG, hepatic venous pressure gradient; IV, intravenous; MRI, magnetic resonance imaging; TIPS, transjugular intrahepatic portosystemic shunt.

Adapted from Toubia N, Sanyal AJ. Portal hypertension and variceal hemorrhage. Med Clin N Am 2008;92(3):551–74; with permission.

decades. Nevertheless, mortality is still around 15% to 20% within the first 6 weeks of an index bleed.[25]

Screening and surveillance

All cirrhotic patients should be screened for varices at the time of diagnosis to identify patients for prophylactic treatment to prevent variceal progression or bleeding.[26] Transplant candidates should be screened for varices during the course of their transplant evaluation.

The gold standard for variceal screening or surveillance is endoscopy. In the past, varices were classified as small (minimally elevated veins above the esophageal mucosal surface), medium (tortuous veins occupying < one-third of the esophageal lumen), or large (occupying > one-third of the esophageal lumen). However, because recommendations for bleeding prophylaxis of medium and large varices are the same,[27] the Baveno I consensus recommended that varices be classified simply as small or large, by semiquantitative morphologic assessment or by quantitative size (ie, varices <5 mm diameter are small; varices >5 mm diameter are large).[28]

In patients without varices on initial endoscopy, surveillance endoscopy should be repeated after 2 to 3 years. The risk of developing varices of any grade after a negative index endoscopy is approximately 9% per year, whereas the development of moderate or large varices and subsequent variceal bleeding in these patients is less than 10% at 3 years.[29,30]

In patients with small varices on initial endoscopy, surveillance endoscopy should be repeated every 2 years. The expected increase in size to moderate or large varices and subsequent variceal bleeding is 10% to 15% per year.

In patients with advanced cirrhosis or red wale marks, a 6-month to 1-year interval should be recommended.[29,30] In this group of patients, the risk of bleeding is high, at 30% in larger varices over a 2-year period (**Box 1**).[27]

The endoscopic pill videocapsule has been evaluated as an alternative to endoscopy for variceal screening. It allows for the identification of esophageal varices and red wale marks,[31–33] but has limited ability to assess variceal size.[34] It is not useful in assessing gastric varices or portal gastropathy. At this time, pill endoscopy cannot be recommended to screen for varices.

Box 1
Risk factors for variceal hemorrhage

1. Severity of chronic liver disease
   - Child-Turcotte-Pugh (CTP) class C > class B > class A
2. Portal pressure
   - Hepatic venous pressure gradient (HVPG) greater than 12 mm Hg
3. Size of varices
   - Large varices > small varices
4. Endoscopic stigmata of hemorrhage
   - Stigmata present > stigmata absent
   - Stigmata: red wales, cherry-red spots, hematocystic spots, diffuse erythema
5. Ascites
   - Tense ascites > nontense ascites or no ascites

Adapted from Toubia N, Sanyal AJ. Portal hypertension and variceal hemorrhage. Med Clin N Am 2008;92(3):551–74; with permission.

Preprimary prophylaxis
There is no evidence to support preprimary prophylaxis in cirrhotics without varices at screening.[26]

Primary prophylaxis
In patients with small varices, primary prophylaxis with a nonselective β-blocker (such as propranolol, nadolol, or carvedilol) is recommended in all patients with CTP class B to C or for small varices with red signs, because the bleeding risk is similar to that of larger varices.[26,27,35,36] Apart from reducing bleeding risk, β-blockers may also reduce the rate of growth of small varices.[37]

For patients with large varices, either nonselective β-blockers or endoscopic variceal ligation (EVL) are recommended for primary prophylaxis. The choice of treatment depends on local resources and expertise, patient preference, characteristics, potential side-effects, and contraindications.[26] Prophylaxis with β-blockers should aim to reduce the heart rate by 25% from baseline or to 60 beats/min[35] or in centers where measurement is available, a decrease in HVPG of at least 20% from baseline or to 12 mm Hg or less.[26] Isosorbide mononitrate administration alone or in combination with β-blocker therapy to further lower the risk for initial bleed is not supported by available evidence.[26,38]

Although EVL is associated with complications, such as bleeding from postbanding ulcers, it should be offered to patients with large varices who have contraindications or intolerance to β-blockers.[27,39] Several trials have compared EVL with β-blockers as a first-line option for primary prophylaxis of variceal bleeding.[40-55] Two meta-analyses have been performed: the first included 8 trials totaling 596 patients,[56] and the second included 12 studies with 839 patients.[36] In both, EVL was associated with a small but significant lower incidence of first variceal hemorrhage without reduction in mortality. The results are the same even when only peer-reviewed published trials or high-quality trials are analyzed.[57] If selected, EVL should be performed every 3 to 4 weeks until variceal obliteration. After successful eradication, serial endoscopy should be performed every 6 months, and varices should be rebanded on recurrence.

Secondary prophylaxis
Acute variceal bleeding requires prompt resuscitation to achieve hemodynamic stability and mechanical ventilation, if necessary. Judicious transfusion guided by hemoglobin and hematocrit levels avoids further increases in portal pressure and rebleeding.[58] Transfusion targets are a hematocrit of 24% or a hemoglobin of 7 to 8 g/dL, although transfusion should be individualized, considering comorbidities, patient age, hemodynamic status, and ongoing bleeding.[26] Prophylactic antibiotics improve survival.[26,59] Vasoconstrictors such as somatostatin or its analogues (eg, terlipressin, if available, or octreotide) should be started as soon as possible to reduce blood flow to the splanchnic vasculature, decreasing portal pressure. Coagulopathy and thrombocytopenia need correction with transfusion and vitamin K. Precipitants of bleeding, such as infection (eg, SBP), portal vein occlusion (eg, from HCC or a thrombosis), or noncompliance to primary prophylaxis should be excluded.

EVL is superior to injection sclerotherapy in secondary prophylaxis,[60] with combination EVL and β-blockade more effective than EVL alone.[61] After an index esophageal variceal bleed, all patients should be β-blocked and undergo EVL every 2 to 3 weeks until the varices are obliterated.[26] However, recent evidence suggests that combining pharmacologic and endoscopic treatment confers no additional benefit, if HVPG remains greater than 12 mm Hg or HVPG reduction less than 20%.[62] These findings suggest that patients with a high rebleeding risk (eg, Child class C, high portal pressure, HVPG nonresponders to pharmacologic therapy) may benefit from transjugular intrahepatic portosystemic shunt (TIPS) insertion instead.[62,63]

In untreated patients, the risk of variceal rebleeding is 60% at 1 year and mortality from each rebleeding episode nearly 20%.[64] Salvage therapy with a TIPS is effective in patients who rebleed despite adequate secondary prophylaxis.[65] Although TIPS reduces the risk of rebleeding, until recently survival advantage over first-line medical and endoscopic therapy had not been established.[66,67] However, a recent randomized study of 63 patients with acute variceal bleed indicated early TIPS within 24 to 72 hours of bleeding should be considered in patients at high risk of treatment failure (ie, CTP class C score <14 or CTP class B with active bleeding) after initial pharmacologic and endoscopic therapy.[68] In this study, patients undergoing TIPS insertion had reductions in both treatment failure and mortality. Studies of TIPS placement in LT candidates are limited. Long-term data have shown that survival is not affected by the insertion of a TIPS.[69] Migration and embedded stents have been reported to complicate LT.[70,71] Current recommendations are that the stent be placed as close as possible to the hepatic vein/inferior vena cava ostium and should extend the shortest possible distance into the main portal vein, to avoid complicating the portal to portal vein anastomoses during transplantation.[72]

Balloon tamponade, although effective, has a limited role in acute variceal bleeding because other more effective and safer modalities are available (eg, vasoconstrictors, sclerotherapy, EVL).[73] It is associated with significant side-effects and hemostasis is transient; varices often rebleed when the balloon is deflated.[74] However, it is indicated if all other measures to control variceal bleeding have failed. Self-expanding metallic stents have recently been deployed in the endoscopic treatment of bleeding from post-EVL banding ulcers and in the management of acute variceal bleeding.[75–77] The stent can be placed without fluoroscopy, because it has a distal balloon that when inflated ensures proper location in the cardia. It is left in situ for 2 to 14 days, after which it can be retrieved by endoscopy with a hook system. More success has been reported in controlling bleeding esophageal than bleeding gastric varices, and it has also been rarely reported to cause minor ulcerations.[76] In the future, self-expanding metallic stents may be an option in patients with uncontrolled variceal hemorrhage.

Gastric varices are responsible for 5% to 10% of bleeding episodes in cirrhotic patients, with a higher mortality than esophageal variceal hemorrhage.[78] Endoscopic therapy with tissue adhesive cyanoacrylate has been recommended for bleeding from isolated gastric varices and for gastroesophageal varices (GOVs) extending beyond the cardia,[26] although this substance is not universally available. EVL or tissue adhesive can be used to control bleeding from GOV type I.[26] Patients who have gastric varices may bleed despite lowering HVPG to les than 12 mm Hg because preferential drainage of the superior mesenteric vein via the short and posterior gastric veins results in formation of gastric varices.[79] Cyanoacrylate is more effective than band ligation or alcohol injection in achieving initial hemostasis.[80–82] Although not common, major complications can arise with injection sclerotherapy using tissue adhesives. These complications include early polymerization, which leads to needle adhesion to the varix, embolization (including pulmonary embolization), abscess formation, esophageal or gastric perforation with peritoneal cavity extravasation, and splenic infarction,[81,83–88] TIPS is effective, with a 90% success rate, especially when accompanied by embolization of the collateral feeding vessels.[89,90]

HCC Screening

HCC screening and surveillance are recommended in all cirrhotic patients, regardless of cause. Regular HCC surveillance improves survival and detects earlier disease.[91–94]

It is also recommended in noncirrhotic patients with chronic HBV at high risk for HCC (ie, those with a family history of HCC, Africans age >20 years, Asian men age >40 years, Asian women age >50 years, or any carrier age >40 with persistent of intermittent alanine transaminase increase or HBV DNA >2000 IU/mL).[95]

There are additional issues related to surveillance for HCC in LT candidates. First, the identification of HCC in the United States may permit increased priority on UNOS if the patient fulfills Milan criteria. Second, detection of HCC identifies patients who may benefit from treatment or bridging therapies while awaiting transplantation. Third, surveillance ensures the candidate's HCC remains within transplant criteria; failing this, the patient would have to be delisted because transplant may not be beneficial to the patient because of a higher rate of recurrence.

Screening tools and interval
The American Association for the Study of Liver Diseases recommends HCC screening and 6-monthly surveillance by ultrasound. Although α-fetoprotein may lack both sensitivity and specificity, it remains part of the surveillance strategy at most centers.[96–98]

Once an initial screening test is abnormal or there is an enhanced suspicion that a patient may have HCC, accurate imaging is important for diagnosis and staging. The most reliable diagnostic tests are triple-phase, helical computed tomography and triple-phase, dynamic, contrast-enhanced magnetic resonance imaging.[99,100] The diagnosis of HCC can be reliably made based on imaging and generally does not require biopsy confirmation. A single, dynamic technique showing typical intense arterial uptake followed by washout of contrast in the venous-delayed phases has been validated for accuracy.[101–103] Biopsy should be reserved for patients with equivocal radiological findings because of the risk of bleeding and tumor seeding of the biopsy track. At least 2 positive stains for glypican 3, heat shock protein 70, or glutamine synthetase on histology specimens, if available, also confirms the diagnosis for HCC, in case of doubt.[104]

HCC treatment of the transplant candidate
Neoadjuvant treatment options for nonresectable HCC may bridge patients to LT before they exceed standard listing criteria. The indications, outcomes, and future of LT for HCC are discussed in greater detail in the article by Levi elsewhere in this issue.

Radiofrequency ablation (RFA) uses a high-frequency alternating current to destroy tumor tissue. RFA for tumors smaller than 2 cm is considered to be a curative option, with recurrence rates similar to that of resection, even in patients with cirrhosis.[105] RFA is more efficacious than other modalities and is now the therapy for choice for locoregional ablation of small tumors.[106,107] Some studies have also suggested that RFA may be more effective than transarterial chemoembolization (TACE) because of its greater ability to induce complete tumor necrosis.[108,109] Minor complications (eg, pain) from RFA are common, but more serious complications such as hemorrhage, portal vein thrombosis, visceral perforation, acute liver decompensation, and death have been known to occur.[110] One concern is the potential for needle-tract seeding, although this is infrequent.[111] Percutaneous ablation is cost-effective if the expected waiting time for LT is expected to be longer than 6 months.[112]

TACE is the direct injection of a chemotherapeutic agent (eg, doxorubicin mixed with lipiodol) into the hepatic artery, followed by arterial embolization with a gelatin sponge or microspheres. TACE confers a survival benefit in patients with noncurable, intermediate-stage HCC with good synthetic liver function.[113,114] Outcomes from studies that looked at the use of TACE in the pretransplant setting have reported variable results in dropout rates, survival, or disease recurrence.[115–118] Patients who respond to TACE with reduction in tumor burden have been reported to have better posttransplant survivals.[119,120] However, TACE may enhance tumor growth via the stimulation of growth factors (eg, vascular endothelial growth factor and basic fibroblast growth factor),[121,122] result in less tumor necrosis,[123] or, from collateral liver damage, even precipitate acute decompensation in cirrhotic patients.[124]

Nevertheless, TACE may be effective bridging therapy in selected patients until LT.[125]

Ascites

In cirrhotic patients, the production of vasoactive mediators (eg, nitric oxide, endothelin) results in vasodilatation that leads to the activation of the renin-angiotensin system. Activation of this system results in sodium retention and, in turn, ascites (**Fig. 1**).[126] Ascites is the most common complication of cirrhosis, after HE and variceal bleeds.[127] Once ascites develops, survival is only 50% at 5 years; its onset should prompt consideration for LT.[128]

Initial evaluation of any cirrhotic patient with new onset ascites should include paracentesis to confirm its transudative nature, and to exclude SBP. A serum-ascites albumin gradient of 1.1 g/dL or greater confirms ascites from portal hypertension with 97% accuracy.[129,130]

General and pharmacologic measures

Patients with ascites should be prescribed a low-sodium (ie, 88 mmol or 2 g/d) diet. Assuming nonurinary sodium excretion in an afebrile patient to be less than 10 mmol/d, the goal of treatment is to achieve a urinary sodium excretion of greater than 78 mmol/d (88 mmol intake/d − 10 mmol nonurinary excretion/d). Compliance can be assessed with a random spot urine sodium-potassium concentration. A ratio greater than 1 correlates with a 24-h urinary sodium excretion greater than 78 mmol/d with 90% accuracy and suggests dietary compliance.[131] Fluid restriction is recommended when serum sodium is less than 120 to 125 mmol/L, although most cirrhotic patients with chronic hyponatremia show neurologic symptoms only at serum sodium levels less than 110 mmol/L or if the decline in serum sodium levels has been rapid.[132]

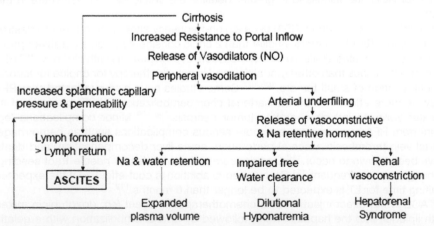

Fig. 1. Pathophysiology of ascites in cirrhosis. (*Reprinted from* Sandhu BS, Sanyal AJ. Management of ascites in cirrhosis. Clin Liver Dis 2005;9:715–32; with permission.)

The usual diuretic combination for mild to moderate ascites is spirinolactone 100 mg and furosemide 40 mg as a single morning dose. This approach achieves natriuresis and maintains normokalemia.[132] Weight and renal function should be monitored while the patient is on diuretic therapy to detect renal impairment, electrolyte imbalance, or dehydration with overly brisk diuresis. Diuretics can be increased simultaneously every 3 to 5 days, maintaining the 100 mg:40 mg ratio, aiming for a weight loss of about 0.5 kg per day in patients without peripheral edema, up to a maximum of spironolactone 400 mg and furosemide 160 mg/d.[132] In patients who are unable to tolerate spironolactone because of tender gynecomastia, amiloride 10 to 40 mg/d may be substituted, although it is a less effective diuretic.

A combined approach of salt restriction and diuretic therapy is effective in 90% of patients in controlling ascites. Diuretics should be withheld in patients with uncontrolled or recurrent HE, serum sodium less than 120 mmol/L despite fluid restriction, or increasing serum creatinine level greater than 2.0 mg/dL (180 μmol/L).[132]

In patients with hypervolemic hyponatremia, fluid restriction has been the standard of care but is seldom effective because fluid intake often cannot be consistently restricted to less than 1 L/d.[132,133] Aquaretic drugs that selectively block V2-arginine vasopressin receptors in the renal collecting ducts have been used to good effect in the treatment of hyponatremia in various causes (eg, SIADH [syndrome of inappropriate antidiuretic hormone hypersecretion]). A pivotal phase 3 randomized, controlled trial has led to the approval of tolvaptan in the United States for the management of severe hypervolemic hyponatremia (<125 mmol/L) associated with cirrhosis.[134] Tolvaptan, starting with an initial dose of 15 mg/d, is titrated progressively to 30 and 60 mg/d, according to serum sodium response. Rapid increases in serum sodium concentration (>8–10 mmol/d) should be avoided to prevent occurrence of osmotic demyelination syndrome. Concomitant treatment with drugs that are either potent inhibitors (eg, clarithromycin, ketoconazole, itraconazole) or inducers (eg, dexamethasone, efavirenz, nevirapine, phenytoin) of the cytochrome P450 3A should be avoided. However, the optimal duration of treatment with tolvaptan is unknown and it has limited long-term safety data. Conivaptan is licensed in some countries for short-term intravenous treatment.[133]

Invasive measures

Refractory ascites is defined as ascites that cannot be mobilized by maximal medical therapy or its early recurrence after therapeutic paracentesis.[135] Approximately 10% of cirrhotic patients with ascites have refractory ascites. Patients with refractory ascites have lower pretransplant survival (50% mortality within 6 months; 75% within 1 year) compared with patients with diuretic-responsive ascites.[136]

Refractory ascites can be effectively controlled by serial paracentesis. A requirement for large-volume (≥5 L) paracenteses more frequently than every fortnight implies noncompliance with a sodium-restricted diet.[132] In large-volume paracentesis, an intravenous infusion of 6 to 8 g of albumin for each liter of fluid drained may reduce the risk of renal dysfunction associated with large-volume fluid shifts.[137,138]

TIPS is more effective in controlling refractory ascites than serial paracentesis with albumin and prevents the development of hepatorenal syndrome (HRS).[139–142] However, data on its effects on transplant-free survival are conflicting. The use of TIPS in patients with MELD greater than 18 is potentially hazardous, because there is a 60% mortality by 3 months after TIPS placement.[143] TIPS is contraindicated in patients with severe liver failure (serum bilirubin >5 mg/dL, INR >2 or CTP score >11, HE ≥ grade 2), bacterial or fungal infection, progressive renal failure, HCC, or severe cardiopulmonary disease.[133] Patients should have an ejection fraction greater than

60% to avoid precipitating heart failure.[144] TIPS typically converts diuretic-resistant ascites to diuretic-sensitive, and titration of doses to achieve natriuresis after TIPS may be required.[132]

SBP

Bacterial infection is common in hospitalized cirrhotic patients and is a major cause of mortality.[145,146] Infections to which such patients may be susceptible include SBP, urinary tract infections, pneumonia, and bacteremia from invasive procedures.[146,147] SBP is the most common bacterial infection in cirrhotic patients with ascites and is associated with a mortality of about 30%.[148–151] SBP if complicated by renal failure has a mortality of 40% to 100%.[152]

Primary prophylaxis

Primary antibiotic prophylaxis is recommended in cirrhotic patients with a low ascitic fluid protein level (<1.5 g/dL) plus at least one of the following: serum creatinine level 1.2 mg/dL or greater, blood urea nitrogen level 25 mg/dL or greater, serum sodium level 130 mmol/L or less, or CTP score 9 points or greater with serum bilirubin level 3 mg/dL or greater.[153] Its use in these circumstances is associated with a reduced incidence of SBP, HRS, and death.[153–155]

Cirrhotic patients with gastrointestinal hemorrhage require antibiotic prophylaxis, because it improves survival and decreases variceal rebleeding.[156,157]

Appropriate antibiotic choices for primary prophylaxis of SBP include intravenous ceftriaxone or third-generation cephalosporin (in patients with active gastrointestinal hemorrhage), oral norfloxacin, or ciprofloxacin.[158,159]

Diagnosis and treatment

SBP should be suspected, and a diagnostic paracentesis performed, in any cirrhotic patient with ascites who has fever, deteriorating hepatocellular function, nonspecific abdominal pain, unexplained encephalopathy, or deteriorating renal function.

A positive ascitic fluid culture or an increased ascitic fluid polymorphonuclear (PMN) leukocyte cell count 250 per mm^3 (0.25 × 10^9/L) or greater in the absence of an intra-abdominal abscess or perforation confirms the diagnosis of SBP.[160]

Patients with ascitic fluid PMN counts 250 per mm^3 (0.25 × 10^9/L) or greater but with negative fluid cultures have culture-negative neutrocytic ascites (CNNA).[161,162] Patients with CNNA have similar signs, symptoms, and mortality as patients with SBP and should be treated empirically with antibiotics for SBP.[161]

Monomicrobial nonneutrocytic bacterascites is infection detected at the bacterascites stage before there is a neutrophilic response (ie, ascitic fluid PMN count <250 cells/mm^3 (0.25 × 10^9/L), and may spontaneously resolve without antibiotics or a neutrophil response.[163] However, if signs or symptoms of overt infection (eg, fever, abdominal pain) develop, empiric antibiotics are indicated regardless of the ascitic PMN count.

When SBP is suspected, the ascitic fluid should be inoculated in blood culture bottles, which increases the diagnostic yield.[164] Simultaneous blood cultures should be obtained, because they are positive in more than 50% of patients with SBP. Rapid diagnosis also can be made using a urine reagent dipstick to test ascitic fluid. If leukocyte esterase is strongly positive, the diagnosis of SBP is highly likely, although the sensitivity of this bedside test may be less than 50%.[165,166] However, a review of 19 studies found that reagent strips had low sensitivity and high false-negative rates, especially in patients with SBP and low PMN counts (<1000/mm^3).[167]

SBP should be treated empirically with broad-spectrum antibiotics until the results of susceptibility testing are known. Intravenous cefotaxime or another third-generation cephalosporin or amoxicillin-clavunate for 5 days leads to resolution in 90% of cases of SBP.[164,168,169] Other antimicrobial agents that may be effective for the treatment of SBP include ampicillin, cotrimoxazole, norfloxacin, ofloxacin, and ciprofloxacin.[170,171]

Plasma expansion with 20% albumin infusion at 1.5 g/kg at the time of diagnosis and a repeat infusion on day 3 at 1 g/kg lowers the risk of renal failure, and reduces in-hospital mortality and 3-month mortality.[172] Albumin infusion can also improve cardiac function and decrease arterial vasodilatation and has antioxidant properties (effects that are not observed with other volume expanders).[173–175]

Secondary prophylaxis

SBP recurs in up to 70% of patients.[176] Hence, all patients with a previous episode of SBP should be maintained on prophylactic antibiotics.[168] Oral norfloxacin (400 mg/d) or ciprofloxacin (750 mg/wk) or trimethoprim 160 mg-sulfamethoxazole 800 mg (cotrimoxazole) daily can be used as secondary prophylaxis, although daily dosing is preferred to intermittent dosing.[132,133,177,178]

Prolonged or frequent use of antibiotics is associated with the risk of drug resistance and changing microbial cause in SBP.[179–181] A study conducted in 3 tertiary hospitals found that fluoroquinolone-resistant *Escherichia coli* SBP prevalence had increased over a 2-year period because of norfloxacin prophylaxis. However, mortality was related to host factors (such as degree of host immunocompetence) rather than to bacterial virulence or resistance.[182] Cycling antibiotics may be an option to decrease the risk of microbial resistance, although no data are available yet to support this approach.

HRS

HRS is defined as serum creatinine level greater than 1.5 mg/dL, in the absence of shock, volume depletion (ie, no sustained improvement of renal function after 2 days of diuretic withdrawal and volume expansion with albumin at 1 g/kg/d up to a maximum 100 g/d), infection, recent use of nephrotoxic drugs, and parenchymal renal disease (ie, proteinuria <0.5 g/d, hematuria <50 red blood cells per high power field, and normal renal ultrasonography).[183]

In HRS, decreased effective arterial blood volume (caused by splanchnic and systemic vasodilatation) activates the sympathetic nervous system and the renin-angiotensin-aldosterone system, resulting in renal vasoconstriction, diminished renal perfusion, and a decrease in glomerular filtration rate.[184–187] Although there is increased synthesis of vasoactive mediators (eg, cysteinyl leukotrienes, thromboxane A2, F2-isoprostanes, and endothelin-1), which may affect renal blood flow, their exact role in the pathogenesis of HRS remains unknown.[133]

HRS is an ominous event in the progression of cirrhosis.[188] HRS is diagnosed in up to 17% of hospitalized patients with ascites and in more than 50% of cirrhotic patients who die during their hospitalization.[186] An accurate diagnosis of HRS is important. Renal dysfunction from non-HRS causes is treated differently and may have specific management (eg, obstructive uropathy). Second, although HRS may improve with LT alone, chronic renal impairment from other causes does not. Such patients may require combined liver-kidney transplant.[189] Thirdly, the prognosis of the different cause of renal failure in cirrhotic patients differs: patients with HRS have the highest mortality.[190] The management of renal dysfunction in LT patients is described in greater detail in the article by Bunnapradist elsewhere in this issue.

Clinical types

HRS is classified based on its severity and progression.

Type 1 HRS is acute and usually has a precipitant, such as infection or gastrointestinal bleeding. It is rapidly progressive, defined by a serum creatinine level doubling to greater than 2.5 mg/dL in less than 2 weeks.[135] In the absence of LT, median survival is only 2 weeks.

Type 2 HRS runs a more insidious course. Type 2 HRS commonly develops in the setting of refractory ascites and is characterized by a moderate and steady decrease in renal function with avid sodium retention. SBP can convert patients with type 2 HRS to type 1 HRS. In the absence of LT, the median survival is 6 months for type 2 HRS.[152,191]

Treatment

LT is the optimal treatment of both types of HRS.[192,193]

General measures include withdrawal of diuretics and nephrotoxic drugs, and avoiding overly aggressive fluid resuscitation. Precipitants such as SBP and gastrointestinal bleeding should be specifically excluded.

Specific therapy with vasoconstrictors is of benefit. Combination terlipressin and albumin (1 g/kg on day 1 then 40 g/d) is beneficial as pharmacologic treatment of HRS, and the evidence for its use in HRS is supported by both nonrandomized and randomized controlled trials.[184,194–200] Terlipressin is initiated at 1 mg every 4 to 6 hours and increased to maximum 2 mg every 4 to 6 hours if there is no reduction in serum creatinine level of 25% or greater compared with baseline at day 3 of therapy. Treatment is maintained till serum creatinine level decreases to less than 1.5 mg/dL. The median time to response is 14 days and recurrence after withdrawal of therapy can be retreated with terlipressin.[133] However, terlipressin is not licensed in some countries, including the United States. Other options include the use of norepinephrine or combination midodrine-octreotide.[201,202] Concomitant albumin infusion is also used with the vasoconstrictors in most of these studies. If selected, the following doses for vasoconstrictors are used: norepinephrine 0.5 to 3 mg/h (continuous infusion) or ornipressin 2 to 6 U/h (continuous infusion), or vasopressin 0.01 to 0.8 U/min (continuous infusion) or octreotide 100 to 200 μg 3 times a day (subcutaneous, or as intravenous 25 μg/h continuous infusion) with midodrine 7.5 to 12.5 mg 3 times a day (by mouth).

TIPS may also be beneficial for HRS treatment, especially in patients with type 2 HRS.[186,203,204] However, no survival benefit has been shown. A prospective study of 14 patients with HRS showed that in 5 of 10 patients who responded to medical therapy (ie, midodrine, octreotide, and albumin) and subsequently underwent TIPS, renal function continued to improve after TIPS.[205] However, TIPS should be reserved for patients who are intolerant of serial paracentesis and who have well-preserved liver function.[72]

Hemodialysis or continuous venous hemofiltration has been used to treat type 1 HRS, although there are no data comparing renal replacement therapy with other treatment options (eg, vasoconstrictors) and data, in general, are scant.[206,207] Patients with type 1 HRS seldom develop severe hyperkalemia, metabolic acidosis, and volume overload requiring emergent renal replacement therapy, particularly in the early stages.[133]

Prophylaxis

HRS is a predictor of poor transplant outcomes with a 65% survival rate for type 1 HRS after LT.[133,192] Approximately 35% of HRS patients may require hemodialysis during transplantation or in the early postoperative period, compared with 5% of non-HRS patients.

Because the onset of HRS portends a poor prognosis, cirrhotic patients should receive antibiotics if variceal bleeding occurs, or albumin infusion on days 1 and 3 and antibiotics in the treatment of SBP, or albumin infusion as large-volume replacement in paracentesis as primary prophylaxis of HRS. Pentoxyfilline (400 mg 3 times a day) in patients with alcoholic hepatitis also reduces HRS rates,[208] as might its use in patients with advanced cirrhosis.[209] Patients who develop HRS should be referred to a transplantation center in a timely manner.

HE

HE is seen in 50% to 70% of patients with cirrhosis.[210] Patients with cirrhosis may experience episodic, persistent, or minimal HE.[211,212] Episodic HE may be precipitated by sepsis, bleeding, or drugs (eg, excessive diuretic use or sedatives). Therapy should be prompt to prevent secondary complications such as aspiration pneumonia. HE is treated with synthetic disaccharide lactulose or lactitol, and nonabsorbable antibiotic rifaximin.[213] Because rifaximin has been found to mitigate recurrent HE, it has been suggested that patients on the transplant waiting list should also receive rifaximin as secondary prophylaxis.[214] Dietary protein-restriction is not routinely advised because most patients are malnourished at presentation.[215,216]

Portopulmonary Hypertension and Hepatopulmonary Syndrome

The management of pulmonary complications in the pre-LT patient is discussed in greater detail in the article by Krowka elsewhere in this issue.

Osteopenia/Osteoporosis

The prevalence of osteoporosis in patients with chronic liver disease may be as high as 10% to 30%, depending on the cause of liver disease.[217,218] Patients with cholestatic disease, who are postmenopausal, or who have been on long-term corticosteroid therapy are at highest risk.[219] In addition, patients with chronic liver disease also have other risk factors for osteoporosis related to their disease, such as hypogonadism, vitamin D insufficiency, excess alcohol consumption, and low body mass index.[220] Osteoporotic or osteopenic patients are at risk of pathologic fractures in the perioperative period.[221] All transplant candidates should be screened for osteopenia/osteoporosis with a bone mineral density at time of transplant evaluation and every 2 years. Hypothyroidism and calcium or vitamin D deficiencies should be excluded and regular exercise encouraged. Oral bisphosphonates should be avoided in patients with esophageal varices because of the risk of ulceration in the esophagus or stomach. Intravenous bisphosphonates (pamidronate or zolendronic acid) 3 to 6 monthly should be advised in LT candidates with esophageal varices who have severe osteoporosis.[222,223] Studies suggest that pre-LT intravenous bisphosphonates may reduce fracturing in the post-LT period.[223]

Vaccination

All patients who have chronic liver disease should be vaccinated against hepatitis A virus (HAV), HBV, pneumococcus, and influenza.[224–227] Because the LT recipient requires high-dose immunosuppression, live or live-attenuated vaccines (eg, varicella zoster or rubella vaccine) 4 weeks before or anytime after transplant are contraindicated. Although the response of cirrhotic patients to active vaccination is impaired, immunization should still be attempted to reduce morbidity and mortality risk with superimposed infection.[228,229] Noncirrhotic patients respond better to vaccination than cirrhotics, and likewise, compensated cirrhotic patients respond better than decompensated cirrhotics.[230–232] The use of immunosuppressants after transplant further reduces antibody response and efforts should be made to vaccinate candidates before rather than after LT.[233] Strategies attempted to improve vaccine response in cirrhotic patients include double-dosing, reduced dosing intervals between shots, or various booster strategies for HBV, pneumococcal, and influenza vaccines.

HAV and HBV vaccination are recommended in patients with chronic liver disease.[234,235] Patients with chronic hepatitis or cirrhosis who acquire superimposed acute HAV or HBV have greater morbidity and mortality.[236–241] Patients with HBV coviral infection (eg, HBV-HCV) have more aggressive disease and are at higher risk of developing cirrhosis or HCC.[242] Because the response to HBV vaccination in cirrhotic patients can be as low as 16% (compared with almost 100% in the normal healthy population),[243–245] double-dose (40 µg) vaccination, closer dosing intervals (0, 1, and 2 months apart), and repeat boosters have all been attempted to improve response rates.[232,246–249]

Pneumococcal and yearly influenza vaccination are also recommended in patients with chronic liver disease. Transplant candidates have been shown to mount immune responses to these vaccinations, albeit not to the extent of healthy individuals.[250–252]

SUMMARY

Care of the LT candidate is one of the most challenging, yet rewarding, aspects of hepatology. Anticipation and intervention for the major complications of advanced liver disease increase the likelihood of survival until transplant.

REFERENCES

1. Kamath PS, Wiesner RH, Malinchoc M, et al. A model to predict survival in patients with end-stage liver disease. Hepatology 2001;33(2):464–70.
2. Wiesner R, Edwards E, Freeman R, et al. Model for end-stage liver disease (MELD) and allocation of donor livers. Gastroenterology 2003;124(1):91–6.
3. Fattovich G, Giustina G, Degos F, et al. Morbidity and mortality in compensated cirrhosis type C: a retrospective follow-up study of 384 patients. Gastroenterology 1997;112(2):463–72.
4. Muhlberger N, Schwarzer R, Lettmeier B, et al. HCV-related burden of disease in Europe: a systematic assessment of incidence, prevalence, morbidity, and mortality. BMC Public Health 2009;9:34.
5. Davis GL, Albright JE, Cook SF, et al. Projecting future complications of chronic hepatitis C in the United States. Liver Transpl 2003;9(4):331–8.
6. El-Serag HB. Hepatocellular carcinoma: recent trends in the United States. Gastroenterology 2004;127(5 Suppl 1):S27–34.
7. Poynard T, McHutchison J, Manns M, et al. Impact of pegylated interferon alfa-2b and ribavirin on liver fibrosis in patients with chronic hepatitis C. Gastroenterology 2002;122(5):1303–13.
8. Shiffman ML, Hofmann CM, Thompson EB, et al. Relationship between biochemical, virological, and histological response during interferon treatment of chronic hepatitis C. Hepatology 1997;26(3):780–5.
9. Fried MW, Hadziyannis SJ. Treatment of chronic hepatitis C infection with peginterferons plus ribavirin. Semin Liver Dis 2004;24(Suppl 2):47–54.
10. Samuel D, Bizollon T, Feray C, et al. Interferon-alpha 2b plus ribavirin in patients with chronic hepatitis C after liver transplantation: a randomized study. Gastroenterology 2003;124(3):642–50.

11. Shergill AK, Khalili M, Straley S, et al. Applicability, tolerability and efficacy of preemptive antiviral therapy in hepatitis C-infected patients undergoing liver transplantation. Am J Transplant 2005;5(1):118–24.

12. Wiesner RH, Sorrell M, Villamil F. Report of the first International Liver Transplantation Society expert panel consensus conference on liver transplantation and hepatitis C. Liver Transpl 2003;9(11):S1–9.

13. Heathcote EJ, Shiffman ML, Cooksley WG, et al. Peginterferon alfa-2a in patients with chronic hepatitis C and cirrhosis. N Engl J Med 2000;343(23): 1673–80.

14. Hadziyannis SJ, Sette H Jr, Morgan TR, et al. Peginterferon-alpha2a and ribavirin combination therapy in chronic hepatitis C: a randomized study of treatment duration and ribavirin dose. Ann Intern Med 2004;140(5):346–55.

15. Perrillo RP, Wright T, Rakela J, et al. A multicenter United States-Canadian trial to assess lamivudine monotherapy before and after liver transplantation for chronic hepatitis B. Hepatology 2001;33(2):424–32.

16. Villeneuve JP, Condreay LD, Willems B, et al. Lamivudine treatment for decompensated cirrhosis resulting from chronic hepatitis B. Hepatology 2000;31(1): 207–10.

17. Yao FY, Bass NM. Lamivudine treatment in patients with severely decompensated cirrhosis due to replicating hepatitis B infection. J Hepatol 2000;33(2): 301–7.

18. Fontana RJ, Hann HW, Perrillo RP, et al. Determinants of early mortality in patients with decompensated chronic hepatitis B treated with antiviral therapy. Gastroenterology 2002;123(3):719–27.

19. Kim WR, Terrault NA, Pedersen RA, et al. Trends in waiting list registration for liver transplantation for viral hepatitis in the United States. Gastroenterology 2009;137(5):1680–6.

20. Groszmann RJ, Garcia-Tsao G, Bosch J, et al. Beta-blockers to prevent gastroesophageal varices in patients with cirrhosis. N Engl J Med 2005;353(21): 2254–61.

21. D'Amico G, Pagliaro L, Bosch J. The treatment of portal hypertension: a meta-analytic review. Hepatology 1995;22(1):332–54.

22. D'Amico G, Luca A. Natural history. Clinical-haemodynamic correlations. Prediction of the risk of bleeding. Baillieres Clin Gastroenterol 1997;11(2):243–56.

23. D'Amico G, Garcia-Tsao G, Pagliaro L. Natural history and prognostic indicators of survival in cirrhosis: a systematic review of 118 studies. J Hepatol 2006;44(1): 217–31.

24. McCormick PA. Pathophysiology and prognosis of oesophageal varices. Scand J Gastroenterol Suppl 1994;207:1–5.

25. Carbonell N, Pauwels A, Serfaty L, et al. Improved survival after variceal bleeding in patients with cirrhosis over the past two decades. Hepatology 2004;40(3):652–9.

26. de Franchis R. Revising consensus in portal hypertension: report of the Baveno V consensus workshop on methodology of diagnosis and therapy in portal hypertension. J Hepatol 2010;53(4):762–8.

27. North Italian Endoscopic Club for the Study and Treatment of Esophageal Varices. Prediction of the first variceal hemorrhage in patients with cirrhosis of the liver and esophageal varices. A prospective multicenter study. N Engl J Med 1988;319(15):983–9.

28. de Franchis R, Pascal JP, Ancona E, et al. Definitions, methodology and therapeutic strategies in portal hypertension. A Consensus Development Workshop,

Baveno, Lake Maggiore, Italy, April 5 and 6, 1990. J Hepatol 1992;15(1–2): 256–61.

29. Merli M, Nicolini G, Angeloni S, et al. Incidence and natural history of small esophageal varices in cirrhotic patients. J Hepatol 2003;38(3):266–72.

30. de Franchis R. Evaluation and follow-up of patients with cirrhosis and oesophageal varices. J Hepatol 2003;38(3):361–3.

31. Eisen GM, Eliakim R, Zaman A, et al. The accuracy of PillCam ESO capsule endoscopy versus conventional upper endoscopy for the diagnosis of esophageal varices: a prospective three-center pilot study. Endoscopy 2006;38(1):31–5.

32. Lapalus MG, Dumortier J, Fumex F, et al. Esophageal capsule endoscopy versus esophagogastroduodenoscopy for evaluating portal hypertension: a prospective comparative study of performance and tolerance. Endoscopy 2006;38(1):36–41.

33. Bosch J, Thabut D, Albillos A, et al. Recombinant factor VIIa for variceal bleeding in patients with advanced cirrhosis: a randomized, controlled trial. Hepatology 2008;47(5):1604–14.

34. Frenette C, Kuldau JG, Hillebrand D, et al. Comparison of esophageal pill endoscopy and conventional endoscopy for variceal screening. Hepatology 2006;44(Suppl 1):445A.

35. D'Amico G, Pagliaro L, Bosch J. Pharmacological treatment of portal hypertension: an evidence-based approach. Semin Liver Dis 1999;19(4):475–505.

36. Garcia-Pagan JC, Bosch J. Endoscopic band ligation in the treatment of portal hypertension. Nat Clin Pract Gastroenterol Hepatol 2005;2(11):526–35.

37. Merkel C, Marin R, Angeli P, et al. A placebo-controlled clinical trial of nadolol in the prophylaxis of growth of small esophageal varices in cirrhosis. Gastroenterology 2004;127(2):476–84.

38. Garcia-Pagan JC, Morillas R, Banares R, et al. Propranolol plus placebo versus propranolol plus isosorbide-5-mononitrate in the prevention of a first variceal bleed: a double-blind RCT. Hepatology 2003;37(6):1260–6.

39. Lim EJ, Gow PJ, Angus PW. Endoscopic variceal ligation for primary prophylaxis of esophageal variceal hemorrhage in pre-liver transplant patients. Liver Transpl 2009;15(11):1508–13.

40. Lo GH, Chen WC, Chen MH, et al. Endoscopic ligation vs. nadolol in the prevention of first variceal bleeding in patients with cirrhosis. Gastrointest Endosc 2004;59(3):333–8.

41. Schepke M, Kleber G, Nurnberg D, et al. Ligation versus propranolol for the primary prophylaxis of variceal bleeding in cirrhosis. Hepatology 2004;40(1):65–72.

42. Sarin SK, Lamba GS, Kumar M, et al. Comparison of endoscopic ligation and propranolol for the primary prevention of variceal bleeding. N Engl J Med 1999;340(13):988–93.

43. Lui HF, Stanley AJ, Forrest EH, et al. Primary prophylaxis of variceal hemorrhage: a randomized controlled trial comparing band ligation, propranolol, and isosorbide mononitrate. Gastroenterology 2002;123(3):735–44.

44. Jutabha R, Jensen DM, Martin P, et al. Randomized study comparing banding and propranolol to prevent initial variceal hemorrhage in cirrhotics with high-risk esophageal varices. Gastroenterology 2005;128(4):870–81.

45. Thuluvath PJ, Maheshwari A, Jagannath S, et al. A randomized controlled trial of beta-blockers versus endoscopic band ligation for primary prophylaxis: a large sample size is required to show a difference in bleeding rates. Dig Dis Sci 2005; 50(2):407–10.

46. De BK, Ghoshal UC, Das T, et al. Endoscopic variceal ligation for primary prophylaxis of oesophageal variceal bleed: preliminary report of a randomized controlled trial. J Gastroenterol Hepatol 1999;14(3):220–4.

47. Lay CS, Tsai YT, Lee FY, et al. Endoscopic variceal ligation versus propranolol in prophylaxis of first variceal bleeding in patients with cirrhosis. J Gastroenterol Hepatol 2006;21(2):413–9.

48. Psilopoulos D, Galanis P, Goulas S, et al. Endoscopic variceal ligation vs. propranolol for prevention of first variceal bleeding: a randomized controlled trial. Eur J Gastroenterol Hepatol 2005;17(10):1111–7.

49. Norberto L, Polese L, Cillo U, et al. A randomized study comparing ligation with propranolol for primary prophylaxis of variceal bleeding in candidates for liver transplantation. Liver Transpl 2007;13(9):1272–8.

50. Chen CY, Sheu MZ, Tsai TL, et al. Endoscopic variceal ligation with multiple band ligator for prophylaxis of first hemorrhage esophageal varices. Endoscopy 1999;31(Suppl 1):35A.

51. Song H, Shin JW, Kim HI, et al. A prospective randomized trial between the prophylactic endoscopic variceal ligation and propranolol administration for prevention of first bleeding in cirrhotic patients with high-risk esophageal varices. J Hepatol 2000;32(Suppl 2):41A.

52. de la Mora G, Farca-Belsaguy AA, Uribe M, et al. Ligation vs propranolol for primary prophylaxis of variceal bleeding using multiple band ligator and objective measurements of treatment adequacy: preliminary results. Gastroenterology 2000;118:6511A.

53. Drastich P, Lata J, Petrtyl J, et al. Endoscopic variceal band ligation in comparison with propranolol in prophylaxis of first variceal bleeding in patients with liver cirrhosis. J Hepatol 2005;42:202A.

54. Abdelfattah MH, Rashed MA, Elfakhry AA, et al. Endoscopic variceal ligation versus pharmacological treatment for primary prophylaxis of variceal bleeding: a randomized study. J Hepatol 2006;44(Suppl 2):83A.

55. Gheorghe C, Gheorghe L, Vadan R, et al. Prophylactic banding ligation of high risk esophageal varices in patients on the waiting list for liver transplantation: an interim analysis. J Hepatol 2002;36(Suppl 1):38A.

56. Khuroo MS, Khuroo NS, Farahat KL, et al. Meta-analysis: endoscopic variceal ligation for primary prophylaxis of oesophageal variceal bleeding. Aliment Pharmacol Ther 2005;21(4):347–61.

57. Garcia-Tsao G, Sanyal AJ, Grace ND, et al. Prevention and management of gastroesophageal varices and variceal hemorrhage in cirrhosis. Hepatology 2007;46(3):922–38.

58. Castaneda B, Morales J, Lionetti R, et al. Effects of blood volume restitution following a portal hypertensive-related bleeding in anesthetized cirrhotic rats. Hepatology 2001;33(4):821–5.

59. Soares-Welser K, Brezis M, Tur-Kaspa R, et al. Antibiotic prophylaxis for cirrhotic patients with gastrointestinal bleeding. Cochrane Database Syst Rev 2002;(2):CD002907.

60. Escorsell A, Banares R, Garcia-Pagan JC, et al. TIPS versus drug therapy in preventing variceal rebleeding in advanced cirrhosis: a randomized controlled trial. Hepatology 2002;35(2):385–92.

61. de la Pena J, Brullet E, Sanchez-Hernandez E, et al. Variceal ligation plus nadolol compared with ligation for prophylaxis of variceal rebleeding: a multicenter trial. Hepatology 2005;41(3):572–8.

62. Garcia-Pagan JC, Villanueva C, Albillos A, et al. Nadolol plus isosorbide mononitrate alone or associated with band ligation in the prevention of recurrent bleeding: a multicentre randomised controlled trial. Gut 2009;58(8):1144–50.
63. Schepke M. Drugs, ligation or both for the prevention of variceal rebleeding? Gut 2009;58(8):1045–6.
64. de Franchis R, Primignani M. Natural history of portal hypertension in patients with cirrhosis. Clin Liver Dis 2001;5(3):645–63.
65. Sanyal AJ, Freedman AM, Luketic VA, et al. Transjugular intrahepatic portosystemic shunts for patients with active variceal hemorrhage unresponsive to sclerotherapy. Gastroenterology 1996;111(1):138–46.
66. de Franchis R, Primignani M. Endoscopic treatments for portal hypertension. Semin Liver Dis 1999;19(4):439–55.
67. Burroughs AK, Vangeli M. Transjugular intrahepatic portosystemic shunt versus endoscopic therapy: randomized trials for secondary prophylaxis of variceal bleeding: an updated meta-analysis. Scand J Gastroenterol 2002;37(3):249–52.
68. Garcia-Pagan JC, Caca K, Bureau C, et al. Early use of TIPS in patients with cirrhosis and variceal bleeding. N Engl J Med 2010;362(25):2370–9.
69. Guerrini GP, Pleguezuelo M, Maimone S, et al. Impact of TIPS preliver transplantation for the outcome posttransplantation. Am J Transplant 2009;9(1): 192–200.
70. Tripathi D, Therapondos G, Redhead DN, et al. Transjugular intrahepatic portosystemic stent-shunt and its effects on orthotopic liver transplantation. Eur J Gastroenterol Hepatol 2002;14(8):827–32.
71. Hutchins RR, Patch D, Tibballs J, et al. Liver transplantation complicated by embedded transjugular intrahepatic portosystemic shunt: a new method for portal anastomosis–a surgical salvage procedure. Liver Transpl 2000;6(2): 237–8.
72. Boyer TD, Haskal ZJ. The role of transjugular intrahepatic portosystemic shunt (TIPS) in the management of portal hypertension: update 2009. Hepatology 2010;51(1):306.
73. Panes J, Teres J, Bosch J, et al. Efficacy of balloon tamponade in treatment of bleeding gastric and esophageal varices. Results in 151 consecutive episodes. Dig Dis Sci 1988;33(4):454–9.
74. Avgerinos A, Armonis A. Balloon tamponade technique and efficacy in variceal haemorrhage. Scand J Gastroenterol Suppl 1994;207:11–6.
75. Hubmann R, Bodlaj G, Czompo M, et al. The use of self-expanding metal stents to treat acute esophageal variceal bleeding. Endoscopy 2006;38(9):896–901.
76. Wright G, Lewis H, Hogan B, et al. A self-expanding metal stent for complicated variceal hemorrhage: experience at a single center. Gastrointest Endosc 2010; 71(1):71–8.
77. Mishin I, Ghidirim G, Dolghii A, et al. Implantation of self-expanding metal stent in the treatment of severe bleeding from esophageal ulcer after endoscopic band ligation. Dis Esophagus 2010;23(7):E35–8.
78. Sarin SK, Lahoti D, Saxena SP, et al. Prevalence, classification and natural history of gastric varices: a long-term follow-up study in 568 portal hypertension patients. Hepatology 1992;16(6):1343–9.
79. Chao Y, Lin HC, Lee FY, et al. Hepatic hemodynamic features in patients with esophageal or gastric varices. J Hepatol 1993;19(1):85–9.
80. Huang YH, Yeh HZ, Chen GH, et al. Endoscopic treatment of bleeding gastric varices by N-butyl-2-cyanoacrylate (Histoacryl) injection: long-term efficacy and safety. Gastrointest Endosc 2000;52(2):160–7.

81. Lo GH, Lai KH, Cheng JS, et al. A prospective, randomized trial of butyl cyano-acrylate injection versus band ligation in the management of bleeding gastric varices. Hepatology 2001;33(5):1060–4.
82. Sarin SK, Jain AK, Jain M, et al. A randomized controlled trial of cyanoacrylate versus alcohol injection in patients with isolated fundic varices. Am J Gastroen-terol 2002;97(4):1010–5.
83. Chen WC, Hou MC, Lin HC, et al. Bacteremia after endoscopic injection of N-butyl-2-cyanoacrylate for gastric variceal bleeding. Gastrointest Endosc 2001; 54(2):214–8.
84. Bhasin DK, Sharma BC, Prasad H, et al. Endoscopic removal of sclerotherapy needle from gastric varix after N-butyl-2-cyanoacrylate injection. Gastrointest Endosc 2000;51(4 Pt 1):497–8.
85. Wai CT, Sutedja DS, Khor CJ, et al. Esophageal sinus formation as a complica-tion of cyanoacrylate injection. Gastrointest Endosc 2005;61(6):773–5.
86. Hwang SS, Kim HH, Park SH, et al. N-butyl-2-cyanoacrylate pulmonary embo-lism after endoscopic injection sclerotherapy for gastric variceal bleeding. J Comput Assist Tomogr 2001;25(1):16–22.
87. Cheng PN, Sheu BS, Chen CY, et al. Splenic infarction after histoacryl injection for bleeding gastric varices. Gastrointest Endosc 1998;48(4):426–7.
88. Cheng HC, Cheng PN, Tsai YM, et al. Sclerosant extravasation as a complication of sclerosing endotherapy for bleeding gastric varices. Endoscopy 2004;36(3):239–41.
89. Chau TN, Patch D, Chan YW, et al. "Salvage" transjugular intrahepatic portosys-temic shunts: gastric fundal compared with esophageal variceal bleeding. Gastroenterology 1998;114(5):981–7.
90. Barange K, Peron JM, Imani K, et al. Transjugular intrahepatic portosystemic shunt in the treatment of refractory bleeding from ruptured gastric varices. Hep-atology 1999;30(5):1139–43.
91. Zhang BH, Yang BH, Tang ZY. Randomized controlled trial of screening for hepatocellular carcinoma. J Cancer Res Clin Oncol 2004;130(7):417–22.
92. McMahon BJ, Bulkow L, Harpster A, et al. Screening for hepatocellular carci-noma in Alaska natives infected with chronic hepatitis B: a 16-year population-based study. Hepatology 2000;32(4 Pt 1):842–6.
93. Wong LL, Limm WM, Severino R, et al. Improved survival with screening for hepatocellular carcinoma. Liver Transpl 2000;6(3):320–5.
94. Bolondi L, Sofia S, Siringo S, et al. Surveillance programme of cirrhotic patients for early diagnosis and treatment of hepatocellular carcinoma: a cost effective-ness analysis. Gut 2001;48(2):251–9.
95. Lok AS, McMahon BJ. Chronic hepatitis B: update 2009. Hepatology 2009; 50(3):661–2.
96. Bruix J, Sherman M. Management of hepatocellular carcinoma: an update. Hep-atology 2011;53(3):1020–2.
97. Singal A, Volk ML, Waljee A, et al. Meta-analysis: surveillance with ultrasound for early-stage hepatocellular carcinoma in patients with cirrhosis. Aliment Pharma-col Ther 2009;30(1):37–47.
98. Lok AS, Sterling RK, Everhart JE, et al. Des-gamma-carboxy prothrombin and alpha-fetoprotein as biomarkers for the early detection of hepatocellular carci-noma. Gastroenterology 2010;138(2):493–502.
99. Choi D, Kim SH, Lim JH, et al. Detection of hepatocellular carcinoma: combined T2-weighted and dynamic gadolinium-enhanced MRI versus combined CT during arterial portography and CT hepatic arteriography. J Comput Assist To-mogr 2001;25(5):777–85.

100. Arguedas MR, Chen VK, Eloubeidi MA, et al. Screening for hepatocellular carcinoma in patients with hepatitis C cirrhosis: a cost-utility analysis. Am J Gastroenterol 2003;98(3):679–90.

101. Forner A, Vilana R, Ayuso C, et al. Diagnosis of hepatic nodules 20 mm or smaller in cirrhosis: prospective validation of the noninvasive diagnostic criteria for hepatocellular carcinoma. Hepatology 2008;47(1):97–104.

102. Sangiovanni A, Manini MA, Iavarone M, et al. The diagnostic and economic impact of contrast imaging techniques in the diagnosis of small hepatocellular carcinoma in cirrhosis. Gut 2010;59(5):638–44.

103. Khalili K, Kim TY, Jang HJ, et al. Implementation of AASLD HCC practice guidelines in North America: 2 years of experience. Hepatology 2008;48(Suppl 1):362A.

104. Pathologic diagnosis of early hepatocellular carcinoma: a report of the international consensus group for hepatocellular neoplasia. Hepatology 2009;49(2):658–64.

105. Livraghi T, Meloni F, Di Stasi M, et al. Sustained complete response and complications rates after radiofrequency ablation of very early hepatocellular carcinoma in cirrhosis: is resection still the treatment of choice? Hepatology 2008; 47(1):82–9.

106. Lin SM, Lin CJ, Lin CC, et al. Radiofrequency ablation improves prognosis compared with ethanol injection for hepatocellular carcinoma < or =4 cm. Gastroenterology 2004;127(6):1714–23.

107. Shiina S, Teratani T, Obi S, et al. A randomized controlled trial of radiofrequency ablation with ethanol injection for small hepatocellular carcinoma. Gastroenterology 2005;129(1):122–30.

108. Lu DS, Yu NC, Raman SS, et al. Percutaneous radiofrequency ablation of hepatocellular carcinoma as a bridge to liver transplantation. Hepatology 2005;41(5): 1130–7.

109. Martin AP, Goldstein RM, Dempster J, et al. Radiofrequency thermal ablation of hepatocellular carcinoma before liver transplantation–a clinical and histological examination. Clin Transplant 2006;20(6):695–705.

110. Curley SA, Marra P, Beaty K, et al. Early and late complications after radiofrequency ablation of malignant liver tumors in 608 patients. Ann Surg 2004; 239(4):450–8.

111. Mazzaferro V, Battiston C, Perrone S, et al. Radiofrequency ablation of small hepatocellular carcinoma in cirrhotic patients awaiting liver transplantation: a prospective study. Ann Surg 2004;240(5):900–9.

112. Llovet JM, Mas X, Aponte JJ, et al. Cost effectiveness of adjuvant therapy for hepatocellular carcinoma during the waiting list for liver transplantation. Gut 2002;50(1):123–8.

113. Llovet JM, Real MI, Montana X, et al. Arterial embolisation or chemoembolisation versus symptomatic treatment in patients with unresectable hepatocellular carcinoma: a randomised controlled trial. Lancet 2002;359(9319):1734–9.

114. Lo CM, Ngan H, Tso WK, et al. Randomized controlled trial of transarterial lipiodol chemoembolization for unresectable hepatocellular carcinoma. Hepatology 2002;35(5):1164–71.

115. Graziadei IW, Sandmueller H, Waldenberger P, et al. Chemoembolization followed by liver transplantation for hepatocellular carcinoma impedes tumor progression while on the waiting list and leads to excellent outcome. Liver Transpl 2003;9(6):557–63.

116. Oldhafer KJ, Chavan A, Fruhauf NR, et al. Arterial chemoembolization before liver transplantation in patients with hepatocellular carcinoma: marked tumor necrosis, but no survival benefit? J Hepatol 1998;29(6):953–9.

117. Decaens T, Roudot-Thoraval F, Bresson-Hadni S, et al. Impact of pretransplantation transarterial chemoembolization on survival and recurrence after liver transplantation for hepatocellular carcinoma. Liver Transpl 2005;11(7):767–75.
118. Maddala YK, Stadheim L, Andrews JC, et al. Drop-out rates of patients with hepatocellular cancer listed for liver transplantation: outcome with chemoembolization. Liver Transpl 2004;10(3):449–55.
119. Majno PE, Adam R, Bismuth H, et al. Influence of preoperative transarterial lipiodol chemoembolization on resection and transplantation for hepatocellular carcinoma in patients with cirrhosis. Ann Surg 1997;226(6):688–701 [discussion: 701–3].
120. Millonig G, Graziadei IW, Freund MC, et al. Response to preoperative chemoembolization correlates with outcome after liver transplantation in patients with hepatocellular carcinoma. Liver Transpl 2007;13(2):272–9.
121. Sergio A, Cristofori C, Cardin R, et al. Transcatheter arterial chemoembolization (TACE) in hepatocellular carcinoma (HCC): the role of angiogenesis and invasiveness. Am J Gastroenterol 2008;103(4):914–21.
122. Shim JH, Park JW, Kim JH, et al. Association between increment of serum VEGF level and prognosis after transcatheter arterial chemoembolization in hepatocellular carcinoma patients. Cancer Sci 2008;99(10):2037–44.
123. Ravaioli M, Grazi GL, Ercolani G, et al. Partial necrosis on hepatocellular carcinoma nodules facilitates tumor recurrence after liver transplantation. Transplantation 2004;78(12):1780–6.
124. Chan AO, Yuen MF, Hui CK, et al. A prospective study regarding the complications of transcatheter intraarterial lipiodol chemoembolization in patients with hepatocellular carcinoma. Cancer 2002;94(6):1747–52.
125. Alba E, Valls C, Dominguez J, et al. Transcatheter arterial chemoembolization in patients with hepatocellular carcinoma on the waiting list for orthotopic liver transplantation. AJR Am J Roentgenol 2008;190(5):1341–8.
126. Thalheimer U, Triantos CK, Samonakis DN, et al. Infection, coagulation, and variceal bleeding in cirrhosis. Gut 2005;54(4):556–63.
127. Gines P, Quintero E, Arroyo V, et al. Compensated cirrhosis: natural history and prognostic factors. Hepatology 1987;7(1):122–8.
128. Planas R, Montoliu S, Balleste B, et al. Natural history of patients hospitalized for management of cirrhotic ascites. Clin Gastroenterol Hepatol 2006;4(11): 1385–94.
129. Runyon BA, Montano AA, Akriviadis EA, et al. The serum-ascites albumin gradient is superior to the exudate-transudate concept in the differential diagnosis of ascites. Ann Intern Med 1992;117(3):215–20.
130. Poonawala A, Nair SP, Thuluvath PJ. Prevalence of obesity and diabetes in patients with cryptogenic cirrhosis: a case-control study. Hepatology 2000; 32(4 Pt 1):689–92.
131. Stiehm AJ, Mendler MH, Runyon BA. Detection of diuretic-resistance or diuretic-sensitivity by the spot urine Na/K ratio in 729 specimens from cirrhotics with ascites: approximately 90% accuracy as compared to 24-hr urine Na excretion. Hepatology 2002;36:222A.
132. Runyon BA. Management of adult patients with ascites due to cirrhosis: an update. Hepatology 2009;49(6):2087–107.
133. European Association for the Study of the Liver. EASL clinical practice guidelines on the management of ascites, spontaneous bacterial peritonitis, and hepatorenal syndrome in cirrhosis. J Hepatol 2010;53(3): 397–417.

134. Schrier RW, Gross P, Gheorghiade M, et al. Tolvaptan, a selective oral vasopressin V2-receptor antagonist, for hyponatremia. N Engl J Med 2006; 355(20):2099–112.

135. Arroyo V, Gines P, Gerbes AL, et al. Definition and diagnostic criteria of refractory ascites and hepatorenal syndrome in cirrhosis. International Ascites Club. Hepatology 1996;23(1):164–76.

136. Bories P, Garcia Compean D, Michel H, et al. The treatment of refractory ascites by the LeVeen shunt. A multi-centre controlled trial (57 patients). J Hepatol 1986;3(2):212–8.

137. Tito L, Gines P, Arroyo V, et al. Total paracentesis associated with intravenous albumin management of patients with cirrhosis and ascites. Gastroenterology 1990;98(1):146–51.

138. Gines P, Tito L, Arroyo V, et al. Randomized comparative study of therapeutic paracentesis with and without intravenous albumin in cirrhosis. Gastroenterology 1988;94(6):1493–502.

139. Rossle M, Ochs A, Gulberg V, et al. A comparison of paracentesis and transjugular intrahepatic portosystemic shunting in patients with ascites. N Engl J Med 2000;342(23):1701–7.

140. Gines P, Uriz J, Calahorra B, et al. Transjugular intrahepatic portosystemic shunting versus paracentesis plus albumin for refractory ascites in cirrhosis. Gastroenterology 2002;123(6):1839–47.

141. Sanyal AJ, Genning C, Reddy KR, et al. The North American Study for the Treatment of Refractory Ascites. Gastroenterology 2003;124(3):634–41.

142. Salerno F, Merli M, Riggio O, et al. Randomized controlled study of TIPS versus paracentesis plus albumin in cirrhosis with severe ascites. Hepatology 2004; 40(3):629–35.

143. Angermayr B, Cejna M, Karnel F, et al. Child-Pugh versus MELD score in predicting survival in patients undergoing transjugular intrahepatic portosystemic shunt. Gut 2003;52(6):879–85.

144. Azoulay D, Castaing D, Dennison A, et al. Transjugular intrahepatic portosystemic shunt worsens the hyperdynamic circulatory state of the cirrhotic patient: preliminary report of a prospective study. Hepatology 1994;19(1): 129–32.

145. Navasa M, Fernandez J, Rodes J. Bacterial infections in liver cirrhosis. Ital J Gastroenterol Hepatol 1999;31(7):616–25.

146. Fernandez J, Navasa M, Gomez J, et al. Bacterial infections in cirrhosis: epidemiological changes with invasive procedures and norfloxacin prophylaxis. Hepatology 2002;35(1):140–8.

147. Fasolato S, Angeli P, Dallagnese L, et al. Renal failure and bacterial infections in patients with cirrhosis: epidemiology and clinical features. Hepatology 2007; 45(1):223–9.

148. Garcia-Tsao G. Bacterial infections in cirrhosis: treatment and prophylaxis. J Hepatol 2005;42(Suppl 1):S85–92.

149. Caruntu FA, Benea L. Spontaneous bacterial peritonitis: pathogenesis, diagnosis, treatment. J Gastrointestin Liver Dis 2006;15(1):51–6.

150. Toledo C, Salmeron JM, Rimola A, et al. Spontaneous bacterial peritonitis in cirrhosis: predictive factors of infection resolution and survival in patients treated with cefotaxime. Hepatology 1993;17(2):251–7.

151. Trikudanathan G, Ahmad I, Devuni D, et al. Prediction of in-hospital mortality in spontaneous bacterial peritonitis (SBP) using integrated Model for End-stage Liver Disease (iMELD) score. Clin Gastroenterol Hepatol 2011;9(2):186.

152. Follo A, Llovet JM, Navasa M, et al. Renal impairment after spontaneous bacterial peritonitis in cirrhosis: incidence, clinical course, predictive factors and prognosis. Hepatology 1994;20(6):1495–501.
153. Fernandez J, Navasa M, Planas R, et al. Primary prophylaxis of spontaneous bacterial peritonitis delays hepatorenal syndrome and improves survival in cirrhosis. Gastroenterology 2007;133(3):818–24.
154. Runyon BA. Low-protein-concentration ascitic fluid is predisposed to spontaneous bacterial peritonitis. Gastroenterology 1986;91(6):1343–6.
155. Terg R, Fassio E, Guevara M, et al. Ciprofloxacin in primary prophylaxis of spontaneous bacterial peritonitis: a randomized, placebo-controlled study. J Hepatol 2008;48(5):774–9.
156. Bernard B, Grange JD, Khac EN, et al. Antibiotic prophylaxis for the prevention of bacterial infections in cirrhotic patients with gastrointestinal bleeding: a meta-analysis. Hepatology 1999;29(6):1655–61.
157. Hou MC, Lin HC, Liu TT, et al. Antibiotic prophylaxis after endoscopic therapy prevents rebleeding in acute variceal hemorrhage: a randomized trial. Hepatology 2004;39(3):746–53.
158. Grange JD, Roulot D, Pelletier G, et al. Norfloxacin primary prophylaxis of bacterial infections in cirrhotic patients with ascites: a double-blind randomized trial. J Hepatol 1998;29(3):430–6.
159. Fernandez J, Ruiz del Arbol L, Gomez C, et al. Norfloxacin vs ceftriaxone in the prophylaxis of infections in patients with advanced cirrhosis and hemorrhage. Gastroenterology 2006;131(4):1049–56 [quiz: 1285].
160. Hoefs JC, Canawati HN, Sapico FL, et al. Spontaneous bacterial peritonitis. Hepatology 1982;2(4):399–407.
161. Runyon BA, Hoefs JC. Culture-negative neutrocytic ascites: a variant of spontaneous bacterial peritonitis. Hepatology 1984;4(6):1209–11.
162. Runyon BA, Antillon MR. Ascitic fluid pH and lactate: insensitive and nonspecific tests in detecting ascitic fluid infection. Hepatology 1991;13(5):929–35.
163. Runyon BA. Monomicrobial nonneutrocytic bacterascites: a variant of spontaneous bacterial peritonitis. Hepatology 1990;12(4 Pt 1):710–5.
164. Rimola A, Salmeron JM, Clemente G, et al. Two different dosages of cefotaxime in the treatment of spontaneous bacterial peritonitis in cirrhosis: results of a prospective, randomized, multicenter study. Hepatology 1995;21(3):674–9.
165. Castellote J, Lopez C, Gornals J, et al. Rapid diagnosis of spontaneous bacterial peritonitis by use of reagent strips. Hepatology 2003;37(4):893–6.
166. Nousbaum JB, Cadranel JF, Nahon P, et al. Diagnostic accuracy of the Multistix 8 SG reagent strip in diagnosis of spontaneous bacterial peritonitis. Hepatology 2007;45(5):1275–81.
167. Nguyen-Khac E, Cadranel JF, Thevenot T, et al. Review article: the utility of reagent strips in the diagnosis of infected ascites in cirrhotic patients. Aliment Pharmacol Ther 2008;28(3):282–8.
168. Rimola A, Garcia-Tsao G, Navasa M, et al. Diagnosis, treatment and prophylaxis of spontaneous bacterial peritonitis: a consensus document. International Ascites Club. J Hepatol 2000;32(1):142–53.
169. Ricart E, Soriano G, Novella MT, et al. Amoxicillin-clavulanic acid versus cefotaxime in the therapy of bacterial infections in cirrhotic patients. J Hepatol 2000;32(4):596–602.
170. Angeli P, Guarda S, Fasolato S, et al. Switch therapy with ciprofloxacin vs. intravenous ceftazidime in the treatment of spontaneous bacterial peritonitis in patients with cirrhosis: similar efficacy at lower cost. Aliment Pharmacol Ther 2006;23(1):75–84.

171. Navasa M, Follo A, Llovet JM, et al. Randomized, comparative study of oral ofloxacin versus intravenous cefotaxime in spontaneous bacterial peritonitis. Gastroenterology 1996;111(4):1011–7.
172. Sort P, Navasa M, Arroyo V, et al. Effect of intravenous albumin on renal impairment and mortality in patients with cirrhosis and spontaneous bacterial peritonitis. N Engl J Med 1999;341(6):403–9.
173. Fernandez J, Navasa M, Garcia-Pagan JC, et al. Effect of intravenous albumin on systemic and hepatic hemodynamics and vasoactive neurohormonal systems in patients with cirrhosis and spontaneous bacterial peritonitis. J Hepatol 2004;41(3):384–90.
174. Fernandez J, Monteagudo J, Bargallo X, et al. A randomized unblinded pilot study comparing albumin versus hydroxyethyl starch in spontaneous bacterial peritonitis. Hepatology 2005;42(3):627–34.
175. Quinlan GJ, Martin GS, Evans TW. Albumin: biochemical properties and therapeutic potential. Hepatology 2005;41(6):1211–9.
176. Tito L, Rimola A, Gines P, et al. Recurrence of spontaneous bacterial peritonitis in cirrhosis: frequency and predictive factors. Hepatology 1988;8(1):27–31.
177. Gines P, Rimola A, Planas R, et al. Norfloxacin prevents spontaneous bacterial peritonitis recurrence in cirrhosis: results of a double-blind, placebo-controlled trial. Hepatology 1990;12(4 Pt 1):716–24.
178. Singh N, Gayowski T, Yu VL, et al. Trimethoprim-sulfamethoxazole for the prevention of spontaneous bacterial peritonitis in cirrhosis: a randomized trial. Ann Intern Med 1995;122(8):595–8.
179. Campillo B, Richardet JP, Kheo T, et al. Nosocomial spontaneous bacterial peritonitis and bacteremia in cirrhotic patients: impact of isolate type on prognosis and characteristics of infection. Clin Infect Dis 2002;35(1):1–10.
180. Cholongitas E, Papatheodoridis GV, Lahanas A, et al. Increasing frequency of Gram-positive bacteria in spontaneous bacterial peritonitis. Liver Int 2005; 25(1):57–61.
181. Park YH, Lee HC, Song HG, et al. Recent increase in antibiotic-resistant microorganisms in patients with spontaneous bacterial peritonitis adversely affects the clinical outcome in Korea. J Gastroenterol Hepatol 2003;18(8):927–33.
182. Cereto F, Herranz X, Moreno E, et al. Role of host and bacterial virulence factors in Escherichia coli spontaneous bacterial peritonitis. Eur J Gastroenterol Hepatol 2008;20(9):924–9.
183. Salerno F, Gerbes A, Gines P, et al. Diagnosis, prevention and treatment of hepatorenal syndrome in cirrhosis. Gut 2007;56(9):1310–8.
184. Stadlbauer V, Wright GA, Banaji M, et al. Relationship between activation of the sympathetic nervous system and renal blood flow autoregulation in cirrhosis. Gastroenterology 2008;134(1):111–9.
185. Gines P, Schrier RW. Renal failure in cirrhosis. N Engl J Med 2009;361(13): 1279–90.
186. Dagher L, Moore K. The hepatorenal syndrome. Gut 2001;49(5):729–37.
187. Ginès P, Cárdenas A, Schrier RW. Liver disease and the kidney. In: Schrier RW, editor. Diseases of the kidney & urinary tract. vol. 3. 8th edition. Philadelphia: Lippincott Williams & Wilkins; 2006. p. 2179–205.
188. Gines A, Escorsell A, Gines P, et al. Incidence, predictive factors, and prognosis of the hepatorenal syndrome in cirrhosis with ascites. Gastroenterology 1993; 105(1):229–36.
189. Papafragkakis H, Martin P, Akalin E. Combined liver and kidney transplantation. Curr Opin Organ Transplant 2010;15(3):263–8.

190. Martin-Llahi M, Guevara M, Torre A, et al. Prognostic importance of the cause of renal failure in patients with cirrhosis. Gastroenterology 2011;140(2):488–96. e484.
191. Salerno F, Gerbes A, Gines P, et al. Diagnosis, prevention and treatment of hepatorenal syndrome in cirrhosis. Postgrad Med J 2008;84(998):662–70.
192. Gonwa TA, Morris CA, Goldstein RM, et al. Long-term survival and renal function following liver transplantation in patients with and without hepatorenal syndrome—experience in 300 patients. Transplantation 1991;51(2):428–30.
193. Gonwa TA, Klintmalm GB, Levy M, et al. Impact of pretransplant renal function on survival after liver transplantation. Transplantation 1995;59(3):361–5.
194. Moreau R, Lebrec D. The use of vasoconstrictors in patients with cirrhosis: type 1 HRS and beyond. Hepatology 2006;43(3):385–94.
195. Gluud LL, Christensen K, Christensen E, et al. Systematic review of randomized trials on vasoconstrictor drugs for hepatorenal syndrome. Hepatology 2010; 51(2):576–84.
196. Moreau R, Durand F, Poynard T, et al. Terlipressin in patients with cirrhosis and type 1 hepatorenal syndrome: a retrospective multicenter study. Gastroenterology 2002;122(4):923–30.
197. Fabrizi F, Dixit V, Martin P. Meta-analysis: terlipressin therapy for the hepatorenal syndrome. Aliment Pharmacol Ther 2006;24(6):935–44.
198. Gluud LL, Kjaer MS, Christensen E. Terlipressin for hepatorenal syndrome. Cochrane Database Syst Rev 2006;(4):CD005162.
199. Sanyal AJ, Boyer T, Garcia-Tsao G, et al. A randomized, prospective, double-blind, placebo-controlled trial of terlipressin for type 1 hepatorenal syndrome. Gastroenterology 2008;134(5):1360–8.
200. Martin-Llahi M, Pepin MN, Guevara M, et al. Terlipressin and albumin vs albumin in patients with cirrhosis and hepatorenal syndrome: a randomized study. Gastroenterology 2008;134(5):1352–9.
201. Angeli P, Volpin R, Gerunda G, et al. Reversal of type 1 hepatorenal syndrome with the administration of midodrine and octreotide. Hepatology 1999;29(6):1690–7.
202. Duvoux C, Zanditenas D, Hezode C, et al. Effects of noradrenalin and albumin in patients with type I hepatorenal syndrome: a pilot study. Hepatology 2002;36(2): 374–80.
203. Brensing KA, Textor J, Perz J, et al. Long term outcome after transjugular intrahepatic portosystemic stent-shunt in non-transplant cirrhotics with hepatorenal syndrome: a phase II study. Gut 2000;47(2):288–95.
204. Guevara M, Gines P, Bandi JC, et al. Transjugular intrahepatic portosystemic shunt in hepatorenal syndrome: effects on renal function and vasoactive systems. Hepatology 1998;28(2):416–22.
205. Wong F, Pantea L, Sniderman K. Midodrine, octreotide, albumin, and TIPS in selected patients with cirrhosis and type 1 hepatorenal syndrome. Hepatology 2004;40(1):55–64.
206. Keller F, Heinze H, Jochimsen F, et al. Risk factors and outcome of 107 patients with decompensated liver disease and acute renal failure (including 26 patients with hepatorenal syndrome): the role of hemodialysis. Ren Fail 1995;17(2): 135–46.
207. Capling RK, Bastani B. The clinical course of patients with type 1 hepatorenal syndrome maintained on hemodialysis. Ren Fail 2004;26(5):563–8.
208. Akriviadis E, Botla R, Briggs W, et al. Pentoxifylline improves short-term survival in severe acute alcoholic hepatitis: a double-blind, placebo-controlled trial. Gastroenterology 2000;119(6):1637–48.

209. Lebrec D, Thabut D, Oberti F, et al. Pentoxifylline does not decrease short-term mortality but does reduce complications in patients with advanced cirrhosis. Gastroenterology 2010;138(5):1755–62.

210. Riordan SM, Williams R. Treatment of hepatic encephalopathy. N Engl J Med 1997;337(7):473–9.

211. Ferenci P, Lockwood A, Mullen K, et al. Hepatic encephalopathy–definition, nomenclature, diagnosis, and quantification: final report of the working party at the 11th World Congresses of Gastroenterology, Vienna, 1998. Hepatology 2002;35(3):716–21.

212. Bajaj JS. Review article: the modern management of hepatic encephalopathy. Aliment Pharmacol Ther 2010;31(5):537–47.

213. Bass NM, Mullen KD, Sanyal A, et al. Rifaximin treatment in hepatic encephalopathy. N Engl J Med 2010;362(12):1071–81.

214. Cardenas A, Gines P. Management of patients with cirrhosis awaiting liver transplantation. Gut 2011;60(3):412–21.

215. Cordoba J, Lopez-Hellin J, Planas M, et al. Normal protein diet for episodic hepatic encephalopathy: results of a randomized study. J Hepatol 2004;41(1):38–43.

216. Kondrup J, Muller MJ. Energy and protein requirements of patients with chronic liver disease. J Hepatol 1997;27(1):239–47.

217. Carey EJ, Balan V, Kremers WK, et al. Osteopenia and osteoporosis in patients with end-stage liver disease caused by hepatitis C and alcoholic liver disease: not just a cholestatic problem. Liver Transpl 2003;9(11):1166–73.

218. Guichelaar MM, Malinchoc M, Sibonga J, et al. Bone metabolism in advanced cholestatic liver disease: analysis by bone histomorphometry. Hepatology 2002;36(4 Pt 1):895–903.

219. Menon KV, Angulo P, Weston S, et al. Bone disease in primary biliary cirrhosis: independent indicators and rate of progression. J Hepatol 2001;35(3):316–23.

220. Collier JD, Ninkovic M, Compston JE. Guidelines on the management of osteoporosis associated with chronic liver disease. Gut 2002;50(Suppl 1):i1–9.

221. Trautwein C, Possienke M, Schlitt HJ, et al. Bone density and metabolism in patients with viral hepatitis and cholestatic liver diseases before and after liver transplantation. Am J Gastroenterol 2000;95(9):2343–51.

222. Reid IR, Brown JP, Burckhardt P, et al. Intravenous zoledronic acid in postmenopausal women with low bone mineral density. N Engl J Med 2002;346(9):653–61.

223. Reeves HL, Francis RM, Manas DM, et al. Intravenous bisphosphonate prevents symptomatic osteoporotic vertebral collapse in patients after liver transplantation. Liver Transpl Surg 1998;4(5):404–9.

224. Centers for Disease Control and Prevention (CDC). Recommended adult immunization schedule–United States, 2011. MMWR Morb Mortal Wkly Rep 2011;60(4):1–4.

225. Gaeta GB, Stornaiuolo G, Precone DF, et al. Immunogenicity and safety of an adjuvanted influenza vaccine in patients with decompensated cirrhosis. Vaccine 2002;20(Suppl 5):B33–35.

226. Cheong HJ, Song JY, Park JW, et al. Humoral and cellular immune responses to influenza vaccine in patients with advanced cirrhosis. Vaccine 2006;24(13):2417–22.

227. McCashland TM, Preheim LC, Gentry MJ. Pneumococcal vaccine response in cirrhosis and liver transplantation. J Infect Dis 2000;181(2):757–60.

228. Guidelines for vaccination of solid organ transplant candidates and recipients. Am J Transplant 2004;4(Suppl 10):160–3.

229. Arguedas MR, McGuire BM, Fallon MB. Implementation of vaccination in patients with cirrhosis. Dig Dis Sci 2002;47(2):384–7.
230. Arguedas MR, Johnson A, Eloubeidi MA, et al. Immunogenicity of hepatitis A vaccination in decompensated cirrhotic patients. Hepatology 2001;34(1):28–31.
231. Smallwood GA, Coloura CT, Martinez E, et al. Can patients awaiting liver transplantation elicit an immune response to the hepatitis A vaccine? Transplant Proc 2002;34(8):3289–90.
232. Dominguez M, Barcena R, Garcia M, et al. Vaccination against hepatitis B virus in cirrhotic patients on liver transplant waiting list. Liver Transpl 2000;6(4):440–2.
233. Idilman R, Colantoni A, De Maria N, et al. Impaired antibody response rates after high dose short interval hepatitis B virus vaccination of immunosuppressed individuals. Hepatogastroenterology 2003;50(49):217–21.
234. Stark K, Gunther M, Neuhaus R, et al. Immunogenicity and safety of hepatitis A vaccine in liver and renal transplant recipients. J Infect Dis 1999;180(6): 2014–7.
235. Arslan M, Wiesner RH, Poterucha JJ, et al. Safety and efficacy of hepatitis A vaccination in liver transplantation recipients. Transplantation 2001;72(2):272–6.
236. Keeffe EB. Is hepatitis A more severe in patients with chronic hepatitis B and other chronic liver diseases? Am J Gastroenterol 1995;90(2):201–5.
237. Papachristou AA, Dumas AS, Katsouyannopoulos VC. Dissociation of alanine aminotransferase values in acute hepatitis A patients with and without past experience to the hepatitis B virus. Epidemiol Infect 1991;106(2):397–402.
238. Vento S, Garofano T, Renzini C, et al. Fulminant hepatitis associated with hepatitis A virus superinfection in patients with chronic hepatitis C. N Engl J Med 1998;338(5):286–90.
239. Yao G. Clinical spectrum and natural history of viral hepatitis in a 1988 Shanghai epidemic. In: Hollinger FB, Lemon SM, Margolis H, editors. Viral hepatitis and liver disease. Baltimore (MD): Lippincott Williams & Wilkins; 1991. p. 76–8.
240. Fukumoto Y, Okita K, Konishi T, et al. Hepatitis A infection in chronic carriers of hepatitis B virus. In: Sung JL, Chen DS, editors. Viral hepatitis and hepatocellular carcinoma. Amsterdam: Excerpta Medica; 1990. p. 43–8.
241. Feray C, Gigou M, Samuel D, et al. Hepatitis C virus RNA and hepatitis B virus DNA in serum and liver of patients with fulminant hepatitis. Gastroenterology 1993;104(2):549–55.
242. Mohamed Ael S, al Karawi MA, Mesa GA. Dual infection with hepatitis C and B viruses: clinical and histological study in Saudi patients. Hepatogastroenterology 1997;44(17):1404–6.
243. Poland GA, Jacobson RM. Clinical practice: prevention of hepatitis B with the hepatitis B vaccine. N Engl J Med 2004;351(27):2832–8.
244. Carey W, Pimentel R, Westveer MK, et al. Failure of hepatitis B immunization in liver transplant recipients: results of a prospective trial. Am J Gastroenterol 1990;85(12):1590–2.
245. Chalasani N, Smallwood G, Halcomb J, et al. Is vaccination against hepatitis B infection indicated in patients waiting for or after orthotopic liver transplantation? Liver Transpl Surg 1998;4(2):128–32.
246. Bonazzi PR, Bacchella T, Freitas AC, et al. Double-dose hepatitis B vaccination in cirrhotic patients on a liver transplant waiting list. Braz J Infect Dis 2008;12(4): 306–9.
247. Macedo G, Maia JC, Gomes A, et al. Efficacy of a reinforced protocol of HBV vaccination in cirrhotic patients waiting for orthotopic liver transplantation. Transplant Proc 2000;32(8):2641.

248. Pascasio JM, Aoufi S, Gash A, et al. Response to a vaccination schedule with 4 doses of 40 microg against hepatitis B virus in cirrhotic patients evaluated for liver transplantation. Transplant Proc 2008;40(9):2943–5.
249. Arslan M, Wiesner RH, Sievers C, et al. Double-dose accelerated hepatitis B vaccine in patients with end-stage liver disease. Liver Transpl 2001;7(4):314–20.
250. Kumar D, Chen MH, Wong G, et al. A randomized, double-blind, placebo-controlled trial to evaluate the prime-boost strategy for pneumococcal vaccination in adult liver transplant recipients. Clin Infect Dis 2008;47(7):885–92.
251. Gaeta GB, Pariani E, Amendola A, et al. Influenza vaccination in patients with cirrhosis and in liver transplant recipients. Vaccine 2009;27(25–26):3373–5.
252. Soesman NM, Rimmelzwaan GF, Nieuwkoop NJ, et al. Efficacy of influenza vaccination in adult liver transplant recipients. J Med Virol 2000;61(1):85–93.

Management of Renal Dysfunction in Patients Receiving a Liver Transplant

Christine Lau, MD[a], Paul Martin, MD[b], Suphamai Bunnapradist, MD[a,*]

KEYWORDS

- Renal failure • Liver-kidney transplant • Liver transplant

Renal dysfunction in orthotopic liver transplant (OLT) recipients is a common occurrence with a reported prevalence between 17% to 95% depending on the study.[1,2] Both preoperative and postoperative acute kidney injury (AKI) are associated with poor outcomes and increased mortality.[3–5] The causes of renal dysfunction differ in the preoperative and postoperative periods. Reducing risk factors for development of renal dysfunction and management of AKI and chronic kidney disease (CKD) may improve the long-term outcomes of liver transplant recipients.

PREOPERATIVE RENAL DYSFUNCTION
Prerenal Azotemia

Prerenal azotemia results from hypoperfusion to the kidneys and is the most common cause of renal dysfunction in patients with end-stage liver disease (ESLD).[6] Cirrhotic patients have multiple potential risk factors that can contribute to prerenal azotemia, including hypovolemia from diuretic use, diarrhea from lactulose, and gastrointestinal hemorrhage. Medications that affect the hemodynamics of renal vasculature, such as nonsteroidal antiinflammatory drugs (NSAIDs), can present as prerenal azotemia by causing afferent arteriole vasoconstriction in the glomerulus and decreased renal blood flow.

The hepatorenal syndrome (HRS) is a functional prerenal azotemia unique to patients with liver failure. HRS is typically seen only in the presence of ascites and can be

The authors have nothing to disclose

[a] Kidney and Pancreas Transplant Program, Division of Nephrology, Department of Medicine, David Geffen School of Medicine at UCLA, 1033 Gayley Avenue, Suite 208, Los Angeles, CA 90024, USA
[b] Division of Hepatology, Department of Medicine, University of Miami, 1500 NW 12th Avenue, Suite 1101, Miami, FL 33136, USA
* Corresponding author. 1033 Gayley Avenue, Suite 208, Los Angeles, CA 90024.
E-mail address: bunnapradist@mednet.ucla.edu

precipitated by spontaneous bacterial peritonitis and other infections, overvigorous diuresis, and large-volume paracentesis. The pathophysiology of HRS is complex, reflecting splanchnic and systemic vasodilation caused by portal hypertension. Systemic vasodilation leads to decreased effective circulatory volume and activation of the renin-angiotensin-aldosterone system (RAAS). The compensatory vasoconstrictive effects of the RAAS hormones can cause renal ischemia and HRS. In addition, decreased effective circulatory volume increases sodium and water retention by the kidneys, worsening ascites and edema. The 2 types of HRS are differentiated based on their time course. Type I HRS is defined as a doubling of the initial serum creatinine to a level greater than 2.5 mg/dL in less than a 2-week period, whereas type II HRS is characterized by ascites that is resistant to diuretics with moderate renal dysfunction that is slowly progressive.[7] Development of HRS suggests a poor prognosis, with a median survival time of 2 weeks in type I HRS and 6 months in type II HRS.[8] The diagnosis of hepatorenal syndrome is one of exclusion, and true intravascular volume depletion must be ruled out before the diagnosis can be made (**Box 1**).

Treatment of hepatorenal syndrome remains challenging, and there is only a small body of evidence supporting specific measures. Most treatments are based on the theory that administration of vasoconstrictors ameliorates arterial vasodilation and increases effective circulatory volume and renal blood flow (**Box 2**). An Italian report in 1999 noted reversal of HRS in 5 patients treated with midodrine, octreotide, and albumin compared with no improvement in 8 patients treated with a dopamine infusion.[9] Treatment with midodrine, octreotide, and albumin was also associated with improved short-term mortality in a more recent case control study examining 102 individuals with HRS type I and 60 with type II.[10] There are data supporting the use of terlipressin, a synthetic analogue of lysine-vasopressin in HRS. A randomized, double-blind, placebo-controlled prospective trial examining the effects of terlipressin on HRS resulted in reversal of renal dysfunction in 34% of treated group versus 13% in a placebo group.[11] However, terlipressin is not yet available in the United States. A small, uncontrolled study in 7 patients with HRS showed that transjugular intrahepatic portosystemic shunt (TIPS) improved renal function and renal plasma flow with decreased plasma renin activity, aldosterone, and norepinephrine in 6 patients. However, use of TIPS needs to be carefully considered in a decompensated cirrhotic because of the risk of precipitating more overt hepatocellular failure and aggravating renal failure. Guidelines on management of portal hypertension published by the American Association for the Study of Liver Diseases do not recommend TIPS for treatment of HRS based on current evidence.[12]

Box 1
Diagnostic criteria for hepatorenal syndrome

- Presence of cirrhosis with ascites
- Serum creatinine greater than 1.5 mg/dL
- No improvement of creatinine after 2 days of fluid or albumin challenge and withdrawal of diuretics
- Absence of shock
- No recent administration of nephrotoxic medications
- Lack of intrinsic kidney disease as shown by bland urinalysis and normal renal ultrasound

Data from Guevara M, Gines P. Hepatorenal syndrome. Dig Dis 2005;23:47.

| Box 2 |
| Management of hepatorenal syndrome |

1. Rule out intravascular depletion with a fluid (1.5 L of normal saline infusion) or albumin (1 g/ kg per day for 2 days with doses divided into 3–4 doses/d, maximum 100 g per day) challenge.

2. If there is no improvement in renal function, start treatment with vasoconstrictors, such as midodrine and octreotide or terlipressin, plus albumin. Start midodrine 7.5 mg orally 3 times daily and octreotide 100 µg subcutaneously 3 times daily, or start terlipressin 0.5 mg intravenously every 6 hours if available. Give 25 to 50 g of albumin daily.

3. Titrate midodrine and octreotide to raise mean arterial pressure (MAP) by at least 15 mm Hg. Midodrine can be increased up to 15 mg 3 times daily and octreotide to 200 µg 3 times daily.

4. Titrate terlipressin to decrease the creatinine by at least 25% by doubling the dose every 2 days for a maximum dose of 12 mg/d.

5. Continue treatment until reversal of HRS (creatinine <1.5 mg/dL). Treatment should be restarted if HRS recurs.

6. Treatment can be stopped if there is no response in the first 3 days or if creatinine does not decrease by at least 50% in the first 7 days at maximum doses. Albumin can be discontinued if serum albumin exceeds 4.5 g/dL or there are signs of volume overload.

Intrinsic Renal Disease

Patients with ESLD are also at risk for intrinsic renal disease (**Table 1** and **Box 3**). Acute tubular necrosis (ATN) is the most common intrinsic renal disease in cirrhotic patients and can be precipitated by systemic hypotension, antibiotics, intravenous (IV) contrast, or prolonged ischemia such as with HRS or shock. Patients at highest risk for developing contrast-induced nephropathy (CIN) include those with preexisting renal dysfunction, diabetes, or volume depletion. A retrospective analysis showed that the incidence of CIN in hospitalized cirrhotic patients was 25% with presence of ascites noted as a significant risk factor.[13] The exact mechanism of CIN is not well understood but may involve renal vasoconstriction and tubular injury caused by generation of oxygen free radicals. Use of nonionic agents, whether low or iso-osmolar, may diminish risk of CIN in high-risk patients. Patients who are at risk for development of CIN should be given isotonic saline or bicarbonate IV fluids before and after the study unless contraindicated. Evidence for use of N-acetylcysteine in protecting against CIN is conflicting,[14–16] but, given its low toxicity and cost, most clinicians give it starting the day before the study.

AIN is another potential cause of AKI in the cirrhotic patient. Causes of AIN include drug hypersensitivity reaction, infection, immune-mediated diseases, and glomerular disease, although many cases remain idiopathic. Patients with ESLD receive multiple antibiotics, many of which have been implicated in AIN. The most common drugs associated with AIN include penicillins, cephalosporins, sulfonamides, and NSAIDs.[17] The classic triad of rash, fever, and eosinophilia is seen in less than 30% of patients but is usually seen in drug-induced AIN. Sterile pyuria and eosinophiliuria also suggest AIN. After the diagnosis is made, the offending medication should be discontinued. Glucocorticoids may be used if renal dysfunction does not improve after discontinuation of the drug, although there are no randomized controlled studies to prove their benefit.

Secondary immunoglobulin A (IgA) nephropathy has been associated with cirrhosis, particularly alcoholic, but its significance in contributing to renal dysfunction is unclear.[18] An observational study of renal biopsies obtained at the time of liver transplantation in 30 patients with hepatitis C–related cirrhosis suggested that the

Table 1
Diagnostic criteria and management of intrinsic renal disease

Renal Disease	Diagnostic Criteria	Risk Factors	Treatment
Acute tubular necrosis	Bland urinalysis, fractional excretion of sodium >1%	Hypotension, nephrotoxic medications, intravenous contrast, prolonged ischemia caused by HRS or shock	Supportive care to treat underlying cause
Acute interstitial nephritis	Classic triad of rash, fever, and eosinophilia; sterile pyuria, eosinophiliuria	β-Lactam antibiotics, cephalosporins, sulfonamides, NSAIDs, infection	Discontinue offending agent
Immunoglobulin A nephropathy	Microscopic hematuria, proteinuria occasionally	Cirrhosis, particularly alcoholic	Supportive care
Membranous nephropathy	Proteinuria, hypocomplementemia, subepithelial deposits on kidney biopsy	Hepatitis B and C infections	Antiviral medications (lamivudine, interferon α)
Membranoproliferative glomerulonephritis/ cryoglubulinemia	Proteinuria, dysmorphic red cells on urinalysis, hypocomplementemia, positive cryocrit, subendothelial deposits on kidney deposit with immune complex deposition	Hepatitis B and C infections	Antiviral medications (interferon α, ribavirin)

Box 3
Evaluation of intrinsic renal disease

1. Rule out prerenal azotemia by checking fractional excretion of sodium and/or fractional excretion of urea (both low in prerenal azotemia).

2. Consider exposure to nephrotoxic agents, such as antibiotics and IV contrast, or hypotensive episodes that can cause ATN.

3. Urinalysis for pyuria, eosinophils, microscopic hematuria, dysmorphic red blood cells, red blood cell casts, and proteinuria to rule out acute interstitial nephritis (AIN) and vasculitides.

4. Send serologic work-up (C3, C4, cryocrit) to rule out glomerulonephritis if urinalysis is concerning for glomerular disease.

5. Consider renal biopsy if cause is unclear.

6. Administer N-acetylcysteine 1200 mg orally twice a day for 48 hours with IV fluids if patient requires a computed tomography study with IV contrast. Ideally, 2 doses should be given before administration of contrast.

7. Evaluate need for dialysis and supportive therapies.

incidence of IgA nephropathy was 23%.[19] Impaired transport of IgA immune complexes from blood to bile by the Kupffer cells in the liver is believed to be the cause of increased IgA deposition in the kidneys.[20] Treatment options remain limited, even in primary IgA nephropathy.

Glomerulonephritis can complicate patients with chronic hepatitis B and C infections. Patients with hepatitis C virus (HCV) may develop mixed cryoglobulinemia with an associated membranoproliferative glomerulonephritis (MPGN).[21] The incidence of MPGN was found to be 40% in patients with HCV who underwent intraoperative renal biopsy at the time of liver transplantation.[19] Cryoglobulinemic vasculitis is seen in less than 10% of patients with HCV, and one-third of those with cryoglobulinemia have renal manifestations with MPGN. Most HCV patients with cryoglobulinemia do not exhibit clinical manifestations, but approximately one-third have arthralgias, purpura, and asthenia.[22] Serologic markers show low C3 and C4 levels with increased rheumatoid factor and cryoglobulins.[23] Treatment of hepatitis C with antiviral medications, including pegylated interferon α and ribavirin, and achievement of virologic response has been shown to improve cryoglobulinemia and renal dysfunction.[24,25] Rituximab has also been reported to decrease cryoglobulins, rheumatoid factor, and proteinuria in 6 patients with hepatitis C–associated cryoglobulinemia.[26]

Hepatitis B virus (HBV) can be associated with membranous nephropathy, MPGN, and polyarteritis nodosa. Previous studies have shown that hepatitis B envelope antigen (HBeAg) is present in the subepithelial deposits seen in HBV-associated membranous nephropathy (HBVMN).[27] Spontaneous remission of nephrotic syndrome has been reported in 30% to 60% of patients, and seroconversion to anti-HBeAg is associated with remission of proteinuria. Treatment with interferon α showed reduction in proteinuria and HBV DNA levels in 8 of 15 patients treated. All of the treatment responders were noted to have HBVMN, whereas the nonresponders mostly had MPGN.[28] Lamivudine has also been used to treat HBVMN. A case control trial of 10 patients treated with lamivudine compared with 12 control patients found that the treatment group had reduction in proteinuria and resolution of HBV DNA.[29] In the control group, 42% subsequently developed severe renal dysfunction requiring dialysis, whereas none in the treatment group required renal replacement after 3 years of follow-up. Although there are no randomized clinical studies examining treatment of hepatitis B–associated glomerulonephritis, antiviral therapy is indicated in patients with replicating HBV and glomerulonephritis.

Estimating Glomerular Filtration Rate

The assessment of renal function in patients with ESLD is challenging because of reduced muscle mass, the substrate for creatinine, leading to a spuriously low serum creatinine despite a decreased estimated glomerular filtration rate (eGFR). Increased bilirubin levels also falsely lower serum creatinine by affecting the assay. A 24-hour urine collection for creatinine clearance has been shown to overestimate eGFR. The gold standard for measurement of eGFR is inulin or iohexol clearance, but these tests are cumbersome. Cystatin C has emerged as an alternative to estimate glomerular filtration rate (GFR). It is a low-molecular-weight protein that is produced by all nucleated cells. Cystatin C is freely filtered by the glomerulus but neither reabsorbed nor secreted. It is catabolized completely in the proximal tubule, and its serum concentration has been shown to estimate GFR at least as accurately as serum creatinine.[30] The serum concentration of cystatin C is independent of muscle mass and not affected by serum bilirubin levels.[31] Further studies in patients with ESLD to assess the accuracy of cystatin C in predicting eGFR are needed. Lack of availability has limited its use to date. The inability to accurately estimate GFR also contributes to untoward effects from medications. Many medications are excreted by the kidneys and require dose adjustment based on eGFR, and they may be administered at inappropriately high doses in cirrhotics because of the inaccuracy of serum creatinine.

Role of Renal Replacement Therapy

Renal replacement therapy (RRT), such as hemodialysis (HD), is often required in sicker OLT candidates as they become more overtly decompensated. For patients who required RRT before surgery, 35% survived to liver transplant or discharge, whereas 65% died while waiting for transplant in the hospital, but the 1-year mortality after transplantation in those who started RRT was 30% compared with 9.7% for patients who did not need RRT before transplantation.[5] Indications for RRT in patients with ESLD are similar to those for other patients (eg, acidemia, electrolyte derangements, volume overload, and uremia refractory to medical management). However, there are some key differences in patients with ESLD. Respiratory alkalosis typically develops in cirrhotic patients and can cause a compensatory metabolic acidosis, which may be mistaken for acidemia unless a blood gas analysis is performed. Uremic encephalopathy may be difficult to differentiate from hepatic encephalopathy. The hemodynamic stability of patients with ESLD also affects RRT because patients frequently become hypotensive during treatment. Continuous RRT (CRRT), or continuous venovenous hemodialysis (CVVHD), may be required if patients have severe hypotension or cerebral edema. The amount of fluid removed and electrolyte corrections that are achieved with CRRT occur in a 24-hour period versus a 3-hour period with single-pass HD, so hemodynamically unstable patients tolerate CRRT better. However, if rapid adjustments in fluid status or electrolytes are needed, such as in severe acidemia or hyperkalemia, single-pass HD is the preferred modality.

Evaluation for Combined Liver-Kidney Transplant

Since the introduction of the Model of End-stage Liver Disease (MELD) system in 2002, combined liver-kidney transplants (CLKT) have tripled, from 134 patients in 2001 to 399 patients in 2006, reflecting the importance of creatinine in this model of organ allocation.[32] Compared with isolated liver transplant (LT) recipients, CLKT recipients with end-stage renal disease (ESRD) had higher posttransplant survival at 1 year, but CLKT recipients without ESRD fared no better than LT-alone recipients.[33] There is concern that CLKT may be recommended for LT candidates with potentially reversible renal failure (eg, hepatorenal syndrome and ATN). A renal biopsy to assess chronicity of renal dysfunction is the gold standard but is daunting in a cirrhotic, coagulopathic patient. Intraoperative renal biopsy has been proposed as a tool to evaluate necessity of CLKT, but there is currently no consensus or criteria to determine which patients to biopsy.[34] Renal ultrasound to assess kidney size and echogenicity of the cortex can help determine the chronicity of renal dysfunction. Generally, if dialysis has been required for more than a few weeks before LT, renal recovery is less likely following OLT, and CLKT needs to considered. A consensus panel of experts convened in 2007 to discuss indications for CLKT, establish a registry, and recommend standard listing criteria (**Box 4**).[35] An algorithm has been recommended for evaluation and selection of patients for CLKT (**Box 5**).[36]

POSTOPERATIVE RENAL DYSFUNCTION
Immediate Postoperative Period

After surgery, multiple risk factors can cause renal dysfunction in LT recipients. Management of postoperative renal dysfunction is summarized in **Box 6**. ATN can

> **Box 4**
> **Recommendations for CLKT**
>
> Regional Review Boards determine listing for CLKT with automatic exceptions for:
>
> 1. Patients with end-stage renal disease with cirrhosis and symptomatic portal hypertension or hepatic vein wedge pressure with gradient greater than 10 mm Hg
>
> 2. Patients with ESLD and CKD with GFR less than or equal to 30 mL/min
>
> 3. Patients with AKI, including HRS, with creatinine greater than or equal to 2.0 mg/dL and dialysis dependence for greater than or equal to 8 weeks
>
> 4. Patients with ESLD and evidence of CKD with renal biopsy showing greater than 30% glomerulosclerosis or fibrosis
>
> Other indications for granting exceptions include comorbidities such as diabetes, hypertension, or other preexisting renal disease, along with proteinuria, kidney size, and duration of creatinine greater than or equal to 2.0 mg/dL.
>
> *Data from* Eason JD, Gonwa TA, Davis CL, et al. Proceedings of Consensus Conference on Simultaneous Liver Kidney Transplantation (SLK). Am J Transplant 2008;8:2243.

result from induction of anesthesia, surgical technique, hemodynamic instability requiring use of vasopressors, intraoperative bleeding, and large volume of transfused blood products. A single-center study involving 250 LTs found that a higher transfusion requirement of packed red blood cells (3.8 L vs 2.29 L) was associated with early-onset renal dysfunction.[37] More patients with early renal dysfunction had hypotension (20.9% vs 7.7%) compared with patients who developed late renal dysfunction. A Spanish study of 184 OLT recipients found that prolonged treatment with dopamine, pretransplant AKI, low serum albumin, and severity of graft dysfunction all contributed to early postoperative renal dysfunction.[38] In this same study, the piggyback technique during the anhepatic phase significantly reduced the probability of AKI compared with the standard technique (with or without venovenous bypass).[39] Efforts to minimize risk factors for renal dysfunction during and immediately after surgery by stabilizing hemodynamics, minimizing bleeding and blood transfusion products, and using different surgical techniques are essential.

Delayed introduction of calcineurin inhibitors (CNI) in OLT recipients has been examined in small studies with various induction therapies to preserve renal function, but results are discordant. An open, randomized, multicenter trial evaluated daclizumab induction with delayed tacrolimus (started on postoperative day 5) versus standard tacrolimus (started on postoperative day 0) alone and found no benefit in renal function with delayed administration of tacrolimus.[40] Both groups also received mycophenolate mofetil (MMF) and steroids, and patient and graft survival rates were comparable. However, another study using the same protocol did suggest significant renal benefit for daclizumab induction with delayed tacrolimus at 6 months of follow-up (eGFR 75.4 mL/min/1.73 m^2 vs 69.5 mL/min/1.73 m^2) without affecting rejection rates.[41]

Long-term Postoperative Period

Although CNIs have lowered rates of acute rejection and improved patient and graft outcomes, they are also associated with nephrotoxicity, hyperglycemia, hyperlipidemia, and hypertension. CNIs can cause AKI by afferent arteriole vasoconstriction producing prerenal ischemia, and prolonged ischemia can lead to ATN. Chronic nephrotoxicity caused by CNIs is reflected in tubular atrophy, interstitial fibrosis, and glomerulosclerosis on kidney biopsy.[42] CNIs are also associated with thrombotic microangiopathy

Box 5
Evaluation and selection of potential patients for CLKT

1. Clinical assessment:

   a. Past medical history: history of diabetes, hypertension, or CKD, baseline serum creatinine levels, urinalysis

   b. History of present illness: current medications (diuretics, NSAIDs, lactulose), gastrointestinal (GI) issues (nausea, vomiting, diarrhea), paracentesis, infections (peritonitis, urinary tract infection), recent use of IV contrast

   c. Physical examination: assessment of volume status, edema, ascites, 24-hour urine output

2. Laboratory evaluation:

   a. Serum creatinine and electrolytes, cystatin C

   b. Spot urine creatinine, sodium, and protein to calculate fractional excretion of sodium and estimate the amount of proteinuria per day

   c. Urinalysis and sediment for hematuria, proteinuria, white blood cells, red blood cells, and casts

   d. Serology for antibodies, complement, cryoglobulinemia, and rheumatoid factor in patients with proteinuria, active sediment, and hepatitis B or C infections

3. Glomerular filtration measurement:

   a. Creatinine clearance by 24-hour urine collection

   b. Cockgroft-Gault and Modification of Diet in Renal Disease formulas

   c. Inulin, iohexol, or I125-iothalamate clearance

4. Renal ultrasound to assess kidney size, echogenicity of the cortex, and to exclude hydronephrosis

5. Renal biopsy:

   a. Suspect glomerular disease, tubular injury, or inflammation based on history and laboratory evaluation

   b. Assess degree of tubular atrophy, interstitial fibrosis, glomerulosclerosis, and arteriosclerosis

6. Management of renal failure:

   a. Correction of prerenal factors, hypovolemia, and other offending agents; discontinue diuretics and nephrotoxic drugs, give IV hydration and albumin; evaluate for GI bleeding

   b. Treatment of hepatorenal syndrome

   c. Treatment of infection

   d. RRT if necessary

7. List for CLKT if:

   a. Patients with end-stage renal disease with cirrhosis and symptomatic portal hypertension or hepatic vein wedge pressure with gradient greater than 10 mm Hg

   b. Patients with ESLD and CKD with GFR less than or equal to 30 mL/min

   c. Patients with AKI, including HRS, with creatinine greater than or equal to 2.0 mg/dL and dialysis dependence for greater than or equal to 8 weeks

   d. Patients with ESLD and evidence of CKD with renal biopsy showing greater than 30% glomerulosclerosis or fibrosis

Data from Papafragkakis H, Martin P, Akalin E. Combined liver and kidney transplantation. Curr Opin Organ Transplant 2011;15:263.

Box 6
Management of postoperative renal dysfunction

1. Consider delayed use or withdrawal of calcineurin inhibitor if patient has baseline renal dysfunction.

2. If patient has AKI associated with hemolytic anemia and thrombocytopenia, the differential diagnosis includes thrombotic microangiopathy (TMA), which may require initiation of plasmapheresis.

3. Monitor blood glucose and blood pressure on a regular basis, and treat aggressively based on goals for patients not receiving transplants.

4. If patient has unexplained kidney disease, consider checking BK virus in blood and urine. If positive, consider kidney biopsy to evaluate for viral inclusion bodies. Treatment strategies include decreasing immunosuppression and giving IV immunoglobulin, leflunomide, or cidofovir if patient has definite BK nephropathy.

5. Patients who develop ESRD may be candidates for kidney transplants and should be referred for evaluation.

(TMA), which can cause renal dysfunction. Several studies have been performed to assess delayed and minimized use of CNIs to decrease risk of renal dysfunction.

Regimens that minimize the use of CNIs by addition of, or substitution with, MMF or mammalian target of rapamycin (mTOR) inhibitors have been studied to assess a potential renal benefit in patients receiving OLT. A prospective randomized trial evaluated whether switching from a CNI to MMF or an mTOR inhibitor in patients with CKD improved renal function.[43] Eight patients who had baseline eGFR less than 30 mL/min had improved eGFR by 63% after 1 year. Overall, the mean eGFR of the cohort improved from 31 mL/min to 42 mL/min at 1 year of follow-up. A study in 19 OLT recipients more than 1 year after transplantation assessed renal function after addition of MMF and taper of the cyclosporine dose.[44] The eGFR increased from 40 mL/min to 64 mL/min but with an acute rejection rate of 29%. A Spanish group studied the effect of switching from a CNI to everolimus and found that renal function improved at 1 year without an increased risk of rejection.[45] Creatinine clearance improved from 54.64 mL/min to 64.46 mL/min in 21 patients. The timing of conversion to MMF or mTOR inhibitor is also an issue that has not been determined. Schleicher and colleagues[46] examined 57 OLT recipients and divided them into 4 groups, early versus late conversion with recipients who had impaired or normal renal function. Patients who had the greatest benefit were converted to MMF or mTOR inhibitor early (<3 months after transplant) with impaired renal function. A study assessing reduction of side effects of standard-dose tacrolimus versus reduced-dose tacrolimus with MMF in recipients with normal renal function found a lower incidence of renal dysfunction in the reduced-dose tacrolimus group.[47] For OLT recipients with renal dysfunction, consideration can be given to minimizing the dose of CNI or switching to MMF or mTOR inhibitor early.

TMA of the kidneys has also been associated with CNI use and renal dysfunction in transplant recipients. TMA is a syndrome characterized by hemolytic anemia, thrombocytopenia, renal dysfunction, fevers, and, occasionally, neurologic deficits. On biopsy, arteriolar thrombi with intimal swelling and fibrinoid necrosis of the vessel wall are seen.[48] Mortality is high: 50% at 3 years in patients with TMA having renal transplants.[49] The association between CNI and TMA may be related to direct endothelial injury.[50] Kidney biopsies performed in nonrenal transplant recipients who had prolonged AKI after transplant or sudden unexplained AKI found a prevalence of 13% in patients receiving LTs.[51] Patients with TMA in this cohort also had the lowest long-term kidney survival compared with other causes of renal dysfunction. Empiric treatment of posttransplant TMA includes therapeutic plasma exchange and discontinuation or exchange of CNI. A case series of patients having renal transplants showed that, after switching from cyclosporine to tacrolimus, 81% of recipients had good graft function 1 year after an episode of TMA.[52] However, in bone marrow transplant recipients, response rates to plasma exchange have been reported to be less than 50%.[48]

New-onset diabetes mellitus after transplant (NODAT) and hypertension also contribute to renal dysfunction in LT recipients. Review of the Organ Procurement and Transplantation Network (OPTN)/United Network for Organ Sharing (UNOS) database revealed that the incidence of NODAT in LT recipients was 26.4%.[53] Risk factors for development of NODAT included older age, African American race, hepatitis C infection, tacrolimus use, steroids on discharge, and high body mass index. Hypertension has also been shown to be associated with CNI use.[54] Renal insufficiency, NODAT, and posttransplant hypertension have all been identified as risk factors for mortality after LT.[55] Although there are no formal transplant studies recommending blood pressure goals, results from large studies summarized in the Joint National Committee on Prevention, Detection, Evaluation, and Treatment of High Blood Pressure have been extrapolated for liver transplant recipients.[56] Goal blood pressure for patients with renal dysfunction is less than 125/75 mm Hg and, for all other patients, is less than 130/80 mm Hg. First-line therapy includes lifestyle modification, such as weight loss and low-sodium diet. Pharmacologic therapies include initiation of calcium channel blockers initially in patients without proteinuria. Use of nondihydropyridine calcium channel blockers, such as verapamil or diltiazem, can increase CNI levels. Recipients with proteinuria should be started on angiotensin-converting enzyme (ACE) inhibitors or angiotensin receptor blockers (ARB) with close monitoring of potassium and renal function. Diabetic nephropathy presents initially with microalbuminuria, and efforts to minimize proteinuria with ACE inhibitors or ARB have been shown to retard progression of renal disease in patients not receiving transplants.

Polyomavirus infection, notably BK virus, can occur with immunosuppression because it remains latent in B-lymphocytes and the kidney after primary infection. Its role in nephropathy of patients receiving renal transplants is well established. However, it is unclear whether BK virus also causes nephropathy in LT recipients. A study in 41 patients after OLT showed a prevalence of BK viruria in 24.2%, but presence or absence of viruria was not associated with a decline in eGFR.[57] An analysis of patients receiving nonrenal solid organ transplants with unexplained chronic renal dysfunction showed that 15% had BK viruria.[58] Although the significance of BK virus and kidney dysfunction in LT recipients is not known at this time, it is a possibility that should be considered if renal disease remains unexplained.

OLT recipients who develop ESRD are potentially candidates for subsequent kidney transplantation. Renal transplant listings for prior OLT recipients have grown substantially between 1995 and 2008, with a 330% increase in listings.[59] In 2008, 124 kidney-after-liver transplantations were performed in the United States, which comprised 0.9% of all kidney transplants.[60] Kidney transplantation does provide a survival benefit compared with remaining on dialysis after OLT.[59] Overall graft survival in kidney-after-liver recipients was less than kidney-alone recipients at 1, 3, and 5 years, but death-censored graft survival was similar between the 2 groups.[60]

SUMMARY

Renal dysfunction is common in patients with ESLD. A 24-hour urine collection or cystatin C are better alternatives to estimate GFR rather than serum creatinine. Before surgery, the most common causes of renal dysfunction are prerenal azotemia and ATN. Efforts to keep patients hemodynamically stable and refrain from using nephrotoxic agents are important. Hepatitis B and C are known to cause glomerulonephritis, which may be treatable if recognized early. A CLKT can be considered in patients whose renal function will likely not recover. After surgery, consideration can be given to reducing exposure to CNI. Aggressive control of NODAT and blood pressure management may aid in slowing progression of CKD. TMA and BK virus are also potential contributors to nephropathy, which is often seen in renal and bone marrow transplant recipients. A kidney-after-liver transplantation can be beneficial in OLT recipients who develop ESRD.

REFERENCES

1. Barri YM, Sanchez EQ, Jennings LW, et al. Acute kidney injury following liver transplantation: definition and outcome. Liver Transpl 2009;15:475.
2. Ojo AO, Held PJ, Port FK, et al. Chronic renal failure after transplantation of a non-renal organ. N Engl J Med 2003;349:931.
3. Gonwa TA, McBride MA, Anderson K, et al. Continued influence of preoperative renal function on outcome of orthotopic liver transplant (OLTX) in the US: where will MELD lead us? Am J Transplant 2006;6:2651.
4. Fraley DS, Burr R, Bernardini J, et al. Impact of acute renal failure on mortality in end-stage liver disease with or without transplantation. Kidney Int 1998;54:518.
5. Wong LP, Blackley MP, Andreoni KA, et al. Survival of liver transplant candidates with acute renal failure receiving renal replacement therapy. Kidney Int 2005;68:362.
6. Garcia-Tsao G, Parikh CR, Viola A. Acute kidney injury in cirrhosis. Hepatology 2008;48:2064.
7. Salerno F, Gerbes A, Gines P, et al. Diagnosis, prevention and treatment of hepatorenal syndrome in cirrhosis. Gut 2007;56:1310.
8. Guevara M, Gines P. Hepatorenal syndrome. Dig Dis 2005;23:47.
9. Angeli P, Volpin R, Gerunda G, et al. Reversal of type 1 hepatorenal syndrome with the administration of midodrine and octreotide. Hepatology 1999;29:1690.
10. Skagen C, Einstein M, Lucey MR, et al. Combination treatment with octreotide, midodrine, and albumin improves survival in patients with type 1 and type 2 hepatorenal syndrome. J Clin Gastroenterol 2009;43:680.
11. Sanyal AJ, Boyer T, Garcia-Tsao G, et al. A randomized, prospective, double-blind, placebo-controlled trial of terlipressin for type 1 hepatorenal syndrome. Gastroenterology 2008;134:1360.
12. Boyer TD, Haskal ZJ. The role of transjugular intrahepatic portosystemic shunt in the management of portal hypertension. Hepatology 2005;41:386.
13. Lodhia N, Kader M, Mayes T, et al. Risk of contrast-induced nephropathy in hospitalized patients with cirrhosis. World J Gastroenterol 2009;15:1459.
14. Alonso A, Lau J, Jaber BL, et al. Prevention of radiocontrast nephropathy with N-acetylcysteine in patients with chronic kidney disease: a meta-analysis of randomized, controlled trials. Am J Kidney Dis 2004;43:1.
15. Isenbarger DW, Kent SM, O'Malley PG. Meta-analysis of randomized clinical trials on the usefulness of acetylcysteine for prevention of contrast nephropathy. Am J Cardiol 2003;92:1454.
16. Marenzi G, Assanelli E, Marana I, et al. N-acetylcysteine and contrast-induced nephropathy in primary angioplasty. N Engl J Med 2006;354:2773.
17. Michel DM, Kelly CJ. Acute interstitial nephritis. J Am Soc Nephrol 1998;9:506.

18. Pouria S, Feehally J. Glomerular IgA deposition in liver disease. Nephrol Dial Transplant 1999;14:2279.
19. McGuire BM, Julian BA, Bynon JS Jr, et al. Brief communication: glomerulonephritis in patients with hepatitis C cirrhosis undergoing liver transplantation. Ann Intern Med 2006;144:735.
20. Amore A, Coppo R, Roccatello D, et al. Experimental IgA nephropathy secondary to hepatocellular injury induced by dietary deficiencies and heavy alcohol intake. Lab Invest 1994;70:68.
21. Roccatello D, Fornasieri A, Giachino O, et al. Multicenter study on hepatitis C virus-related cryoglobulinemic glomerulonephritis. Am J Kidney Dis 2007;49:69.
22. Perico N, Cattaneo D, Bikbov B, et al. Hepatitis C infection and chronic renal diseases. Clin J Am Soc Nephrol 2009;4:207.
23. Mackelaite L, Alsauskas ZC, Ranganna K. Renal failure in patients with cirrhosis. Med Clin North Am 2009;93:855.
24. Alric L, Plaisier E, Thebault S, et al. Influence of antiviral therapy in hepatitis C virus-associated cryoglobulinemic MPGN. Am J Kidney Dis 2004;43:617.
25. Misiani R, Bellavita P, Fenili D, et al. Interferon alfa-2a therapy in cryoglobulinemia associated with hepatitis C virus. N Engl J Med 1994;330:751.
26. Roccatello D, Baldovino S, Rossi D, et al. Long-term effects of anti-CD20 monoclonal antibody treatment of cryoglobulinaemic glomerulonephritis. Nephrol Dial Transplant 2004;19:3054.
27. Bhimma R, Coovadia HM. Hepatitis B virus-associated nephropathy. Am J Nephrol 2004;24:198.
28. Conjeevaram HS, Hoofnagle JH, Austin HA, et al. Long-term outcome of hepatitis B virus-related glomerulonephritis after therapy with interferon alfa. Gastroenterology 1995;109:540.
29. Tang S, Lai FM, Lui YH, et al. Lamivudine in hepatitis B-associated membranous nephropathy. Kidney Int 2005;68:1750.
30. Hojs R, Bevc S, Ekart R, et al. Serum cystatin C-based equation compared to serum creatinine-based equations for estimation of glomerular filtration rate in patients with chronic kidney disease. Clin Nephrol 2008;70:10.
31. Orlando R, Mussap M, Plebani M, et al. Diagnostic value of plasma cystatin C as a glomerular filtration marker in decompensated liver cirrhosis. Clin Chem 2002;48:850.
32. Tanriover B, Mejia A, Weinstein J, et al. Analysis of kidney function and biopsy results in liver failure patients with renal dysfunction: a new look to combined liver kidney allocation in the post-MELD era. Transplantation 2008;86:1548.
33. Locke JE, Warren DS, Singer AL, et al. Declining outcomes in simultaneous liver-kidney transplantation in the MELD era: ineffective usage of renal allografts. Transplantation 2008;85:935.
34. Chopra A, Cantarovich M, Bain VG. Simultaneous liver and kidney transplants: optimizing use of this double resource. Transplantation 2011;91:1305.
35. Eason JD, Gonwa TA, Davis CL, et al. Proceedings of Consensus Conference on Simultaneous Liver Kidney Transplantation (SLK). Am J Transplant 2008;8:2243.
36. Papafragkakis H, Martin P, Akalin E. Combined liver and kidney transplantation. Curr Opin Organ Transplant 2011;15:263.
37. Lebron Gallardo M, Herrera Gutierrez ME, Seller Perez G, et al. Risk factors for renal dysfunction in the postoperative course of liver transplant. Liver Transpl 2004;10:1379.
38. Cabezuelo JB, Ramirez P, Rios A, et al. Risk factors of acute renal failure after liver transplantation. Kidney Int 2006;69:1073.

39. Cabezuelo JB, Ramirez P, Acosta F, et al. Does the standard vs piggyback surgical technique affect the development of early acute renal failure after orthotopic liver transplantation? Transplant Proc 2003;35:1913.
40. Calmus Y, Kamar N, Gugenheim J, et al. Assessing renal function with daclizumab induction and delayed tacrolimus introduction in liver transplant recipients. Transplantation 2010;89:1504.
41. Yoshida EM, Marotta PJ, Greig PD, et al. Evaluation of renal function in liver transplant recipients receiving daclizumab (Zenapax), mycophenolate mofetil, and a delayed, low-dose tacrolimus regimen vs. a standard-dose tacrolimus and mycophenolate mofetil regimen: a multicenter randomized clinical trial. Liver Transpl 2005;11:1064.
42. Flechner SM, Kobashigawa J, Klintmalm G. Calcineurin inhibitor-sparing regimens in solid organ transplantation: focus on improving renal function and nephrotoxicity. Clin Transplant 2008;22:1.
43. Herlenius G, Felldin M, Norden G, et al. Conversion from calcineurin inhibitor to either mycophenolate mofetil or sirolimus improves renal function in liver transplant recipients with chronic kidney disease: results of a prospective randomized trial. Transplant Proc 2010;42:4441.
44. Cantarovich M, Tzimas GN, Barkun J, et al. Efficacy of mycophenolate mofetil combined with very low-dose cyclosporine microemulsion in long-term liver-transplant patients with renal dysfunction. Transplantation 2003;76:98.
45. Castroagudin JF, Molina E, Romero R, et al. Improvement of renal function after the switch from a calcineurin inhibitor to everolimus in liver transplant recipients with chronic renal dysfunction. Liver Transpl 2009;15:1792.
46. Schleicher C, Palmes D, Utech M, et al. Timing of conversion to mammalian target of rapamycin inhibitors is crucial in liver transplant recipients with impaired renal function at transplantation. Transplant Proc 2010;42:2572.
47. Boudjema K, Camus C, Saliba F, et al. Reduced-dose tacrolimus with mycophenolate mofetil vs. standard-dose tacrolimus in liver transplantation: a randomized study. Am J Transplant 2011;11:965.
48. Batts ED, Lazarus HM. Diagnosis and treatment of transplantation-associated thrombotic microangiopathy: real progress or are we still waiting? Bone Marrow Transplant 2007;40:709.
49. Reynolds JC, Agodoa LY, Yuan CM, et al. Thrombotic microangiopathy after renal transplantation in the United States. Am J Kidney Dis 2003;42:1058.
50. Ruggenenti P. Post-transplant hemolytic-uremic syndrome. Kidney Int 2002;62:1093.
51. Schwarz A, Haller H, Schmitt R, et al. Biopsy-diagnosed renal disease in patients after transplantation of other organs and tissues. Am J Transplant 2010;10:2017.
52. Zarifian A, Meleg-Smith S, O'Donovan R, et al. Cyclosporine-associated thrombotic microangiopathy in renal allografts. Kidney Int 1999;55:2457.
53. Kuo HT, Sampaio MS, Ye X, et al. Risk factors for new-onset diabetes mellitus in adult liver transplant recipients, an analysis of the Organ Procurement and Transplant Network/United Network for Organ Sharing database. Transplantation 2010;89:1134.
54. Perez MJ, Garcia DM, Taybi BJ, et al. Cardiovascular risk factors after liver transplantation: analysis of related factors. Transplant Proc 2011;43:739.
55. Watt KD, Pedersen RA, Kremers WK, et al. Evolution of causes and risk factors for mortality post-liver transplant: results of the NIDDK long-term follow-up study. Am J Transplant 2010;10:1420.
56. Guckelberger O. Long-term medical comorbidities and their management: hypertension/cardiovascular disease. Liver Transpl 2009;15(Suppl 2):S75.

57. Salama M, Boudville N, Speers D, et al. Decline in native kidney function in liver transplant recipients is not associated with BK virus infection. Liver Transpl 2008;14:1787.

58. Barton TD, Blumberg EA, Doyle A, et al. A prospective cross-sectional study of BK virus infection in non-renal solid organ transplant recipients with chronic renal dysfunction. Transpl Infect Dis 2006;8:102.

59. Srinivas TR, Stephany BR, Budev M, et al. An emerging population: kidney transplant candidates who are placed on the waiting list after liver, heart, and lung transplantation. Clin J Am Soc Nephrol 2010;5:1881.

60. Gonwa TA, McBride MA, Mai ML, et al. Kidney transplantation after previous liver transplantation: analysis of the Organ Procurement Transplant Network database. Transplantation 2011;92(1):31–5.

Medical Management of the Liver Transplant Recipient

R. Todd Stravitz, MD[a],*, Daniel E. Carl, MD[b],
Diane M. Biskobing, MD[c]

KEYWORDS

- Liver transplantation • Complications • Calcineurin inhibitors
- Posttransplant malignancy

Although approximately 65% of orthotopic liver transplant (OLT) recipients survive 10 years after transplantation, they experience an increased risk and accelerated course of atherosclerotic cardiovascular disease and malignancy, which account for the vast majority of late deaths.[1,2] Most of the increased risk of nongraft-related morbidity can be ascribed to the long-term use of immunosuppressive medications (**Table 1**).[3] Unfortunately, few studies address the optimal medical management of OLT recipients. Therefore, this article provides guidelines to improve the management of OLT recipients based on a limited foundation of evidence-based medicine, often extrapolated from studies in renal transplant recipients.

HYPERTENSION

Whereas hypertension is uncommon in patients with decompensated cirrhosis, de novo hypertension after OLT affects more than 50% of recipients,[4–6] often within the first several months after transplant.[7,8] Clinical hypertension, defined as blood pressure greater than 140/90 mm Hg, develops in 50% to 75% of patients within the first 6 postoperative months,[3,6] and the incidence of clinical hypertension in OLT recipients may be as high as 75% to 80%.[5]

The authors have nothing to disclose.
[a] Section of Hepatology, Division of Gastroenterology, Hepatology, and Nutrition, Hume-Lee Transplant Center, Virginia Commonwealth University, PO Box 980341, Richmond, VA 23298-0341, USA
[b] Division of Nephrology, Virginia Commonwealth University, Richmond, VA, USA
[c] Division of Endocrinology, Virginia Commonwealth University, Richmond, VA, USA
* Corresponding author. 1200 East Broad Street, Richmond, VA 23298.
E-mail address: RSTRAVIT@VCU.EDU

Clin Liver Dis 15 (2011) 821–843
doi:10.1016/j.cld.2011.08.007
1089-3261/11/$ – see front matter © 2011 Elsevier Inc. All rights reserved.

Table 1
Relative risk of adverse metabolic effects of common immunosuppressive agents in orthotopic liver transplant recipients

Adverse Effect	CYA	TAC	SIR	MMF	CS
Hypertension	+++	++	–	–	+
Renal insufficiency	+++	++	–	–	–
Diabetes mellitus	–	+	–	–	++
Proteinuria	–	–	+	–	–
Hypercholesterolemia	+	–	++	–	+
Hypertriglyceridemia	–	+	+++	–	+
Osteoporosis	++	+	–	–	+++

Abbreviations: CS, corticosteroids; CYA, cyclosporine A; MMF, mycophenolate mofetil; SIR, sirolimus; TAC, tacrolimus.

The two most important factors contributing to post-OLT hypertension include a reversal of the cirrhotic hemodynamic state and the initiation of immunosuppressive agents, principally the calcineurin inhibitors (CNIs). OLT reverses the circulatory derangements of advanced cirrhosis (low systemic venous resistance, elevated cardiac output, low mean arterial pressure, and renal arteriolar vasoconstriction) within days, with restoration of normal hemodynamics within 6 months.[8,9] CNIs play an integral role in the immunosuppressant regimen post OLT, and both cyclosporine A (CYA) and tacrolimus (TAC) increase blood pressure in a dose-related manner by increasing peripheral vascular resistance.[10,11] These changes following OLT may be more pronounced than after transplantation of other solid organs.[12] Acutely, CNIs induce reversible vasoconstriction of both the afferent and efferent arterioles within the glomerulus temporally related to peak serum concentrations.[13,14] The mechanisms by which CNIs cause systemic and renal vasoconstriction are multifactorial, but include increase in thromboxane, angiotensin II, and endothelin activity, the activation of the sympathetic nervous system, and the inhibition of nitric oxide synthesis.[15–17] Renal blood flow decreases,[11] increasing sodium reabsorption and decreasing natriuresis, further contributing to hypertension.[18] CYA may have a greater adverse effect on blood pressure than TAC,[19,20] and in healthy volunteers CYA but not TAC has been shown to increase muscle sympathetic nerve activity even at high doses.[17] Glucocorticoids exacerbate CNI-induced hypertension by mineralocorticoid effects, expanding blood volume, and possibly by increasing systemic venous resistance.[21]

There are no guidelines for surveillance practices for post-OLT hypertension. By consensus,[22] treatment for hypertension has been recommended at a blood pressure greater than 140/90 mm Hg with a treatment goal of less than 140/90 mm Hg, or less than 130/80 mm Hg in patients with diabetes or chronic kidney disease. Because OLT recipients on CNIs might be considered de facto to have chronic kidney disease, a threshold blood pressure of 130/80 seems to be a reasonable indication for, and a goal of, therapy. Lifestyle modifications, including weight loss, sodium restriction, and alcohol and tobacco abstinence, should be advocated first, followed by early administration of an antihypertensive agent.

The optimal antihypertensive agent for OLT recipients remains undefined, due to a paucity of clinical trials. Practitioners should consider the underlying pathophysiology of CNI-induced hypertension as well as certain antihypertensive drug interactions with CNIs (**Table 2**). Coexisting medical problems should also be considered;

Table 2
Useful antihypertensive agents in orthotopic liver transplant recipients: advantages and disadvantages

Antihypertensive Agent	Advantages	Disadvantages
Calcium-channel blockers	Decreases CNI-induced vasoconstriction	Edema, tachycardia, headache Cytochrome P450 interactions[a]
β-Blockers	Decreases left ventricular hypertrophy Decreases CNI headache	Impotence, bronchospasm
ACE inhibitors	Renal sparing effect in diabetics Decreases CNI-induced renal fibrosis	Hyperkalemia, azotemia, acidosis
ATII receptor antagonists	Decreases CNI-induced vasoconstriction	Hyperkalemia
α-Adrenergic agonists (clonidine)	?Decreases CNI-induced neurogenic renal vasoconstriction	Sedation
Thiazide diuretics	Decreases hypervolemia	Hyperlipidemia

Abbreviations: ACE, angiotensin-converting enzyme; ATII, angiotensin II; CNI, calcineurin inhibitors.
[a] Cytochrome P450 interactions with CNI result from competition for metabolism, and are greatest for diltiazem, verapamil, and nicardipine, and least for nifedipine and amlodipine.

for example, angiotensin-converting enzyme (ACE) inhibitors and angiotensin receptor blockers (ARBs) are drugs of choice in diabetics without significant hyperkalemia, and β-blockers should be considered as first-line agents in patients with coronary artery disease. Calcium-channel blockers (CCBs) have become antihypertensive agent of choice for many OLT recipients within the first year of transplant because of their ability to attenuate vasoconstriction. Because nondihydropyridine CCBs, such as verapamil and diltiazem, compete with CNIs for metabolism by cytochrome P450 3A4, thereby risking toxicity, dihydropyridine CCBs (amlodipine or nifedipine) are preferred. A significant number of OLT recipients develop side effects of CCBs, including edema, headaches, and tachycardia.[2,23] CNIs activate the renin-angiotensin-aldosterone (RAA) axis, suggesting that ACE inhibitors and ARBs may have a physiologic advantage in OLT recipients. Clonidine, a centrally acting α-adrenergic agonist, also has been used effectively to treat posttransplant hypertension, and is particularly useful in patients whose hypertension is mediated from excessive sympathetic nervous system activation.

Few studies have compared CCBs with other therapy in hypertensive OLT recipients. In recipients with hypertension who were intolerant or poorly controlled by amlodipine, those randomized to receive lisinopril achieved a greater reduction in blood pressure than those randomized to receive bisoprolol.[24] In addition, this study showed that increasing the daily dose of amlodipine from 5 to 10 mg was generally ineffective in achieving a goal systolic blood pressure of less than 140 mm Hg. A different study prospectively randomized 30 patients with post-OLT hypertension to carvedilol or nifedipine, and concluded that control of blood pressure was equivalent.[25]

RENAL DYSFUNCTION

The true incidence of chronic kidney disease (CKD) after OLT is unknown, due to a lack of uniform definition. From a database of nonrenal transplant recipients including nearly 37,000 OLT recipients, the incidence of chronic renal failure (glomerular filtration rate [GFR] <30 mL/min/1.73 m^2) at 5 years post transplant was 18.1%, higher than in recipients of heart or lung transplants.[26] In another study, the point prevalence for each stage of CKD in OLT recipients followed for a mean of 5.6 years was 0.9% in stage 5, 3.9% in stage 4, 41.3% in stage 3, 44.8% in stage 2, and the remainder in stage 1; 71% of patients surviving 5 years had a GFR less than 60 mL/min/1.73 m^2.[27] The largest decline in GFR occurs within the first 6 months of transplantation. Severe renal failure (GFR <30 mL/min/1.73 m^2) has been associated with decreased survival in OLT recipients, with the relative risk of death of 3 to 4.[26–28]

Multiple factors contribute to the development of post-OLT CKD. The most important pretransplant variable is renal dysfunction and the hepatorenal syndrome. A direct relationship also exists between acute kidney injury (AKI) in the immediate postoperative period and the future development of CKD.[29] Cirrhotic patients are particularly susceptible to AKI because of the underlying decreased effective renal perfusion and exposure to multiple insults that can lead to ischemic renal tubular injury, such as prolonged hypotension, sepsis, nephrotoxic agents, antibiotics, and radiocontrast. Other demographic and comorbid variables that have been implicated in the development of CKD include older age, female sex, preexisting diabetes and/or hypertension, vascular disease, hyperbilirubinemia, and hypoalbuminemia.[26,30,31] In the posttransplant period, risk factors for CKD include older age, diabetes, hypertension, and hepatitis C virus (HCV) infection,[26,32] the latter due to glomerular deposition of immune complexes. In HCV-positive OLT recipients who underwent routine kidney biopsies at surgery, more than 80% revealed evidence of an immune complex glomerulonephritis despite most having normal serum creatinine.[33] Although BK virus nephropathy is an important cause of CKD in the renal transplant population, a possible role BK infection in OLT recipients with CKD has not been defined.[34]

The most important posttransplant contributor to CKD in OLT recipients is CNI exposure. As already noted, acute exposure to CNIs causes a reversible, dose-related vasoconstriction of the afferent and efferent arterioles, causing azotemia. Long-term exposure to CNIs results in chronic nephropathy characterized by a slow decline in GFR and subnephrotic-range proteinuria, with progressive interstitial fibrosis, arteriosclerosis, glomerulosclerosis, and tubular atrophy.[35] These changes are considered irreversible. The underlying mechanisms that lead to CNI-induced chronic nephropathy are not well understood, but include increased oxidative stress,[36] the elaboration of fibrogenic cytokines such as transforming growth factor β,[37] activation of the RAA system,[38] and the development of thrombotic microangiopathy.[14]

OLT recipients should be evaluated and possibly treated for CKD once GFR drops below 60 mL/min/1.73 m^2. The management of CKD after OLT should include vigorous management of hypertension, bone mineral homeostasis, and anemia. Specific guidelines for treating CKD in the OLT population are lacking, however. Immunosuppressive induction protocols with delayed introduction of CNIs have met with mixed success[39,40] and concerns of increased risk of acute cellular rejection. In the longer term, the management of CKD in OLT recipients usually involves management of comorbidities, such as diabetes and hypertension. Agents considered "renoprotective" such as ACE inhibitors and ARBs should be strongly considered in nonhyperkalemic recipients, because ACE inhibitors reduces microalbuminuria, and blockade of the RAA system slows progression of CKD in renal transplant recipients.[41] Indeed, RAA axis inhibition in animal models downregulates fibrogenesis in kidneys with CNI toxicity.[38]

In patients with established chronic CNI nephropathy, CKD progression can stabilize or even improve by decreasing CNI exposure, often substituting a less nephrotoxic agent such as sirolimus (SIR) or mycophenolate mofetil (MMF). In 42 OLT recipients with CKD or severe dyslipidemia, complete conversion from a CNI to MMF (1.5 g/d) improved renal function in 89% and resulted in only one case of acute cellular rejection.[42] Although other uncontrolled studies have noted variable degrees of improved renal function with CNI conversion to MMF monotherapy, many also noted an increase in acute cellular rejection; consequently, MMF monotherapy is not generally advocated.[43] Protocols minimizing CNI with the coadministration of MMF appear to stabilize or improve renal function, with a lower risk of precipitating rejection.[44] Studies with conversion of CNIs to SIR have also reported stabilization of renal function.[45–47] However, a threshold of renal failure may exist (creatinine clearance <30 mL/min) beyond which conversion to SIR may not only fail to prevent progression but also increase the risk of adverse outcomes.[46] Furthermore, experience with SIR has revealed a high incidence of adverse side effects including nephrotoxicity characterized by proteinuria; concern has also been raised about the adequacy of immunosuppression under SIR monotherapy.[47,48]

OLT recipients with end-stage renal disease should be evaluated for kidney transplantation. Mortality is high in OLT recipients maintained on chronic hemodialysis, but improves by approximately 50% in OLT recipients who receive sequential kidney transplant compared with those maintained on hemodialysis.[49] Although an initial transient increase in mortality has been observed after renal transplantation in recipients of other solid organs including the liver, the relative risk of mortality decreases to

0.56 by 5 years after renal transplantation compared with that of patients who continue on hemodialysis.[26]

DIABETES MELLITUS

Recent studies have shown a 15% to 38% incidence of posttransplant diabetes mellitus (PTDM) within 1 year after OLT,[50,51] with the majority of patients (64%–81%) diagnosed within the first 3 postoperative months. Thereafter, both the incidence of PTDM and degree of hyperglycemia decline as doses of corticosteroids and TAC are decreased.[50,52] HCV infection confers an additional risk for diabetes mellitus both pretransplant and posttransplant[53]; HCV-positive recipients not previously known to be diabetic have a 42% to 64% incidence of PTDM compared with 19% to 28% in HCV-negative patients.[50,54] PTDM has been associated with an accelerated risk of cardiovascular disease, infections, neuropsychiatric complications, and acute rejection,[55,56] but the impact on mortality remains unclear.[54] Graft fibrosis in patients transplanted for HCV who develop PTDM is accelerated compared with nondiabetics,[57] probably due to concomitant nonalcoholic fatty liver disease.

Impaired glucose tolerance (IGT) and/or insulin resistance occur frequently in patients with cirrhosis, and are important risk factors for developing PTDM.[50] Additional independent risk factors for PTDM include recipient age older than 50 years, African American race, body mass index (BMI; weight in kilograms divided by height in meters squared, ie, kg/m^2) greater than 25, HCV infection, higher Child-Pugh score at transplant, donor age older than 60 years, TAC usage, and corticosteroid use at time of discharge.[50,51] The use of high-dose corticosteroids in the early post-OLT period worsens insulin resistance[53] and is responsible for the highest incidence of PTDM within the first 3 months after OLT.[50] In addition, the weight gain associated with corticosteroid use exacerbates insulin resistance even after discontinuation of steroids.[53] The use of CNIs, particularly TAC, increases the risk of PTDM,[50,53,58] due to direct toxicity on pancreatic β cells.[59] A recent study has suggested a low incidence of PTDM in OLT recipients under SIR immunosuppression in comparison with SIR plus CNI.[60] As noted, a strong association between HCV infection, insulin resistance, and the development of PTDM has been demonstrated.[50,61]

Surveillance for diabetes and IGT (**Fig. 1**) should be performed before OLT to identify those at highest risk for developing PTDM. Transplant candidates with IGT or diabetes should be counseled about lifestyle modification and, if indicated, those with diabetes should be started on pharmacologic therapy prior to OLT (see **Fig. 1**). Individualization of the initial immunosuppressive regimen should be considered in such patients, with preference for corticosteroid-sparing and TAC-sparing regimens.[62] Monitoring for PTDM should begin immediately after transplant, with regular fasting plasma glucose levels (eg, weekly for the first month, and at 3, 6, and 12 months post OLT)[63] and hemoglobin A1C every 3 months in high-risk patients. After the first year post OLT, monitoring for PTDM should be tailored according to the presence of the aforementioned risk factors but yearly at a minimum, more frequently in those with underlying IGT. Treatment should be initiated in OLT recipients meeting criteria for diabetes (see **Fig. 1**).[63]

For most OLT recipients, lifestyle and immunosuppressive regimen modification fails to achieve glucose goals within 2 to 3 months, and pharmacologic therapy becomes mandatory. The decision whether to begin insulin versus other hypoglycemic agents should be based on the glucose level and hemoglobin A1C (see **Fig. 1**).[62,64] Mild hyperglycemia and a hemoglobin A1C less than 9% should prompt consideration of one of several hypoglycemic agents (**Table 3**). Hypoglycemic

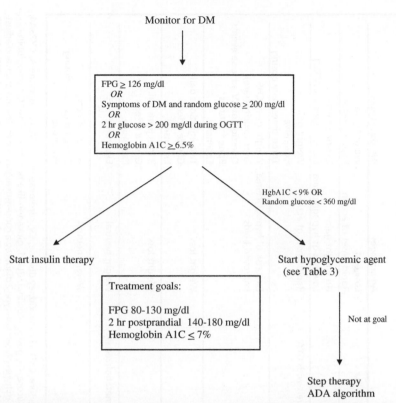

Fig. 1. Screening and treatment algorithm for posttransplant diabetes mellitus in orthotopic liver transplant recipients. ADA, American Diabetes Association; DM, diabetes mellitus; FPG, fasting plasma glucose; Hbg, hemoglobin; OGTT, oral glucose tolerance test. (*Adapted from* Wilkinson A, Davidson J, Dotta F, et al. Guidelines for the treatment and management of new-onset diabetes after transplantation. Clin Transplant 2005;19(3):291–8, with permission; and Nathan DM, Buse JB, Davidson MB, et al. Medical management of hyperglycemia in type 2 diabetes: a consensus algorithm for the initiation and adjustment of therapy: a consensus statement of the American Diabetes Association and the European Association for the Study of Diabetes. Diabetes Care 2009;32(1):193–203; with permission.)

medications should be selected on the basis of patient characteristics, efficacy in hemoglobin A1C reduction, medication interactions, side effects, and cost (see **Table 3**). Combination hypoglycemic therapy followed by an oral agent and insulin should be instituted in a stepwise fashion if control of diabetes remains unattainable. In recipients with more severe hyperglycemia (hemoglobin A1C >9%, glucose >360 mg/dL, signs of metabolic decompensation such as ketosis or weight loss), insulin therapy should be initiated immediately.[65] Corticosteroid therapy tends to cause afternoon hyperglycemia; consequently, a morning dose of NPH insulin may be preferred because it shares the same time course of action as prednisone, can rapidly ameliorate hyperglycemia, and is easily adjusted for tapering doses of prednisone.[66] In recipients who do not respond adequately to morning NPH insulin, multiple insulin injections are required. Regular self-monitoring of blood glucose and management of dyslipidemia should accompany these measures, and patients should be screened annually for diabetic complications such as retinopathy and nephropathy.

Table 3
Common hypoglycemic agents: potential interactions, advantages and disadvantages in liver transplant recipients

Antidiabetic Class	Expected Decrease in HbA1C with Monotherapy (%)	Interactions	Advantages	Disadvantages
Sulfonylureas	1–2	↑ CYA levels	Low cost Rapid onset of action	Weight gain Hypoglycemia
Metformin	1–2	—	No weight gain Low risk of hypoglycemia	GI side effects Lactic acidosis (in CKD)
Meglitinides	0.5–1.5	↑ Glinide levels with CYA	Rapid onset of action	Weight gain Expensive Three times daily dosing
Thiazolidine-diones	0.5–1.4	—	Low risk of hypoglycemia Improved lipids	Weight gain, CHF Liver toxicity (rare) Question of CV adverse events Bone fractures Expensive
GLP-1 agonist	0.5–1.0	—	Weight loss	Two injections daily GI side effects Expensive
Amylin analogs	0.5–1.0	—	Weight loss	3 injections daily GI side effects Expensive
DPP-4 inhibitors	0.5–0.8	Hepatically metabolized by CYP3A4	Weight neutral	Expensive
α-Glucosidase inhibitors	0.5–0.8	—	Weight neutral	GI side effects Three times daily dosing Expensive

Abbreviations: ADA, American Diabetes Association; CHF, congestive heart failure; CKD, chronic kidney disease; CV, cardiovascular; CYA, cyclosporine A; CYP3A4, cytochrome P-450 3A4; DPP-4, dipeptidyl peptidase-4; FPG, fasting plasma glucose; GI, gastrointestinal; GLP-1, glucagon–like peptide-1; HbA1C, hemoglobin A₁c.

Adapted from Nathan DM, Buse JB, Davidson MB, et al. Medical management of hyperglycemia in type 2 diabetes: a consensus algorithm for the initiation and adjustment of therapy: a consensus statement of the American Diabetes Association and the European Association for the Study of Diabetes. Diabetes Care 2009;32(1):193–203, with permission; and Rakel A, Karelis AD. New-onset diabetes after transplantation: risk factors and clinical impact. Diabetes Metab 2011;37(1):1–14, with permission.

HYPERLIPIDEMIA

Hyperlipidemia occurs in one-third to one-half of OLT recipients, and contributes cardiovascular ischemic events.[4,67] Mixed hyperlipidemia predominates, but isolated hypercholesterolemia and hypertriglyceridemia also occur after OLT, depending on genetic factors and the immunosuppression regimen. Risk factors for hyperlipidemia after OLT include its presence before transplant; risk factors for isolated hypertriglyceridemia also include posttransplant renal dysfunction and the metabolic syndrome.[67] Although diet, obesity, and diabetes contribute to the high incidence of hyperlipidemia after OLT, the choice of immunosuppressive drug plays the most defining role. CYA predominantly causes hypercholesterolemia by inhibiting sterol 27-hydroxylase, the initiating enzyme in an alternative pathway of bile acid biosynthesis from cholesterol, as well as by binding to the low-density lipoprotein (LDL) receptor, impairing its ability to take up LDL cholesterol (LDL-C) into hepatocytes.[68,69] TAC usually has minimal effects on serum cholesterol, but can increase triglycerides when associated with PTDM.[4,20] SIR affects serum lipids most dramatically[70] by decreasing peripheral tissue hydrolysis and increasing hepatic synthesis of lipoproteins.[71]

A lipid panel should be obtained regularly in all OLT recipients, especially early after transplantation and after a change in immunosuppression. The relative contribution of hyperlipidemia to cardiovascular morbidity and mortality has admittedly not been well studied in OLT recipients, and levels at which to initiate therapy and target levels of therapy remain undefined. As in the nontransplant population, correction of LDL-C should be the primary target of lipid-lowering therapy in OLT recipients.[72] In OLT recipients with low or medium cardiovascular risk, correction of high-density lipoprotein cholesterol (HDL-C) and triglycerides, which contribute less to cardiovascular risk, may not be reasonable considering the increasing probability of drug interactions. The addition of a fibric acid derivative to a statin in recipients on CYA poses a particular risk of rhabdomyolysis, because CYA and statins compete for metabolism by cytochrome P450 3A4, and fibrates potentiate the myotoxicity of statins.[73] Of interest, despite metabolism by the same cytochrome P450, statins do not usually increase CYA levels.[74] Although certain statins (eg, pravastatin and fluvastatin) may be less likely than others to adversely interact with CYA and other drugs,[73,75] there are no convincing data to suggest that one statin is safer than another.

Therapeutic lifestyle changes, such as exercise and dietary modification, remain essential adjuncts to treat hyperlipidemic OLT recipients. As for PTDM, individualization of a hyperlipidemic OLT recipient's immunosuppressive regimen should be considered, specifically, changing the immunosuppressive regimen from SIR or CYA to TAC,[76] or to dose reduction. As in the nontransplant population, statins remain the treatment of choice in OLT recipients with isolated hypercholesterolemia or mixed hyperlipidemia. The threshold at which LDL-C should prompt initiation of a statin should also be individualized. In recipients with moderate or high cardiovascular risk (2 or more risk factors, known coronary artery or peripheral vascular disease, diabetes), statins in standard doses should be considered when LDL-C exceeds 100 mg/dL. In patients with intolerance to statins or who do not achieve the therapeutic goal of lowering LDL-C by 30% to 40%, ezetimibe can be added safely. Ezetimibe inhibits cholesterol absorption from the intestinal lumen, and synergistically lowers serum cholesterol with statins while having no significant effect on immunosuppressive levels.[77] In addition, ezetimibe has few drug interactions and a negligible risk of hepatotoxicity.[78] Bile acid sequestrants bind immunosuppressive agents and other medications within the gut lumen, and therefore have been largely abandoned in transplant recipients.

Mild to moderate hypertriglyceridemia confers a modest cardiovascular risk to non-transplant subjects, and treatment in OLT recipients should therefore be through dietary modification, exercise, weight loss, control of PTDM, and fish oil supplements (2–8 g/d). By contrast, severe hypertriglyceridemia increases cardiovascular risk in the nontransplant population, and levels greater than 1000 mg/dL also may cause acute pancreatitis, and therefore should prompt consideration of adding a fibric acid derivative (gemfibrozil or fenofibrate). Fibrates and fish oil do not have important drug interactions with CYA.[74] In the nontransplant population, low HDL-C (<40 mg/dL for men; <50 mg/dL for women) also contributes to cardiovascular risk, but has not been studied in OLT recipients. OLT recipients with moderate to severe cardiovascular risk and low HDL-C may be given niacin, with the understanding that the sustained-release form has been associated with hepatotoxicity.[79] Despite these recommendations, there are no data demonstrating decreased cardiovascular events or improved mortality in OLT recipients treated for hyperlipidemia. Even in renal transplants, two recent Cochrane reviews failed to demonstrate improvements in cardiovascular mortality in patients treated with statins or fish oil.

METABOLIC BONE DISEASE

Low bone mineral density (BMD) as diagnosed by bone densitometry (DEXA) is defined as a T-score (the number of standard deviations from peak young, healthy, adult BMD) of −1.0 to −2.5 and osteoporosis as a T-score of less than −2.5.[80] Low BMD and osteoporosis or fracture before OLT are the most significant risk factors for fracture after OLT.[81] The prevalence of osteoporosis in patients awaiting OLT is 20% to 43% in patients with cirrhosis of mixed etiology, and higher in patients with cholestatic liver diseases; between 7% and 35% have had osteoporotic fractures.[81,82] In contrast to the general population, the prevalence of osteoporosis before OLT is similar between men, premenopausal women, and postmenopausal women. After OLT, the highest rate of bone loss occurs within the first 3 to 4 months, due to physical inactivity and a higher use of corticosteroid. In a 15 year study, 82% of patients displayed a rapid decline in BMD 4 months after OLT (**Fig. 2**),[82] with an overall initial rate of bone loss between 15% and 18%.[83] More recent studies report less vigorous bone loss of between 0% and 5% within the first year after OLT,[84] possibly due to changes in the use of immunosuppressive drugs, increased awareness, and treatment of osteoporosis risk factors pretransplant. In untreated patients, the bone loss seen early after OLT improves over the next several years (see **Fig. 2**),[82,85] but BMD of lumbar spine and femoral neck often remains below pretransplant levels for several years after surgery.[85,86] Within the first year of OLT, up to 40% of recipients will have an osteoporotic fracture, many of which are asymptomatic vertebral fractures.[81,83]

Contributors to low BMD in patients with cirrhosis include hypogonadism, malnutrition, low BMI, physical inactivity, and vitamin D deficiency.[86,87] Although osteomalacia is rare, vitamin D deficiency is present in up to two-thirds of cirrhotics and 96% of transplant candidates, and contributes to low BMD and an increased fracture risk.[88] The etiology of the underlying liver disease pre-OLT also contributes to the severity and prevalence of low BMD after OLT. Patients with cholestatic liver diseases (primary biliary cirrhosis and primary sclerosing cholangitis) often have the lowest BMD of all OLT candidates because of decreased bone formation, thought to be secondary to toxic effects of bilirubin on osteoblasts and low insulin-like growth factor levels.[89] Patients with autoimmune hepatitis may have low BMD due to corticosteroid

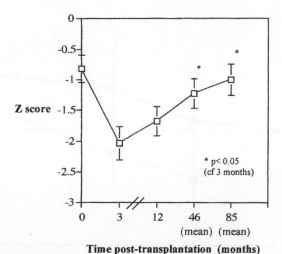

Fig. 2. Natural history of decline and recovery of bone mineral density after orthotopic liver transplantation for mixed liver diseases. (*From* Feller RB, McDonald JA, Sherbon KJ, et al. Evidence of continuing bone recovery at a mean of 7 years after liver transplantation. Liver Transpl Surg 1999;5(5):408; with permission.)

treatment.[87] BMI before OLT also correlates both with BMD and fracture risk after OLT.[90] Independent risk factors for early posttransplant bone loss include a shorter duration of liver disease, primary sclerosing cholangitis (PSC), and higher posttransplant direct bilirubin.[82] Independent predictors of post-OLT fractures include pretransplant fracture, low BMD, increasing age, primary biliary cirrhosis, and glucocorticoid doses used after OLT.[81]

Immunosuppressive agents play a major role in the further decline in BMD after OLT. The duration and total exposure of OLT recipients to corticosteroids directly correlates with the incidence of post-OLT fractures. In vitro and in vivo studies also suggest that TAC and CYA directly increase bone resorption,[87] possibly less so with TAC.[91] A recent study compared TAC alone versus TAC plus corticosteroid, and found similar rates of osteoporosis.[92] Animal and small studies in OLT recipients have suggested minimal if any effect of SIR or MMF on BMD.[93,94]

All patients being evaluated for OLT should be screened by DEXA, and should be counseled about adequate vitamin D and calcium intake, weight-bearing exercise, nutritional repletion, alcohol use, and smoking cessation.[80] A significant number of men awaiting OLT have hypogonadism,[86] and should be screened with a free testosterone level and repleted. In cirrhotic patients with osteoporosis or a fracture history, bisphosphonate therapy should be started before OLT.[89] Considering the accelerated bone loss in the first year after OLT, prophylactic bisphosphonate therapy should probably be administered to patients with low bone mass (T-score between −1 and −2.5). Bisphosphonates, which are antibone resorptive agents, are the treatment of choice for this purpose. Recently there have been several prospective, randomized trials of bisphosphonates for prevention of post–liver transplant bone loss.[95] Alendronate, ibandronate, zoldronic acid, and pamidronate have all been shown to prevent post-OLT bone loss compared with control groups treated with calcium and vitamin D alone.[84,96–98] Although the dose of zoledronic acid was higher than standard (**Fig. 3**),[96] treatment markedly attenuated loss of BMD compared with treatment with calcium and vitamin D alone. Other studies have also shown a significant

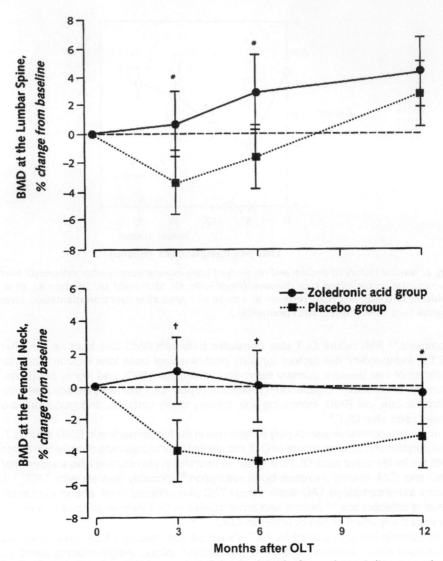

Fig. 3. Change from baseline bone mineral density (BMD) after orthotopic liver transplantation (OLT) in patients randomized to zoledronic acid (at time of OLT and 1, 3, 6, and 9 months post OLT; N = 32) or placebo (N = 30). *P<.05; †P<.001. (*From* Crawford BA, Kam C, Pavlovic J, et al. Zoledronic acid prevents bone loss after liver transplantation: a randomized, double-blind, placebo-controlled trial. Ann Intern Med 2006;144(4):246; with permission.)

decrease in fracture rate in patients treated with ibandronate or zoledronic acid compared with placebo.[96,97] There have been no studies in OLT recipients of other agents used to treat osteoporosis, such as teriparatide or denosumab.

MALIGNANCIES

Malignancies developing after OLT, so-called de novo malignancies, comprise the second most common cause of late mortality behind cardiovascular disease.[99] The cumulative risk of de novo malignancies ranges widely between studies (between 5% and 50%) depending on the definition of malignancy and length of follow-up; however, OLT recipients appear to develop de novo malignancies less frequently than recipients of other solid organs.[100] Risk factors for de novo malignancies include increasing age, male sex, time from transplant, negative Epstein-Barr virus (EBV) antibodies before OLT, heavy alcohol consumption, and total sun exposure.[99] Several malignancies are characteristic of immunosuppressed patients, such virally driven posttransplant lymphoproliferative disorder (PTLD). Others are more common in OLT recipients than age- and sex-matched population controls, including carcinomas of the skin, lung, head and neck, and esophagus. The latter 3 represent the well-established synergistic mutagenicity of heavy alcohol consumption and cigarette smoking. The remainder of common malignancies, including prostate, cervix, and breast, do not develop with higher incidence in OLT recipients in comparison with the general population.[99,101]

Several causes of an increased risk of de novo malignancy after OLT have been proposed. The most important contributor may be high-risk behavior before OLT, such as cigarette and alcohol abuse.[99,102] Although long-term immunosuppression has been hypothesized to the increase risk of malignancy because of "loss of immunovigilance," supporting data remain inconclusive.[103,104] Specific immunosuppressive agents have also been associated with an increased risk of malignancies in some series, but also remain controversial.[105,106] In OLT recipients, the addition of MMF to CNIs has not been shown to increase the development of de novo malignancies.[107] It has been hypothesized that SIR, which has antiproliferative properties, may protect transplant recipients from de novo and recurrent malignancies.[108] However, SIR has not been studied in prospective, randomized trials against other immunosuppressive agents, and therefore cannot be advocated as "chemopreventive."

Skin Cancer

Similar to renal transplant recipients, nonmelanoma skin cancers (NMSC; squamous and basal cell carcinomas) are the most commonly encountered malignancies in OLT recipients, with an incidence of up to 20-fold higher than the age-matched and sex-matched general population,[109] and a mean time to diagnosis of approximately 45 and 20 months from transplant, respectively.[110] In contrast to the general population, squamous cell carcinomas outnumber basal cell carcinomas in solid organ transplant recipients, and are more aggressive and have a greater propensity to recur and metastasize.[111] The risk of developing NMSC after OLT is higher in recipients with fair skin complexion and high total sun exposure. Melanoma has also been reported to occur more frequently after OLT than in the general population,[112] but is less frequently encountered than NMSC. The prevention and optimal surveillance of OLT recipients for NMSC has not been extensively studied. Recently, 120 solid organ recipients were randomized to receive education about sun protection, or education in addition to a broad-spectrum sunscreen.[113] During 2 years of follow-up, the incidence of actinic keratoses and squamous cell carcinoma was significantly lower in those who applied a broad-spectrum sunscreen an average of 5.6 times per week than in those who did not. In addition to advocating the use of sunscreens, routine examinations by a dermatologist should also be performed in any OLT recipient with actinically damaged skin, a previous history of skin neoplasms, and perhaps in those living in areas of high ultraviolet light exposure.

A rare skin malignancy, Kaposi sarcoma (KS), is caused by the human herpes virus type 8 (HHV-8). Most of the data on the relative risk of developing KS after transplant have been from large, solid organ transplant databases not limited to OLT recipients,[111] in whom the relative risk may be 500 compared with the general population. Similar to other oncogenic virally driven posttransplant malignancies, minimization of immunosuppression can cause tumor regression.

Carcinoma of the Oropharynx and Esophagus

The incidence of head and neck cancer after OLT is increased in most series, and particularly after OLT for alcoholic cirrhosis, where the risk may be more than 25-fold higher than for those transplanted for nonalcoholic liver diseases.[114] The incidence of squamous cell carcinoma of the head and neck was 27% versus 5%, respectively, after OLT for alcoholic cirrhosis compared with nonalcoholic cirrhosis, in another retrospective series.[115] Squamous cell carcinoma of the esophagus has also been described, with a relative risk as high as 18.7 compared with the general age-matched and sex-matched population.[112] As for the nontransplant population, cigarette smoking synergistically increases this risk.[102] Although there are no studies exploring the effectiveness of surveillance programs for these tumors after OLT, it seems reasonable to perform a screening upper endoscopy and oropharyngeal examination before transplant, especially in those with alcoholic liver disease, and for new oropharyngeal or swallowing symptoms after transplant. Data in OLT recipients with Barrett esophagus, the precursor of adenocarcinoma, are sparse, but support an increased rate of progression to severe dysplasia.[116]

Lung Cancer

Lung cancer is one of the most common de novo malignancies after OLT behind skin and head and neck carcinomas, with an incidence of approximately 14%.[117,118] The increased risk of lung cancer has been reported to be especially elevated over the general population in women recipients.[101] As for head and neck cancers, patients transplanted for alcoholic liver disease may be particularly vulnerable to lung cancer because of the strong association of alcohol abuse and cigarette smoking.

Colon Cancer

The association between OLT and an increased risk of colorectal carcinoma (CRC) remains controversial, but increasingly probable. A recent meta-analysis of OLT recipients emphasizes the divergent practices of screening for CRC before and surveillance after OLT, hampering comparison between studies.[119] However, the investigators concluded that the relative risk of CRC in all OLT recipients was 2.6 (95% confidence interval [CI] 1.7–2.1) overall, and 1.8 (95% CI 1.1–2.9) for non-PSC OLT recipients, compared with weighted age-matched controls. The incidence of CRC after OLT for PSC is dramatically elevated in patients with ulcerative colitis (UC), approaching 7% within 2 years of transplant.[120] Although not entirely conclusive, these observations support CRC surveillance by colonoscopy in all OLT recipients. The interval of examination should be individualized. There are insufficient data to recommend a surveillance interval for average-risk OLT recipients, but many authorities advocate a shorter than standard-of-practice interval.[99,121,122] Recipients with a pretransplant history of adenomatous polyps should be considered for examination 2 years after transplant and every 3 to 5 years thereafter. Patients without a history of UC who were transplanted for PSC should undergo more intensive surveillance. Finally, patients transplanted for PSC with UC should undergo colonoscopy with random biopsies for dysplasia yearly, with a low threshold for total proctocolectomy.

Lymphoma

Posttransplant non-Hodgkin lymphoma or PTLD has traditionally been considered a de novo malignancy of pediatric solid organ recipients driven by the EBV.[123] In adults, EBV-positive PTLD predominates within the first 18 months of OLT, but EBV-negative cases predominate by 8 years after OLT.[124] The cumulative incidence of PTLD is 5.4% after 15.5 years, and is highest in the first 18 months post transplant in adult transplant recipients. Risk factors for PTLD include infection with HCV, a history of alcohol abuse, increasing age, and relatively high levels of immunosuppression, including after treatment for acute cellular rejection. Although an EBV-negative OLT recipient who receives a solid organ transplant from an EBV-positive donor is at highest risk for EBV-positive PTLD in children, EBV serologies in adult donors and recipients are usually not available; therefore, this risk factor in adults can only be extrapolated from the pediatric experience. The association of HCV infection and an increased risk of PTLD in adults is supported by its well-established ability to induce monoclonal expansion of B lymphocytes, strong association with non-Hodgkin lymphoma in the nontransplant population, and increased prevalence in EBV-negative cases of PTLD.[125] PTLD differs clinically from lymphoma in the nontransplant population by being predominantly B-cell, and having a predilection for infiltration of the liver allograft and other solid organs and the bowel.[126] Reduction of immunosuppression often induces a durable remission of EBV-associated PTLD, with acyclovir or ganciclovir and chemotherapy reserved for refractory cases.[127–129]

Surveillance Programs for De Novo Malignancies

Recent studies have compared the survival in patients undergoing intensive malignancy surveillance programs with those who presented either with symptoms or were incidentally diagnosed.[130,131] Although these studies are subject to bias favoring surveillance, malignancies were diagnosed at earlier stages and survival was improved in those who underwent intensive surveillance. One surveillance protocol performed annual chest and abdominal computed tomography, and urological, gynecologic, and dermatologic examinations, and in addition colonoscopy 3 years post transplant followed by every 5 years thereafter for low-risk patients. Median overall posttransplant survival increased from 3.1 years in the historical controls to 11.3 years after adoption of intensive surveillance.[131] For colon carcinoma, it has been estimated that current surveillance recommendations based on the nontransplant population (to begin surveillance at age 50) would exclude more than 25% of at-risk solid organ recipients[132]; consequently, it may be reasonable to begin surveillance by colonoscopy at a younger age (eg, 40 years). Cost, inconvenience, complications, and X-ray exposure must be considered before advocating intensive surveillance programs, however.

SUMMARY

Liver transplant recipients represent a high-risk population for atherosclerotic cardiovascular disease, CKD, metabolic bone disease, and malignancy. These complications will assume an even greater role in the long-term morbidity and mortality of liver transplant recipients as the prevalence of the metabolic syndrome in patients with chronic liver disease increases. Studies to define optimal surveillance and treatment practices for the metabolic complications of liver transplantation are urgently needed.

REFERENCES

1. Pruthi J, Medkiff KA, Esrason KT, et al. Analysis of causes of death in liver transplant recipients who survived more than 3 years. Liver Transpl 2001;7(9): 811–5.
2. Neal DA, Tom BD, Luan J, et al. Is there disparity between risk and incidence of cardiovascular disease after liver transplant? Transplantation 2004;77(1): 93–9.
3. Rabkin JM, Corless CL, Rosen HR, et al. Immunosuppression impact on long-term cardiovascular complications after liver transplantation. Am J Surg 2002; 183(5):595–9.
4. Guckelberger O, Bechstein WO, Neuhaus R, et al. Cardiovascular risk factors in long-term follow-up after orthotopic liver transplantation. Clin Transplant 1997; 11(1):60–5.
5. Sheiner PA, Magliocca JF, Bodian CA, et al. Long-term medical complications in patients surviving > or = 5 years after liver transplant. Transplantation 2000; 69(5):781–9.
6. Neal DA, Brown MJ, Wilkinson IB, et al. Mechanisms of hypertension after liver transplantation. Transplantation 2005;79(8):935–40.
7. Textor SC. De novo hypertension after liver transplantation. Hypertension 1993; 22(2):257–67.
8. Piscaglia F, Zironi G, Gaiani S, et al. Systemic and splanchnic hemodynamic changes after liver transplantation for cirrhosis: a long-term prospective study. Hepatology 1999;30(1):58–64.
9. Schrier RW, Arroyo V, Bernardi M, et al. Peripheral arterial vasodilation hypothesis: a proposal for the initiation of renal sodium and water retention in cirrhosis. Hepatology 1988;8(5):1151–7.
10. Greenberg ML, Uretsky BF, Reddy PS, et al. Long-term hemodynamic follow-up of cardiac transplant patients treated with cyclosporine and prednisone. Circulation 1985;71(3):487–94.
11. Taler SJ, Textor SC, Canzanello VJ, et al. Hypertension after liver transplantation: a predictive role for pretreatment hemodynamics and effects of isradipine on the systemic and renal circulations. Am J Hypertens 2000;13(3):231–9.
12. Textor SC, Taler SJ, Canzanello VJ, et al. Posttransplantation hypertension related to calcineurin inhibitors. Liver Transpl 2000;6(5):521–30.
13. Ruggenenti P, Perico N, Mosconi L, et al. Calcium channel blockers protect transplant patients from cyclosporine-induced daily renal hypoperfusion. Kidney Int 1993;43(3):706–11.
14. Bloom RD, Reese PP. Chronic kidney disease after nonrenal solid-organ transplantation. J Am Soc Nephrol 2007;18(12):3031–41.
15. Ramzy D, Rao V, Tumiati LC, et al. Role of endothelin-1 and nitric oxide bioavailability in transplant-related vascular injury: comparative effects of rapamycin and cyclosporine. Circulation 2006;114(Suppl 1):I214–9.
16. Binet I, Wallnofer A, Weber C, et al. Renal hemodynamics and pharmacokinetics of bosentan with and without cyclosporine A. Kidney Int 2000;57(1):224–31.
17. Klein IH, Abrahams AC, van ET, et al. Differential effects of acute and sustained cyclosporine and tacrolimus on sympathetic nerve activity. J Hypertens 2010; 28(9):1928–34.
18. Sturrock ND, Lang CC, Struthers AD. Cyclosporin-induced hypertension precedes renal dysfunction and sodium retention in man. J Hypertens 1993; 11(11):1209–16.

19. Margreiter R. Efficacy and safety of tacrolimus compared with cyclosporin microemulsion in renal transplantation: a randomised multicentre study. Lancet 2002;359(9308):741–6.
20. Canzanello VJ, Schwartz L, Taler SJ, et al. Evolution of cardiovascular risk after liver transplantation: a comparison of cyclosporine A and tacrolimus (FK506). Liver Transpl Surg 1997;3(1):1–9.
21. Schacke H, Docke WD, Asadullah K. Mechanisms involved in the side effects of glucocorticoids. Pharmacol Ther 2002;96(1):23–43.
22. Chobanian AV, Bakris GL, Black HR, et al. The seventh report of the Joint National Committee on Prevention, Detection, Evaluation, and Treatment of High Blood Pressure: the JNC 7 report. JAMA 2003;289(19):2560–72.
23. Textor SC, Schwartz L, Wilson DJ, et al. Systemic and renal effects of nifedipine in cyclosporine-associated hypertension. Hypertension 1994;23(Suppl 1):I220–4.
24. Neal DA, Brown MJ, Wilkinson IB, et al. Hemodynamic effects of amlodipine, bisoprolol, and lisinopril in hypertensive patients after liver transplantation. Transplantation 2004;77(5):748–50.
25. Galioto A, Angeli P, Guarda S, et al. Comparison between nifedipine and carvedilol in the treatment of de novo arterial hypertension after liver transplantation: preliminary results of a controlled clinical trial. Transplant Proc 2005;37(2):1245–7.
26. Ojo AO, Held PJ, Port FK, et al. Chronic renal failure after transplantation of a nonrenal organ. N Engl J Med 2003;349(10):931–40.
27. O'Riordan A, Wong V, McCormick PA, et al. Chronic kidney disease post-liver transplantation. Nephrol Dial Transplant 2006;21(9):2630–6.
28. Sharma P, Welch K, Eikstadt R, et al. Renal outcomes after liver transplantation in the model for end-stage liver disease era. Liver Transpl 2009;15(9):1142–8.
29. Campbell MS, Kotlyar DS, Brensinger CM, et al. Renal function after orthotopic liver transplantation is predicted by duration of pretransplantation creatinine elevation. Liver Transpl 2005;11(9):1048–55.
30. Pawarode A, Fine DM, Thuluvath PJ. Independent risk factors and natural history of renal dysfunction in liver transplant recipients. Liver Transpl 2003;9(7):741–7.
31. Guitard J, Ribes D, Kamar N, et al. Predictive factors for chronic renal failure one year after orthotopic liver transplantation. Ren Fail 2006;28(5):419–25.
32. Gonwa TA, Mai ML, Melton LB, et al. End-stage renal disease (ESRD) after orthotopic liver transplantation (OLTX) using calcineurin-based immunotherapy: risk of development and treatment. Transplantation 2001;72(12):1934–9.
33. McGuire BM, Julian BA, Bynon JS, et al. Brief communication: glomerulonephritis in patients with hepatitis C cirrhosis undergoing liver transplantation. Ann Intern Med 2006;144(10):735–41.
34. Randhawa P, Brennan DC. BK virus infection in transplant recipients: an overview and update. Am J Transplant 2006;6(9):2000–5.
35. Fisher NC, Nightingale PG, Gunson BK, et al. Chronic renal failure following liver transplantation: a retrospective analysis. Transplantation 1998;66(1):59–66.
36. Moreno JM, Ruiz MC, Ruiz N, et al. Modulation factors of oxidative status in stable renal transplantation. Transplant Proc 2005;37(3):1428–30.
37. Langham RG, Egan MK, Dowling JP, et al. Transforming growth factor-beta1 and tumor growth factor-beta-inducible gene-H3 in nonrenal transplant cyclosporine nephropathy. Transplantation 2001;72(11):1826–9.

38. Deniz H, Ogutmen B, Cakalagaoglu F, et al. Inhibition of the renin angiotensin system decreases fibrogenic cytokine expression in tacrolimus nephrotoxicity in rats. Transplant Proc 2006;38(2):483–6.
39. Hirose R, Roberts JP, Quan D, et al. Experience with daclizumab in liver transplantation: renal transplant dosing without calcineurin inhibitors is insufficient to prevent acute rejection in liver transplantation. Transplantation 2000;69(2):307–11.
40. Yoshida EM, Marotta PJ, Greig PD, et al. Evaluation of renal function in liver transplant recipients receiving daclizumab (Zenapax), mycophenolate mofetil, and a delayed, low-dose tacrolimus regimen vs. a standard-dose tacrolimus and mycophenolate mofetil regimen: a multicenter randomized clinical trial. Liver Transpl 2005;11(9):1064–72.
41. Artz MA, Hilbrands LB, Borm G, et al. Blockade of the renin-angiotensin system increases graft survival in patients with chronic allograft nephropathy. Nephrol Dial Transplant 2004;19(11):2852–7.
42. Orlando G, Baiocchi L, Cardillo A, et al. Switch to 1.5 grams MMF monotherapy for CNI-related toxicity in liver transplantation is safe and improves renal function, dyslipidemia, and hypertension. Liver Transpl 2007;13(1):46–54.
43. Soliman T, Hetz H, Burghuber C, et al. Short-term induction therapy with anti-thymocyte globulin and delayed use of calcineurin inhibitors in orthotopic liver transplantation. Liver Transpl 2007;13(7):1039–44.
44. Reich DJ, Clavien PA, Hodge EE. Mycophenolate mofetil for renal dysfunction in liver transplant recipients on cyclosporine or tacrolimus: randomized, prospective, multicenter pilot study results. Transplantation 2005;80(1):18–25.
45. Nair S, Eason J, Loss G. Sirolimus monotherapy in nephrotoxicity due to calcineurin inhibitors in liver transplant recipients. Liver Transpl 2003;9(2):126–9.
46. DuBay D, Smith RJ, Qiu KG, et al. Sirolimus in liver transplant recipients with renal dysfunction offers no advantage over low-dose calcineurin inhibitor regimens. Liver Transpl 2008;14(5):651–9.
47. Harper SJ, Gelson W, Harper IG, et al. Switching to sirolimus-based immune suppression after liver transplantation is safe and effective: a single-center experience. Transplantation 2011;91(1):128–32.
48. Cravedi P, Ruggenenti P, Remuzzi G. Sirolimus for calcineurin inhibitors in organ transplantation: contra. Kidney Int 2010;78(11):1068–74.
49. Gonwa TA, Mai ML, Klintmalm GB. Chronic renal failure after transplantation of a nonrenal organ. N Engl J Med 2003;349(26):2563–5.
50. Saliba F, Lakehal M, Pageaux GP, et al. Risk factors for new-onset diabetes mellitus following liver transplantation and impact of hepatitis C infection: an observational multicenter study. Liver Transpl 2007;13(1):136–44.
51. Kuo HT, Sampaio MS, Ye X, et al. Risk factors for new-onset diabetes mellitus in adult liver transplant recipients, an analysis of the Organ Procurement and Transplant Network/United Network for Organ Sharing database. Transplantation 2010;89(9):1134–40.
52. Navasa M, Bustamante J, Marroni C, et al. Diabetes mellitus after liver transplantation: prevalence and predictive factors. J Hepatol 1996;25(1):64–71.
53. Rakel A, Karelis AD. New-onset diabetes after transplantation: risk factors and clinical impact. Diabetes Metab 2011;37(1):1–14.
54. Baid S, Cosimi AB, Farrell ML, et al. Posttransplant diabetes mellitus in liver transplant recipients: risk factors, temporal relationship with hepatitis C virus allograft hepatitis, and impact on mortality. Transplantation 2001;72(6):1066–72.
55. John PR, Thuluvath PJ. Outcome of liver transplantation in patients with diabetes mellitus: a case-control study. Hepatology 2001;34(5):889–95.

56. John PR, Thuluvath PJ. Outcome of patients with new-onset diabetes mellitus after liver transplantation compared with those without diabetes mellitus. Liver Transpl 2002;8(8):708–13.
57. Veldt BJ, Poterucha JJ, Watt KD, et al. Insulin resistance, serum adipokines and risk of fibrosis progression in patients transplanted for hepatitis C. Am J Transplant 2009;9(6):1406–13.
58. Vincenti F, Friman S, Scheuermann E, et al. Results of an international, randomized trial comparing glucose metabolism disorders and outcome with cyclosporine versus tacrolimus. Am J Transplant 2007;7(6):1506–14.
59. van Hooff JP, Christiaans MH, van Duijnhoven EM. Tacrolimus and posttransplant diabetes mellitus in renal transplantation. Transplantation 2005;79(11):1465–9.
60. Vivarelli M, Dazzi A, Cucchetti A, et al. Sirolimus in liver transplant recipients: a large single-center experience. Transplant Proc 2010;42(7):2579–84.
61. Gado-Borrego A, Casson D, Schoenfeld D, et al. Hepatitis C virus is independently associated with increased insulin resistance after liver transplantation. Transplantation 2004;77(5):703–10.
62. Wilkinson A, Davidson J, Dotta F, et al. Guidelines for the treatment and management of new-onset diabetes after transplantation. Clin Transplant 2005;19(3):291–8.
63. Marchetti P. New-onset diabetes after liver transplantation: from pathogenesis to management. Liver Transpl 2005;11(6):612–20.
64. Nathan DM, Buse JB, Davidson MB, et al. Medical management of hyperglycemia in type 2 diabetes: a consensus algorithm for the initiation and adjustment of therapy: a consensus statement of the American Diabetes Association and the European Association for the Study of Diabetes. Diabetes Care 2009; 32(1):193–203.
65. Rodbard HW, Jellinger PS, Davidson JA, et al. Statement by an American Association of Clinical Endocrinologists/American College of Endocrinology consensus panel on type 2 diabetes mellitus: an algorithm for glycemic control. Endocr Pract 2009;15(6):540–59.
66. Clore JN, Thurby-Hay L. Glucocorticoid-induced hyperglycemia. Endocr Pract 2009;15(5):469–74.
67. Gisbert C, Prieto M, Berenguer M, et al. Hyperlipidemia in liver transplant recipients: prevalence and risk factors. Liver Transpl Surg 1997;3(4):416–22.
68. McCashland TM, Donovan JP, Amelsberg A, et al. Bile acid metabolism and biliary secretion in patients receiving orthotopic liver transplants: differing effects of cyclosporine and FK 506. Hepatology 1994;19(6):1381–9.
69. Rayyes OA, Wallmark A, Floren CH. Cyclosporine inhibits catabolism of low-density lipoproteins in HepG2 cells by about 25%. Hepatology 1996;24(3):613–9.
70. Trotter JF, Wachs ME, Trouillot TE, et al. Dyslipidemia during sirolimus therapy in liver transplant recipients occurs with concomitant cyclosporine but not tacrolimus. Liver Transpl 2001;7(5):401–8.
71. Morrisett JD, Abdel-Fattah G, Kahan BD. Sirolimus changes lipid concentrations and lipoprotein metabolism in kidney transplant recipients. Transplant Proc 2003;35(Suppl 3):143S–50S.
72. Grundy SM, Cleeman JI, Merz CN, et al. Implications of recent clinical trials for the National Cholesterol Education Program Adult Treatment Panel III Guidelines. J Am Coll Cardiol 2004;44(3):720–32.
73. Imagawa DK, Dawson S III, Holt CD, et al. Hyperlipidemia after liver transplantation: natural history and treatment with the hydroxy-methylglutaryl-coenzyme A reductase inhibitor pravastatin. Transplantation 1996;62(7):934–42.

74. Asberg A. Interactions between cyclosporin and lipid-lowering drugs: implications for organ transplant recipients. Drugs 2003;63(4):367–78.
75. Goldberg R, Roth D. Evaluation of fluvastatin in the treatment of hypercholesterolemia in renal transplant recipients taking cyclosporine. Transplantation 1996; 62(11):1559–64.
76. Neal DA, Gimson AE, Gibbs P, et al. Beneficial effects of converting liver transplant recipients from cyclosporine to tacrolimus on blood pressure, serum lipids, and weight. Liver Transpl 2001;7(6):533–9.
77. Langone AJ, Chuang P. Ezetimibe in renal transplant patients with hyperlipidemia resistant to HMG-CoA reductase inhibitors. Transplantation 2006;81(5): 804–7.
78. Almutairi F, Peterson TC, Molinari M, et al. Safety and effectiveness of ezetimibe in liver transplant recipients with hypercholesterolemia. Liver Transpl 2009; 15(5):504–8.
79. Vogt A, Kassner U, Hostalek U, et al. Evaluation of the safety and tolerability of prolonged-release nicotinic acid in a usual care setting: the NAUTILUS study. Curr Med Res Opin 2006;22(2):417–25.
80. Watts NB, Bilezikian JP, Camacho PM, et al. American Association of Clinical Endocrinologists Medical Guidelines for Clinical Practice for the diagnosis and treatment of postmenopausal osteoporosis. Endocr Pract 2010;16(Suppl): 31–7.
81. Guichelaar MM, Schmoll J, Malinchoc M, et al. Fractures and avascular necrosis before and after orthotopic liver transplantation: long-term follow-up and predictive factors. Hepatology 2007;46(4):1198–207.
82. Guichelaar MM, Kendall R, Malinchoc M, et al. Bone mineral density before and after OLT: long-term follow-up and predictive factors. Liver Transpl 2006;12(9): 1390–402.
83. Eastell R, Dickson ER, Hodgson SF, et al. Rates of vertebral bone loss before and after liver transplantation in women with primary biliary cirrhosis. Hepatology 1991;14(2):296–300.
84. Atamaz F, Hepguler S, Akyildiz M, et al. Effects of alendronate on bone mineral density and bone metabolic markers in patients with liver transplantation. Osteoporos Int 2006;17(6):942–9.
85. Feller RB, McDonald JA, Sherbon KJ, et al. Evidence of continuing bone recovery at a mean of 7 years after liver transplantation. Liver Transpl Surg 1999;5(5):407–13.
86. Monegal A, Navasa M, Guanabens N, et al. Bone disease after liver transplantation: a long-term prospective study of bone mass changes, hormonal status and histomorphometric characteristics. Osteoporos Int 2001;12(6):484–92.
87. Compston JE. Osteoporosis after liver transplantation. Liver Transpl 2003;9(4): 321–30.
88. Collier J. Bone disorders in chronic liver disease. Hepatology 2007;46(4): 1271–8.
89. Guanabens N, Pares A. Liver and bone. Arch Biochem Biophys 2010;503(1): 84–94.
90. Ninkovic M, Love SA, Tom B, et al. High prevalence of osteoporosis in patients with chronic liver disease prior to liver transplantation. Calcif Tissue Int 2001; 69(6):321–6.
91. Monegal A, Navasa M, Guanabens N, et al. Bone mass and mineral metabolism in liver transplant patients treated with FK506 or cyclosporine A. Calcif Tissue Int 2001;68(2):83–6.

92. Weiler N, Thrun I, Hoppe-Lotichius M, et al. Early steroid-free immunosuppression with FK506 after liver transplantation: long-term results of a prospectively randomized double-blinded trial. Transplantation 2010;90(12):1562–6.
93. Goodman GR, Dissanayake IR, Sodam BR, et al. Immunosuppressant use without bone loss–implications for bone loss after transplantation. J Bone Miner Res 2001;16(1):72–8.
94. Dissanayake IR, Goodman GR, Bowman AR, et al. Mycophenolate mofetil: a promising new immunosuppressant that does not cause bone loss in the rat. Transplantation 1998;65(2):275–8.
95. Kasturi KS, Chennareddygari S, Mummadi RR. Effect of bisphosphonates on bone mineral density in liver transplant patients: a meta-analysis and systematic review of randomized controlled trials. Transpl Int 2010;23(2):200–7.
96. Crawford BA, Kam C, Pavlovic J, et al. Zoledronic acid prevents bone loss after liver transplantation: a randomized, double-blind, placebo-controlled trial. Ann Intern Med 2006;144(4):239–48.
97. Kaemmerer D, Lehmann G, Wolf G, et al. Treatment of osteoporosis after liver transplantation with ibandronate. Transpl Int 2010;23(7):753–9.
98. Monegal A, Guanabens N, Suarez MJ, et al. Pamidronate in the prevention of bone loss after liver transplantation: a randomized controlled trial. Transpl Int 2009;22(2):198–206.
99. Chak E, Saab S. Risk factors and incidence of de novo malignancy in liver transplant recipients: a systematic review. Liver Int 2010;30(9):1247–58.
100. Feng S, Buell JF, Chari RS, et al. Tumors and transplantation: the 2003 Third Annual ASTS State-of-the-Art Winter Symposium. Am J Transplant 2003;3(12):1481–7.
101. Oo YH, Gunson BK, Lancashire RJ, et al. Incidence of cancers following orthotopic liver transplantation in a single center: comparison with national cancer incidence rates for England and Wales. Transplantation 2005;80(6):759–64.
102. Kenngott S, Gerbes AL, Schauer R, et al. Rapid development of esophageal squamous cell carcinoma after liver transplantation for alcohol-induced cirrhosis. Transpl Int 2003;16(9):639–41.
103. Dantal J, Hourmant M, Cantarovich D, et al. Effect of long-term immunosuppression in kidney-graft recipients on cancer incidence: randomised comparison of two cyclosporin regimens. Lancet 1998;351(9103):623–8.
104. Ingvar A, Smedby KE, Lindelof B, et al. Immunosuppressive treatment after solid organ transplantation and risk of post-transplant cutaneous squamous cell carcinoma. Nephrol Dial Transplant 2010;25(8):2764–71.
105. Haagsma EB, Hagens VE, Schaapveld M, et al. Increased cancer risk after liver transplantation: a population-based study. J Hepatol 2001;34(1):84–91.
106. Jonas S, Rayes N, Neumann U, et al. De novo malignancies after liver transplantation using tacrolimus-based protocols or cyclosporine-based quadruple immunosuppression with an interleukin-2 receptor antibody or antithymocyte globulin. Cancer 1997;80(6):1141–50.
107. Lake JR, David KM, Steffen BJ, et al. Addition of MMF to dual immunosuppression does not increase the risk of malignant short-term death after liver transplantation. Am J Transplant 2005;5(12):2961–7.
108. Gutierrez-Dalmau A, Campistol JM. The role of proliferation signal inhibitors in post-transplant malignancies. Nephrol Dial Transplant 2007;22(Suppl 1):i11–6.
109. Herrero JI, Espana A, Quiroga J, et al. Nonmelanoma skin cancer after liver transplantation. Study of risk factors. Liver Transpl 2005;11(9):1100–6.
110. Sanchez EQ, Marubashi S, Jung G, et al. De novo tumors after liver transplantation: a single-institution experience. Liver Transpl 2002;8(3):285–91.

111. Euvrard S, Kanitakis J, Claudy A. Skin cancers after organ transplantation. N Engl J Med 2003;348(17):1681–91.

112. Baccarani U, Adani GL, Serraino D, et al. De novo tumors are a major cause of late mortality after orthotopic liver transplantation. Transplant Proc 2009;41(4): 1303–5.

113. Ulrich C, Jurgensen JS, Degen A, et al. Prevention of non-melanoma skin cancer in organ transplant patients by regular use of a sunscreen: a 24 months, prospective, case-control study. Br J Dermatol 2009;161(Suppl):378–84.

114. Jain A, DiMartini A, Kashyap R, et al. Long-term follow-up after liver transplantation for alcoholic liver disease under tacrolimus. Transplantation 2000;70(9): 1335–42.

115. Duvoux C, Delacroix I, Richardet JP, et al. Increased incidence of oropharyngeal squamous cell carcinomas after liver transplantation for alcoholic cirrhosis. Transplantation 1999;67(3):418–21.

116. Trotter JF, Brazer SR. Rapid progression to high-grade dysplasia in Barrett's esophagus after liver transplantation. Liver Transpl Surg 1999;5(4):332–3.

117. Marques ME, Jimenez RC, Gomez de la CA, et al. Malignancy after liver transplantation: cumulative risk for development. Transplant Proc 2009;41(6): 2447–9.

118. Fraile P, Garcia-Cosmes P, Martin P, et al. Non-skin solid tumors as a cause of morbidity and mortality after liver transplantation. Transplant Proc 2009;41(6): 2433–4.

119. Sint NJ, de Jonge V, Steyerberg EW, et al. Risk of colorectal carcinoma in post-liver transplant patients: a systematic review and meta-analysis. Am J Transplant 2010;10(4):868–76.

120. Higashi H, Yanaga K, Marsh JW, et al. Development of colon cancer after liver transplantation for primary sclerosing cholangitis associated with ulcerative colitis. Hepatology 1990;11(3):477–80.

121. McGuire BM, Rosenthal P, Brown CC, et al. Long-term management of the liver transplant patient: recommendations for the primary care doctor. Am J Transplant 2009;9(9):1988–2003.

122. Sethi A, Stravitz RT. Review article: medical management of the liver transplant recipient—a primer for non-transplant doctors. Aliment Pharmacol Ther 2007; 25(3):229–45.

123. Paya CV, Fung JJ, Nalesnik MA, et al. Epstein-Barr virus-induced posttransplant lymphoproliferative disorders. Transplantation 1999;68(10):1517–25.

124. Kremers WK, Devarbhavi HC, Wiesner RH, et al. Post-transplant lymphoproliferative disorders following liver transplantation: incidence, risk factors and survival. Am J Transplant 2006;6(5 Pt 1):1017–24.

125. Burra P, Buda A, Livi U, et al. Occurrence of post-transplant lymphoproliferative disorders among over thousand adult recipients: any role for hepatitis C infection? Eur J Gastroenterol Hepatol 2006;18(10):1065–70.

126. Ben Ari Z, Amlot P, Lachmanan SR, et al. Posttransplantation lymphoproliferative disorder in liver recipients: characteristics, management, and outcome. Liver Transpl Surg 1999;5(3):184–91.

127. McCarthy M, Ramage J, McNair A, et al. The clinical diversity and role of chemotherapy in lymphoproliferative disorder in liver transplant recipients. J Hepatol 1997;27(6):1015–21.

128. Starzl TE, Nalesnik MA, Porter KA, et al. Reversibility of lymphomas and lymphoproliferative lesions developing under cyclosporin-steroid therapy. Lancet 1984; 1(8377):583–7.

129. Dotti G, Fiocchi R, Motta T, et al. Lymphomas occurring late after solid-organ transplantation: influence of treatment on the clinical outcome. Transplantation 2002;74(8):1095–102.
130. Herrero JI, Alegre F, Quiroga J, et al. Usefulness of a program of neoplasia surveillance in liver transplantation. A preliminary report. Clin Transplant 2009; 23(4):532–6.
131. Finkenstedt A, Graziadei IW, Oberaigner W, et al. Extensive surveillance promotes early diagnosis and improved survival of de novo malignancies in liver transplant recipients. Am J Transplant 2009;9(10):2355–61.
132. Johnson EE, Leverson GE, Pirsch JD, et al. A 30-year analysis of colorectal adenocarcinoma in transplant recipients and proposal for altered screening. J Gastrointest Surg 2007;11(3):272–9.

Management of Recurrent Hepatitis C Infection after Liver Transplantation

Alpna R. Limaye, MD, Roberto J. Firpi, MD*

KEYWORDS

- Hepatitis C • Liver transplant • Recurrent • Management

Chronic hepatitis C virus (HCV) infection affects approximately 3% of the world's population, with cirrhosis caused by chronic HCV the most frequent indication for liver transplantation (LT) in the United States and Europe.[1] Between 1999 and 2007, 37% to 41% of all recipients of LT in the United States had chronic HCV.[2] However, survival of LT recipients with chronic HCV remains lower than that of recipients without HCV. This decreased survival is related to the near-universal recurrence of HCV after transplantation as well as the accelerated course of recurrent HCV after LT.[3] Between 25% and 30% of LT recipients with HCV develop graft cirrhosis, with a median time to recurrent cirrhosis of 8 to 10 years.[4,5] The clinical outcomes of these patients, and the likelihood of graft cirrhosis, are affected by multiple factors, including donor demographics, recipient virological status, posttransplant immunosuppression, and antiviral therapy. This article reviews the natural history and management of HCV following LT.

POSTTRANSPLANT RECURRENCE OF HEPATITIS C
Viral Kinetics

LT recipients with actively replicating HCV experience a rapid reduction in HCV RNA levels on removal of the infected native liver, with a half-life of less than 1 hour.[6] This is followed by a rapid increase in viral load as the new graft is infected by circulating virions. Post-LT viral loads reach pretransplant levels (or more) within 1 to 5 days.[6] A new viral load steady state is achieved within 1 to 3 months, and this new steady state is typically 1 to 2 logs higher than the pre-LT viral load.[6,7] It also seems that those

The authors have nothing to disclose.

Division of Gastroenterology, Hepatology, and Nutrition, Department of Medicine, University of Florida College of Medicine, 1600 South West Archer Road, Room HD 602, PO Box 100214, Gainesville, FL 32610, USA

* Corresponding author.

E-mail address: Roberto.Firpi@medicine.ufl.edu

Clin Liver Dis 15 (2011) 845–858

doi:10.1016/j.cld.2011.08.003

1089-3261/11/$ – see front matter Published by Elsevier Inc.

recipients with higher pre-LT viral loads reach the new post-LT steady state more rapidly[6] and have higher viral loads at 4 months after LT.[8]

Although HCV reinfection is inevitable in viremic LT recipients, the clinical course of these patients is variable. Although reports of spontaneous clearance of HCV after LT have been published,[9] and some LT recipients with HCV experience an indolent course, those who develop graft cirrhosis typically do so rapidly.[4,5] A small percentage of patients experience a severe form of recurrent HCV, fibrosing cholestatic hepatitis, characterized by cholestasis, hepatocyte ballooning, and rapid progression to graft failure.[6,10]

Donor-related and Surgical Predictors of Recurrence

Given the variable, but often aggressive, course of recurrent HCV, factors that predict severe recurrence of HCV and mortality are of major interest. The donor-related factor that is the major predictor of severe recurrence and progression to graft cirrhosis and graft failure is donor age.[11-13] A review of the United Network for Organ Sharing (UNOS) Liver Transplant Registry (LTR) data showed that donor age greater than 50 years was an independent predictor of recipient death or graft failure within 1 year of LT.[14] A smaller study found that donor age less than 30 years predicted improved graft survival in recipients with chronic HCV.[13]

The worldwide donor shortage has prompted the use of so-called extended criteria donors, including donation after cardiac death (DCD) and living-donor LT (LDLT). DCD transplantation may be an independent predictor of decreased graft and overall survival in patients undergoing LT for HCV,[15] although a more recent, smaller study failed to show a statistically significant difference.[16] Use of liver grafts from DCD donors for LT may diminish survival due an increased frequency of ischemic biliary complications and hepatic abscesses.[15] For this reason, many authorities question the wisdom of using organs from DCD donors in HCV-infected recipients.

There have also been concerns regarding the use of LDLT in HCV recipients. A recent retrospective review of the Adult-to-Adult Living Donor Transplantation Cohort showed that patients with HCV who receive living-donor transplants had a higher mortality hazard ratio than those receiving deceased-donor transplants.[17] However, this negative effect is likely related to surgical experience with LDLT, because analyses that take center experience into account do not show a difference in graft and overall survival between patients with HCV receiving living-donor and deceased-donor transplants.[18-21] Although the use of LDLT has become limited because of concerns about donor morbidity and mortality, its use for HCV recipients seems to be supported by the current literature.

Other potential donor-related and surgical factors remain controversial. Concerns about donor graft macrosteatosis have prompted several groups to investigate the effects of donor steatosis on outcomes of LT in patients with HCV. Although a recent study reported more frequent and rapid recurrence of HCV in patients who received grafts with greater than 30% steatosis, protocol biopsies were not used to clearly define an increase in fibrosis progression.[22] Another study in the same year, which used protocol biopsies, did not show an increase in fibrosis progression in HCV-infected recipients who had received mildly to moderately steatotic grafts.[23] Several studies have reported poor outcomes in grafts with prolonged cold ischemic time, particularly in advanced-donor-age grafts,[24,25] and the presence of preservation injury seems to predict rapid HCV recurrence in patients with stage 2 or greater fibrosis on 1-year protocol liver biopsy.[26] Larger prospective studies are needed to determine whether donor grafts with significant steatosis or preservation injury should be avoided in patients with HCV.

Recipient-related Predictors of Recurrence

Multiple recipient-related factors have been suggested as predictors of severe recurrence of HCV, graft failure, and poor patient survival in those undergoing LT for HCV. These factors include advanced age, female gender, coinfection with human immunodeficiency virus (HIV) or cytomegalovirus (CMV), the presence of metabolic syndrome, and high pretransplant HCV viral loads.[27–32] Recent evidence indicates that the presence of the interleukin-28b (IL-28b) TT allele may be associated with more rapid fibrosis (although specific IL-28b genotype did not seem to be predictive of survival).[33]

Immunosuppressive Regimens

The management of post-LT patients with HCV is complicated by the need for balanced immunosuppression to prevent rejection while allowing adequate immune control of HCV replication. Early acute cellular rejection has been shown to be associated with an increased mortality risk in patients who have undergone LT for HCV.[34] However, treatment of acute cellular rejection, including bolused high-dose corticosteroids[35] (mean daily dose of 100 mg daily or greater in the first 42 days after LT), anti-lymphocyte antibodies, and anti–interleukin-2 receptor antibodies,[36] are linked to higher rates of progression to cirrhosis, graft failure, and severe cholestatic HCV recurrence. A recent meta-analysis of randomized controlled trials concluded that steroid-free immunosuppression regimens were associated with fewer episodes of acute rejection, HCV recurrence, and acute graft hepatitis.[37] However, these conclusions are limited by the variability of immunosuppression regimens used in the various trials.

Whether specific immunosuppression regimens differentially affect HCV recurrence outcomes remains controversial. One meta-analysis of 16 randomized controlled trials found that mortality and graft failure at 1 year were significantly reduced in patients who had received tacrolimus compared with cyclosporine (although this study did not specifically address the outcomes in patients with HCV).[38] A subsequent meta-analysis of 5 randomized controlled trials found no difference in mortality, graft survival, acute rejection, or cholestatic hepatitis in patients treated with tacrolimus compared with cyclosporine.[39]

Recent prospective randomized trials have also yielded conflicting results. In the 12-month follow-up analysis of data from a multicenter prospective, randomized trial, one group reported a higher rate of mortality and graft loss in patients who had received tacrolimus compared with cyclosporine, but with similar rates of histologic HCV recurrence in both groups.[40] A subsequent prospective randomized trial comparing tacrolimus monotherapy with combination therapy with tacrolimus, azathioprine, and short-term steroids found slower fibrosis progression in patients receiving triple therapy.[41] In contrast, a recent prospective study with protocol liver biopsies found no differences in severe recurrent HCV (defined as bridging fibrosis, cirrhosis, cholestatic hepatitis, graft failure, or death related to recurrent disease) or overall survival in those receiving cyclosporine compared with those receiving tacrolimus.[42]

There is some evidence that the choice of calcineurin inhibitor may affect the efficacy of antiviral therapy for recurrent HCV. Several recent retrospective studies have shown that patients after LT undergoing antiviral therapy for recurrent HCV are more likely to achieve sustained virological response (SVR) if they are on cyclosporine compared with tacrolimus.[43,44] A recent prospective randomized pilot study showed that a change in immunosuppression from tacrolimus to cyclosporine was associated with higher SVR rates.[45] In addition, it seems that the IL-28b CC genotype in either the donor or the recipient is associated with increased rates of SVR after antiviral therapy for recurrent HCV.[33]

Although preliminary data indicate that switching to cyclosporine may be beneficial when antiviral therapy for recurrent HCV is being considered, there is insufficient evidence that one immunosuppressive regimen is superior to another. It seems that avoidance of more intense immunosuppression might be more important than specific immunosuppressive regimen.

DIAGNOSIS OF POSTTRANSPLANT RECURRENT HCV

The gold standard for diagnosis and staging of recurrent HCV remains the liver biopsy with trichrome staining. Multiple studies have investigated the usefulness of noninvasive testing such as transient elastography[46] and serum biomarkers of fibrosis,[47,48] but, until these noninvasive tests are validated, protocol liver biopsy should be obtained at least yearly to assess recurrent HCV and determine the timing of antiviral therapy.

ANTIVIRAL THERAPY
Pretransplant Antiviral Therapy

The goal of HCV treatment is achieving SVR, which is associated with improved clinical outcomes.[49,50] Achievement of SVR before LT in patients with HCV seems to be associated with lower rates of virological and histologic recurrence.[51] However, the treatment of HCV in the setting of even compensated cirrhosis with pegylated interferon and ribavirin yields SVR rates of only 11% to 22%.[52,53] The likelihood of achieving SVR is even lower in decompensated cirrhotic patients (who comprise most of the patients awaiting liver transplantation).[53] Furthermore, the treatment of patients with decompensated cirrhosis in a pilot study was associated with high rates of serious complications including treatment-related mortality.[54] The evidence to date indicates that HCV treatment with pegylated interferon and ribavirin in Child B or C cirrhosis is associated with unacceptably high risks with a low likelihood of achieving SVR. Treatment of patients with Child A or early Child B cirrhosis should be undertaken only by experienced hepatologists in collaboration with transplant centers.

Preemptive Posttransplant Antiviral Therapy

The decreased rates of complications seen in patients with HCV who achieve SVR led to the theory that treatment of HCV in the early posttransplant period, before histologic recurrence, might be beneficial. Several groups have investigated this so-called preemptive therapy strategy. However, the results have been disappointing, with rates of SVR ranging from 5% to 24%.[55-57] Although one retrospective study indicated that the benefits of preemptive therapy might be seen even in those patients who do not achieve SVR, these results failed to reach statistical significance.

Beyond the question of efficacy is the issue of tolerability. Patients in the immediate posttransplant period (within 3 weeks of transplantation) often lack the cell count stability, renal function, and/or clinical stability to tolerate full-dose HCV therapy.[57] Rates of early discontinuation of therapy in this population are reported to be as high as 37%.[57-59] For this reason, some centers have investigated the use of preemptive therapy 3 to 6 months after LT,[60,61] as well as the use of escalated dosing of pegylated interferon.[60] These strategies seem to be more tolerable, with early discontinuation rates of 11.5% to 13%, but SVR rates remained modest, particularly for patients with genotype 1 (13%–35%).[60,61] A recent meta-analysis failed to identify any studies of preemptive therapy that met inclusion criteria for study quality.[62] Based on the current literature, preemptive therapy should only be considered in those patients at high risk of severe recurrent disease.

Treatment of Established Recurrent HCV

Given the unproven efficacy and limited tolerability of early preemptive therapy, treatment is primarily focused on patients with established histologic HCV recurrence. Most centers advocate treatment of patients with significant histologic recurrence, defined by the International Liver Transplantation Society as grade III to IV (moderate to severe) inflammation or stage II fibrosis.[6] This approach centers on the use of both protocol and clinically indicated liver biopsies to identify patients with significant recurrence. As with any decision to initiate HCV therapy, comorbidities that predict tolerance of pegylated interferon and ribavirin must be taken into consideration. Achievement of SVR in these patients does seem to be durable and associated with improvement in histology, so this should be the goal in all patients with clinically significant post-LT recurrence of HCV.[63]

Early studies of therapy for recurrent HCV used either interferon monotherapy (pegylated interferon α-2a[57] or standard interferon α-2a[64,65]) or interferon (pegylated interferon or standard interferon) plus ribavirin.[66–72] Interferon monotherapy (either standard or pegylated) seems to have limited efficacy. The combination of standard interferon and ribavirin yields SVR rates of 7% to 33%, but tolerance is variable (discontinuation rates of 30%–50%).[66–72] Data after the introduction of pegylated interferon reveal that the combination of pegylated interferon and ribavirin seems to be more effective.

Multiple studies in the past decade have investigated the efficacy and safety of pegylated interferon and ribavirin to treat recurrent HCV (**Table 1**). These studies have reported end-of-treatment response (ETR) rates of 28% to 68% and SVR rates of 23% to 45%.[73–80] Tolerance was variable in these studies, with 1 study reporting all 25 patients completing therapy as intended,[77] but others reporting 20% to 40% of patients requiring discontinuation of therapy secondary to adverse effects.[73–76] In an attempt to synthesize composite data regarding the combination treatment of recurrent HCV, a recent systematic review examined the available literature.[81] A total of 611 patients pooled from 19 trials were included in the analysis (including 2 trials that treated patients in the acute phase of recurrent HCV). The composite SVR in patients treated with pegylated interferon and ribavirin was 30.2%, and 27.6% of patients required discontinuation of therapy secondary to adverse effects.[81] Factors that seemed predictive of achieving SVR included early virological response (at 3 months of treatment), treatment adherence (often entailing the use of growth factors), HCV genotype 2, and low pretreatment HCV viral loads.[81]

Despite the low rates of virological response in patients after LT with recurrent HCV, SVR remains the primary goal, because it does seem to be associated with improved graft survival[63,82–84] and overall patient survival.[84,85] However, evidence exists of histologic benefits in this patient population even in the absence of SVR.[80,86] These data have prompted some to advocate the use of long-term maintenance antiviral therapy in those who do not achieve SVR. An early pilot study evaluated the use of long-term antiviral therapy in those with an ETR, and found improvement of inflammation and fibrosis scores in these patients.[87] A more recent retrospective study showed a slower rate of fibrosis progression in patients who did not achieve SVR but who received at least 6 months of maintenance antiviral therapy.[88] Prospective, controlled data are needed to determine whether this approach results in improved graft and patient survival.

Table 1
Summary of recent data regarding treatment of established recurrent HCV with combination pegylated interferon and ribavirin therapy

Investigators [Reference Number]	Study Year	Study Design	Number of Subjects	Treatment Regimen	Intended Treatment Duration	ETR with ITT Analysis (%)	SVR with ITT Analysis (%)	Histologic Response	Tolerance	Acute Rejection
Sharma et al[73]	2007	Retrospective	35	PEG-IFNα2a 180 μg/d/wk or PEG-IFNα2b 1.5 μg/kg/wk and RBV 800 mg/d	46 wk	54	37	N/A	43% discontinued therapy secondary to AEs	11% with mild to moderate acute rejection
Dumortier et al[74]	2004	Pilot study	20	Escalating dosages: PEG-IFN 0.5 μg/kg/wk for 4 wk, then 1 μg/kg/wk for duration and RBV 400 mg/d for 4 wk, then 1000–1200 mg/d for duration	12 months	55	45	Mean METAVIR score improved from A1.8F2.2 to A03.F1.6 after treatment	20% discontinued therapy secondary to AEs	25% with mild acute rejection (resolved with enhancement of IS regimen)
Oton et al[75]	2006	Prospective observation	55	PEG-IFNα2a 180 μg/kg/wk or PEG-IFNα2b 1.5 μg/kg/wk and weight-dosed RBV (800–1200 mg/d)	Genotype 1 or 4: 48 wk Genotype 2 or 3: 24 wk	65	44	15 cases with data: HAI improved from 7.3 ± 1.6 to 4.2 ± 3.1 after treatment; no difference in fibrosis	29% discontinued therapy secondary to AEs 11% discontinued secondary to nonresponse	0%

Fernandez et al[76]	2006	Prospective observation	47	PEG-IFN 1.5 µg/kg/wk and weight-dosed RBV (600–1000 mg/d)	48 wk	36	23	16 cases with data: improved inflammation and no change in fibrosis in responders. No change in inflammation or fibrosis in nonresponders	21% discontinued therapy secondary to AEs. 32% required RBV dose reduction. 36% required darbepoetin	1 case
Neumann et al[77]	2006	Prospective observation	25	PEG-IFNα2b 1 µg/kg/wk and weight-dosed RBV (400–1000 mg/d)	48 wk	68	36	Fibrosis worsened from mean stage 1.7 to 2.0 after treatment, inflammation improved from mean grade 1.66 to 1.3 after treatment in all subjects	0% discontinued therapy. 52% required IFN dose reduction, and 36% required RBV dose reduction	0%
Mukherjee et al[78]	2006	Prospective observation	32	PEG-IFNα2a 180 µg/kg/wk and RBV 1000–1200 mg/d	48 wk		41	Progressive fibrosis in 75% of sustained responders	16% discontinued therapy secondary to AEs	
Mukherjee et al[79]	2006	Prospective observation	39	PEG-IFNα2b 1.5 µg/kg/wk and RBV 800 mg/d	Genotype 1 or 4: 1 y Genotype 2 or 3: 6 mo	28	33	17 cases with data: improved or stable fibrosis scores in 43% of nonresponders	44% discontinued therapy secondary to AEs	Not reported

(continued on next page)

Table 1
(continued)

Investigators [Reference Number]	Year	Study Design	Number of Subjects	Treatment Regimen	Intended Treatment Duration	ETR with ITT Analysis (%)	SVR with ITT Analysis (%)	Histologic Response	Tolerance	Acute Rejection
Carrion et al[80]	2007	Randomized, controlled trial	54, plus 27 patients with severe recurrence	PEG-IFNα2b 1.5 μg/kg/wk and RBV 800–1200mg/d	48 wk	N/A	48% in treated patients with mild recurrence, vs 18% in patients with severe recurrence, and 0% in control patients	26% of treated patients had improved fibrosis scores	22% of patients with mild recurrence discontinued therapy secondary to AEs (56% of those with severe recurrence)	15% of those with severe recurrence. 0% in mild recurrence

Abbreviations: AE, adverse events; ETR, end-of-treatment response; HAI, hepatic activity index; IFN, interferon; IS, immunosuppression; ITT, intention to treat; PEG, pegylated; RBV, ribavirin.

Direct-acting antiviral therapies for HCV, including the protease inhibitors telaprevir and boceprevir, were recently approved and will be routinely used for the treatment of chronic HCV. It remains to be seen whether the initial promising effects of these drugs on previous nonresponders to standard-of-care therapy[89] will also be seen in patients after LT with recurrent HCV. The potential for drug interactions with the immunosuppressants is a major concern.

RETRANSPLANTATION FOR RECURRENT HCV

As discussed earlier, progression of post-LT recurrent HCV is accelerated, with at least a quarter of patients developing graft cirrhosis, and many of these going on to develop graft failure. Given the limited efficacy and tolerability of post-LT antiviral therapy, the only definitive treatment of these patients is retransplantation (RT). Liver RT, regardless of indication, is associated with decreased graft and patient survival and more rapid progression to graft cirrhosis compared with primary LT.[90] It remains unclear whether the presence of HCV infection is an independent predictor of poor outcomes after RT, because the literature contains studies with conflicting results. Nevertheless, it seems that a history of severe recurrent HCV (with graft failure within the first year after primary LT) or a high MELD (Model for End-stage Liver Disease) score (>28) predicts a poor outcome after RT,[90,91] and therefore should likely not be pursued in these patients. Further studies are required to determine the impact of viral eradication on outcomes after RT, and to delineate the factors that predict improved survival in this population.

REFERENCES

1. World Health Organization. Available at: http://www.who.org. Accessed February 28, 2011.
2. OPTN/SRTR 2009 Annual Report. Chapter IV: liver transplantation in the United States, 1999-2008. Available at: http://optn.transplant.hrsa.gov/ar2009/Chapter_IV_AR_CD.htm. Accessed February 28, 2011.
3. Firpi RJ, Clark V, Soldevila-Pico C, et al. The natural history of hepatitis C cirrhosis after liver transplantation. Liver Transpl 2009;15(9):1063-71.
4. Neumann UP, Berg T, Bahra M, et al. Fibrosis progression after liver transplantation in patients with recurrent hepatitis C. J Hepatol 2004;41(5):830-6.
5. Sanchez-Fueyo A, Restrepo JC, Quinto L, et al. Impact of the recurrence of hepatitis C virus infection after liver transplantation on the long-term viability of the graft. Transplantation 2001;73(1):56-63.
6. Weisner RH, Sorrell M, Villamil F, International Liver Transplantation Society Expert Panel. Report of the first International Liver Transplantation Society expert panel consensus conference on liver transplantation and hepatitis C. Liver Transpl 2003;9(11):S1-9.
7. Powers KA, Ribeiro RM, Patel K, et al. Kinetics of hepatitis C virus reinfection after liver transplantation. Liver Transpl 2006;12(2):207-16.
8. Garcia-Retortillo M, Forns X, Feliu A, et al. Hepatitis C virus kinetics during and immediately after liver transplantation. Hepatology 2002;35(3):680-7.
9. Haque M, Hashim A, Greanya ED, et al. Spontaneous clearance of hepatitis C infection post-liver transplant: a rare but real phenomenon? a case report and review of the literature. Ann Hepatol 2010;9(2):202-6.
10. Sreekumar R, Gonzalez-Koch A, Maor-Kendler Y, et al. Early identification of recipients with progressive histologic recurrence of hepatitis C after liver transplantation. Hepatology 2000;32(5):1125-30.

11. Rayhill SC, Wu YM, Katz DA, et al. Older donor livers show early severe histological activity, fibrosis, and graft failure after liver transplantation for hepatitis C. Transplantation 2007;84(3):331–9.

12. Machicao VI, Bonatti H, Krishna M, et al. Donor age affects fibrosis progression and graft survival after liver transplantation for hepatitis C. Transplantation 2004; 77(1):84–92.

13. Perez-Daga JA, Ramirez-Plaza C, Suarez MA, et al. Impact of donor age on the results of liver transplantation in hepatitis C virus-positive recipients. Transplant Proc 2008;40(9):2959–61.

14. Condron SL, Heneghan MA, Patel K, et al. Effect of donor age on survival of liver transplant recipients with hepatitis C virus infection. Transplantation 2005;80(1): 145–8.

15. Yagci G, Fernandez LA, Knechtle SJ, et al. The impact of donor variables on the outcome of orthotopic liver transplantation for hepatitis C. Transplant Proc 2008; 40(1):219–23.

16. Tao R, Ruppert K, Cruz RJ Jr, et al. Hepatitis C recurrence is not adversely affected by the use of donation after cardiac death liver allografts. Liver Transpl 2010;16(11):1288–95.

17. Olthoff KM, Abecassis MM, Emond JC, et al, A2ALL Study Group. Outcomes for adult living donor liver transplantation: comparison of A2ALL and national experience. Liver Transpl 2011;17(7):789–97.

18. Kuo A, Terrault NA. Is recurrent hepatitis C worse with living donors? Curr Opin Organ Transplant 2009;14(3):240–4.

19. Russo MW, Galanko J, Beavers K, et al. Patient and graft survival in hepatitis C recipients after adult living donor liver transplantation in the United States. Liver Transpl 2004;10(3):340–6.

20. Terrault NA, Shiffman ML, Lok AS, et al, A2ALL Study Group. Outcomes in hepatitis C virus-infected recipients of living donor vs. deceased donor liver transplantation. Liver Transpl 2007;13(1):122–9.

21. Gallegos-Orozco JF, Yosephy A, Noble B, et al. Natural history of post-liver transplantation hepatitis C: a review of factors that may influence its course. Liver Transpl 2009;15(12):1872–81.

22. Briceno J, Ciria R, Pleguezuelo M, et al. Impact of donor graft steatosis on overall outcome and viral recurrence after liver transplantation for hepatitis C virus cirrhosis. Liver Transpl 2009;15(1):37–48.

23. Burra P, Loreno M, Russo FP, et al. Donor livers with steatosis are safe to use in hepatitis C virus-positive recipients. Liver Transpl 2009;15(6):619–28.

24. Reese PP, Sonawane SB, Thomasson A, et al. Donor age and cold ischemia interact to produce inferior 90-day liver allograft survival. Transplantation 2008; 85(12):1737–44.

25. Cassuto JR, Patel SA, Tsoulfas G, et al. The cumulative effects of cold ischemic time and older donor age on liver graft survival. J Surg Res 2008; 148(1):38–44.

26. Michaels A, Dhanasekaran R, Alkhasawneh A, et al. The impact of preservation injury on accelerated hepatitis C recurrence after liver transplantation [abstract: 2]. In: AASLD Abstracts. Hepatology 2010;52(Suppl 4):320A.

27. Charlton M, Ruppert K, Belle SH, et al. Long-term results and modeling to predict outcomes in recipients with HCV infection: results of the NIDDK liver transplantation database. Liver Transpl 2004;10(9):1120–30.

28. Belli LS, Burroughs AK, Burra P, et al. Liver transplantation for HCV cirrhosis: improved survival in recent years and increased severity of recurrent disease

in female recipients: results of a long term retrospective study. Liver Transpl 2007; 13(5):733–40.

29. Lai JC, Vema EC, Brown RS. Hepatitis C virus (HCV) infected females are at higher risk of graft loss after liver transplantation (LT): a multicenter cohort study. Abstract 6, presented November 1, 2009 at the liver meeting 2009: American Association for the Study of Liver Diseases 60th Annual Meeting. Boston (MA).

30. Testilano M, Fernandez JR, Suarez MJ, et al. Survival and hepatitis C virus recurrence after liver transplantation in HIV- and hepatitis C virus-coinfected patients: experience in a single center. Transplant Proc 2009;41(3):1041–3.

31. Duclos-Vallee JC, Feray C, Sebagh M, et al, THEVIC Study Group. Survival and recurrence of hepatitis C after liver transplantation in patients coinfected with human immunodeficiency virus and hepatitis C virus. Hepatology 2008;47(2): 407–17.

32. Burak KW, Kremers WK, Batts KP, et al. Impact of cytomegalovirus infection, year of transplantation, and donor age on outcomes after liver transplantation for hepatitis C. Liver Transpl 2002;8(4):362–9.

33. Charlton MR, Thompson A, Veldt BJ, et al. Interleukin-28B polymorphisms are associated with histological recurrence and treatment response following liver transplantation in patients with hepatitis C virus infection. Hepatology 2011; 53(1):317–24.

34. Charlton M, Seaberg E. Impact of immunosuppression and acute rejection on recurrence of hepatitis C: results of the National Institute of Diabetes and Digestive and Kidney Diseases Liver Transplantation Database. Liver Transpl Surg 1999;5(4 Suppl 1):S107–114.

35. Charlton M, Seaberg E, Wiesner R, et al. Predictors of patient and graft survival following liver transplantation for hepatitis C. Hepatology 1998;28(3):823–30.

36. Nelson DR, Soldevila-Pico C, Reed A, et al. Anti-interleukin-2 receptor therapy in combination with mycophenolate mofetil is associated with more severe hepatitis C recurrence after liver transplantation. Liver Transpl 2001;7(12):1064–70.

37. Sgourakis G, Radtke A, Fouzas I, et al. Corticosteroid-free immunosuppression in liver transplantation: a meta-analysis and meta-regression of outcomes. Transpl Int 2009;22(9):892–905.

38. McAlister VC, Haddad E, Renouf E, et al. Cyclosporin versus tacrolimus as primary immunosuppressant after liver transplantation: a meta-analysis. Am J Transplant 2006;6(7):1578–85.

39. Berenguer M, Royuela A, Zamora J. Immunosuppression with calcineurin inhibitors with respect to the outcomes of HCV recurrence after liver transplantation: results of a meta-analysis. Liver Transpl 2007;13(1):21–9.

40. Levy G, Grazi GL, Sanjuan F, et al. 12-month follow-up analysis of a multi-center, randomized, prospective trial in de novo liver transplant recipients (LIS2T) comparing cyclosporine microemulsion (C2 monitoring) and tacrolimus. Liver Transpl 2006;12(10):1464–72.

41. Manousou P, Samonakis D, Cholongitas E, et al. Outcome of recurrent hepatitis C virus after liver transplantation in a randomized trial of tacrolimus monotherapy versus triple therapy. Liver Transpl 2009;15(12):1783–91.

42. Berenguer M, Aguilera V, San Juan F, et al. Effect of calcineurin inhibitors in the outcome of liver transplantation in hepatitis C virus-positive recipients. Transplantation 2010;90(11):1204–9.

43. Cescon M, Grazi GL, Cucchetti A, et al. Predictors of sustained virological response after antiviral treatment for hepatitis C recurrence following liver transplantation. Liver Transpl 2009;15(7):782–9.

44. Selzner N, Renner EL, Selzner M, et al. Antiviral treatment of recurrent hepatitis C after liver transplantation: predictors of response and long-term outcome. Transplantation 2009;88(10):1214–21.
45. Firpi RJ, Soldevila-Pico C, Morelli GG, et al. The use of cyclosporine for recurrent hepatitis C after liver transplant: a randomized pilot study. Dig Dis Sci 2010;55(1): 196–203.
46. Cholongitas E, Tsochatzis E, Goulis J, et al. Noninvasive tests for evaluation of fibrosis in HCV recurrence after liver transplantation: a systematic review. Transpl Int 2010;23(9):861–70.
47. Carrion JA, Fernandez-Varo G, Bruguera M, et al. Serum fibrosis markers identify patients with mild and progressive hepatitis C recurrence after liver transplantation. Gastroenterology 2010;138(1):147–58.
48. Berres ML, Trautwein C, Schmeding M, et al. Serum chemokine CXC ligand 10 (CXCL 10) predicts fibrosis progression after liver transplantation for hepatitis C infection. Hepatology 2011;53(2):596–603.
49. Bruno S, Stroffolini T, Colombo M, et al. Italian Association of the Study of the Liver Disease (AISF). Sustained virological response to interferon-alpha is associated with improved outcome in HCV-related cirrhosis: a retrospective study. Hepatology 2007;45(3):579–87.
50. Pradat P, Tillmann HL, Sauleda S, et al, HENCORE Group. Long-term follow-up of the hepatitis C HENCORE cohort: response to therapy and occurrence of liver-related complications. J Viral Hepat 2007;14(8):556–63.
51. Nudo CG, Cortes RA, Weppler D, et al. Effect of pretransplant hepatitis C virus RNA status on posttransplant outcome. Transplant Proc 2008;40(5):1449–55.
52. Shiffman ML, Di Bisceglie AM, Lindsay KL, et al. Hepatitis C Antiviral Long-Term Treatment Against Cirrhosis Trial Group. Peginterferon alfa-2a and ribavirin in patient with chronic hepatitis C who have failed prior treatment. Gastroenterology 2004;126(4):1015–23.
53. Iacobellis A, Ippolito A, Andriulli A. Antiviral therapy in hepatitis C virus cirrhotic patients in compensated and decompensated condition. World J Gastroenterol 2008;14(42):6467–72.
54. Crippin JS, McCashland T, Terrault N, et al. A pilot study of the tolerability and efficacy of antiviral therapy in hepatitis C virus-infected patients awaiting liver transplantation. Liver Transpl 2002;8(4):350–5.
55. Singh N, Gayowski T, Wannstedt CF, et al. Interferon-alpha for prophylaxis of recurrent viral hepatitis C in liver transplant recipients: a prospective, randomized, controlled trial. Transplantation 1998;65(1):82–6.
56. Sheiner PA, Boros P, Klion FM, et al. The efficacy of prophylactic interferon alfa-2b in preventing recurrent hepatitis C after liver transplantation. Hepatology 1998 Sep;28(3):831–8.
57. Shergill AK, Khalili M, Straley S, et al. Applicability, tolerability, and efficacy of preemptive antiviral therapy in hepatitis C-infected patients undergoing liver transplantation. Am J Transplant 2005;5(1):118–24.
58. Chalasani N, Manzarbeitia C, Ferenci P, et al, Pegasys Transplant Study Group. Peginterferon alfa-2a for hepatitis C after liver transplantation: two randomized, controlled trials. Hepatology 2005;41(2):289–98.
59. Sugawara Y, Makuuchi M, Matsui Y, et al. Preemptive therapy for hepatitis C virus after living-donor liver transplantation. Transplantation 2004;78(9):1308–11.
60. Zimmermann T, Bocher WO, Biesterfeld S, et al. Efficacy of an escalating dose regimen of pegylated interferon alpha-2-a plus ribavirin in the early phase of HCV reinfection. Transpl Int 2007;20(7):583–90.

61. Castells L, Vargas V, Allende H, et al. Combined treatment with pegylated interferon (alpha-2b) and ribavirin in the acute phase of hepatitis C virus recurrence after liver transplantation. J Hepatol 2005;43(1):53–9.
62. Xirouchakis E, Triantos C, Manousou P, et al. Pegylated-interferon and ribavirin in liver transplant candidates and recipients with HCV cirrhosis: systematic review and meta-analysis of prospective controlled trials. J Viral Hepat 2008;15(10): 699–709.
63. Abdelmalek MF, Firpi RJ, Soldevila-Pico C, et al. Sustained viral response to interferon and ribavirin in liver transplant recipients with recurrent hepatitis C. Liver Transpl 2004;10(2):199–207.
64. Gane EJ, Lo SK, Riordan SM, et al. A randomized study comparing ribavirin and interferon alfa monotherapy for hepatitis C recurrence after liver transplantation. Hepatology 1998;27(5):1403–7.
65. Feray C, Samuel D, Gigou M, et al. An open trial of interferon alfa recombinant for hepatitis C after liver transplantation: antiviral effects and risk of rejection. Hepatology 1995;22(4 Pt 1):1084–9.
66. Ross AS, Bhan AK, Pascual M, et al. Pegylated interferon alpha-2b plus ribavirin in the treatment of post-liver transplant recurrent hepatitis C. Clin Transplant 2004;18(2):166–73.
67. Saab S, Kalmaz D, Gajjar NA, et al. Outcomes of acute rejection after interferon therapy in liver transplant recipients. Liver Transpl 2004;10(7):859–67.
68. Toniutto P, Fabris C, Fumo E, et al. Pegylated versus standard interferon-alpha in antiviral regimens for post-transplant recurrent hepatitis c: comparison of tolerability and efficacy. J Gastroenterol Hepatol 2005;20(4):577–82.
69. Stravitz RT, Shiffman ML, Sanyal AJ, et al. Effects of interferon treatment on liver histology and allograft rejection in patients with recurrent hepatitis C following liver transplantation. Liver Transpl 2004;10(7):850–8.
70. Berenguer M, Palau A, Fernandez A, et al. Efficacy, predictors of response, and potential risks associated with antiviral therapy in liver transplant recipients with recurrent hepatitis C. Liver Transpl 2006;12(7):1067–76.
71. Mukherjee S, Lyden E, McCashland TM, et al. Interferon alpha 2b and ribavirin for the treatment of recurrent hepatitis C after liver transplantation: cohort study of 38 patients. J Gastroenterol Hepatol 2005;20(2):198–203.
72. Bahra M, Neumann UP, Jacob D, et al. Fibrosis progression in hepatitis C positive liver recipients after sustained virologic response to antiviral combination therapy (interferon-ribavirin therapy). Transplantation 2007;83(3):351–3.
73. Sharma P, Marrero JA, Fontana RJ, et al. Sustained virologic response to therapy of recurrent hepatitis C after liver transplantation is related to early virologic response and dose adherence. Liver Transpl 2007;13(8):1100–8.
74. Dumortier J, Scoazec JY, Chevallier P, et al. Treatment of recurrent hepatitis C after liver transplantation: a pilot study of peginterferon alfa-2b and ribavirin combination. J Hepatol 2004;40(4):669–74.
75. Oton E, Barcena R, Moreno-Planas JM, et al. Hepatitis C recurrence after liver transplantation: viral and histologic response to full-dose PEG-interferon and ribavirin. Am J Transplant 2006;6(10):2348–55.
76. Fernandez I, Meneu JC, Colina F, et al. Clinical and histological efficacy of pegylated interferon and ribavirin therapy of recurrent hepatitis C after liver transplantation. Liver Transpl 2006;12(12):1805–12.
77. Neumann U, Puhl G, Bahra M, et al. Treatment of patients with recurrent hepatitis C after liver transplantation with peginterferon alfa-2B plus ribavirin. Transplantation 2006;82(1):43–7.

78. Mukherjee S, Lyden E. Impact of pegylated interferon alfa-2a and ribavirin on hepatic fibrosis in liver transplant patients with recurrent hepatitis C: an open label series. Hepatogastroenterology 2006;53(70):561–5.

79. Mukherjee S, Lyden E. Impact of pegylated interferon alpha-2B and ribavirin on hepatic fibrosis in liver transplant patients with recurrent hepatitis C: an open-label series. Liver Int 2006;26(5):529–35.

80. Carrion JA, Navasa M, Garcia-Retortillo M, et al. Efficacy of antiviral therapy on hepatitis C recurrence after liver transplantation: a randomized controlled study. Gastroenterology 2007;132(5):1746–56.

81. Berenguer M. Systematic review of the treatment of established recurrent hepatitis C with pegylated interferon in combination with ribavirin. J Hepatol 2008; 49(2):274–87.

82. Bizollon T, Pradat P, Mabrut JY, et al. Benefit of sustained virological response to combination therapy on graft survival of liver transplanted patients with recurrent chronic hepatitis C. Am J Transplant 2005;5(8):1909–13.

83. Firpi RJ, Abdelmalek MF, Soldevila-Pico C, et al. Combination of interferon alfa-2b and ribavirin in liver transplant recipients with histological recurrent hepatitis C. Liver Transpl 2002;8(11):1000–6.

84. Picciotto FP, Tritto G, Lanza AG, et al. Sustained virological response to antiviral therapy reduces mortality in HCV reinfection after liver transplantation. J Hepatol 2007;46(3):459–65.

85. Kornberg A, Kupper B, Tannapfel A, et al. Sustained clearance of serum hepatitis C virus-RNA independently predicts long-term survival in liver transplant patients with recurrent hepatitis C. Transplantation 2008;86(3):469–73.

86. Bizollon T, Pradat P, Mabrut JY, et al. Histological benefit of retreatment by pegylated interferon alfa-2b and ribavirin in patients with recurrent hepatitis C virus infection posttransplantation. Am J Transplant 2007;7(2):448–53.

87. Kornberg A, Kupper B, Tannapfel A, et al. Antiviral maintenance treatment with interferon and ribavirin for recurrent hepatitis C after liver transplantation: pilot study. J Gastroenterol Hepatol 2007;22(12):2135–42.

88. Walter T, Scoazec JY, Guillaud O, et al. Long-term antiviral therapy for recurrent hepatitis C after liver transplantation in nonresponders: biochemical, virological, and histological impact. Liver Transpl 2009;15(1):54–63.

89. Pawlotsky JM. The results of phase III clinical trials with telaprevir and boceprevir presented at the Liver Meeting 2010: a new standard of care for hepatitis C virus. Gastroenterology 2011;140(3):746–54.

90. Carrion JA, Navasa M, Forns X. Retransplantation in patients with hepatitis C recurrence after liver transplantation. J Hepatol 2010;53(5):962–70.

91. Burton JR Jr, Sonnenberg A, Rosen HR. Retransplantation for recurrent hepatitis C in the MELD era: maximizing utility. Liver Transpl 2004;10(10 Suppl 2):S59–64.

Recurrent and De Novo Autoimmune Liver Diseases

Flavia Mendes, MD[a], Claudia A. Couto, MD, PhD[b],
Cynthia Levy, MD[c],*

KEYWORDS

- Primary biliary cirrhosis • Primary sclerosing cholangitis
- Autoimmune hepatitis • Recurrence • Liver transplantation

Primary biliary cirrhosis (PBC), primary sclerosing cholangitis (PSC), and autoimmune hepatitis (AIH) each account for approximately 5% of liver transplants per year performed in the United States and Europe.[1–4] Even though outcomes are excellent, with reported 5-year patient and graft survival exceeding 90% and 80%, 80% and 75%, 72% and 65% for PBC,[5–7] PSC,[3,8–10] and AIH,[11,12] respectively, the issue of recurrent autoimmune liver disease after orthotopic liver transplantation (OLT) is increasingly recognized as a cause of graft dysfunction, death, and need for retransplantation. In this article the authors individually review diagnostic criteria, epidemiology, risk factors, and outcomes of recurrent PBC, PSC, and AIH after liver transplantation.

PRIMARY BILIARY CIRRHOSIS

PBC is an organ-specific autoimmune disease characterized by inflammation and destruction of the interlobular and septal bile ducts, eventually leading to biliary cirrhosis. Ursodeoxycholic acid (UDCA) has been shown to improve survival free of liver transplantation but approximately one-third of patients do not respond to UDCA. Among nonresponders, approximately 10% go on to progress to liver failure and require liver transplantation.[13] Overall survival rates after liver transplantation for PBC are excellent, with reported 15-year survival as high as 82%.[4–6,14–23]

The authors have nothing to disclose.

[a] Division of Hepatology, Miami VA Medical Center, 1201 Northwest 16th Street Suite 1101, Miami, FL 33125, USA

[b] Department of Internal Medicine, School of Medicine, Federal University of Minas Gerais, Av Professor Alfredo Balena, 190, Santa Efigenia, 30130100 Belo Horizonte, Minas Gerais, Brazil

[c] Division of Hepatology, Department of Medicine, University of Miami, 1500 NW 12th Avenue, Suite 1101, Miami, FL 33136, USA

* Corresponding author.

E-mail address: clevy@med.miami.edu

Clin Liver Dis 15 (2011) 859–878

doi:10.1016/j.cld.2011.08.008

1089-3261/11/$ – see front matter © 2011 Elsevier Inc. All rights reserved.

liver.theclinics.com

Despite a substantial increase in the overall number of liver transplants performed in the United States over the past decade, the absolute number of liver transplants performed for PBC and waiting-list additions have declined.[24] Similar temporal trends were described in the United Kingdom and the Netherlands, where the proportion of transplants for PBC decreased from 11.7% to 4.5%.[2,4] While part of this decline can be explained by a relative increase in the proportion of transplants performed for other indications, such as hepatitis B–related cirrhosis and hepatocellular carcinoma, the decreased liver-related mortality in patients with PBC and the increase in their age at death suggest that widespread use of UDCA is also a likely explanation.[25]

Recurrent PBC was first described in 1982[26] and has since become a well-recognized entity, affecting roughly a third of recipients. Controversy still exists as regards the best approach to diagnosis and management of recurrence, but it seems clear that recurrent disease only rarely (<2%) affects graft or patient outcomes.

Diagnosis

Given that the typical clinical presentation of PBC is rarely seen in the posttransplant setting, clinicians must rely mainly on histology for diagnosis of recurrent disease.

Histology

A strict diagnostic definition implies the presence of typical florid duct lesion (granulomatous cholangitis) or destructive lymphocytic cholangitis within a dense portal infiltrate and in the absence of acute cellular rejection.[27,28] **Fig. 1** illustrates a classic case

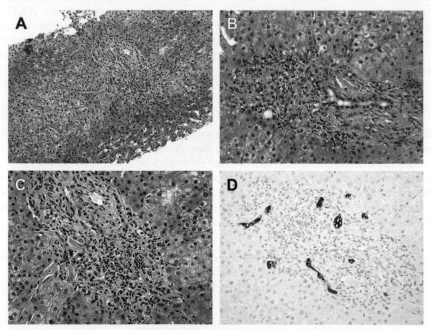

Fig. 1. (*A*) Liver parenchyma with portal inflammatory infiltrate (hematoxylin-eosin [H&E], original magnification ×200). (*B*) Portal area with focally dense chronic inflammatory cell infiltrate closely associated to a bile duct (H&E, original magnification ×600). (*C*) Portal area with epithelioid and lymphoid cells (granuloma). No normal bile duct is present (H&E, original magnification ×600). (*D*) Distorted interlobular bile ducts (CK7 immunostain, original magnification ×600). (*Courtesy of* Dr Monica Garcia, Department of Pathology, University of Miami Miller School of Medicine.)

of recurrent PBC. Other less specific features such as the presence of a dense lymphoplasmacytic portal infiltrate or moderate lymphocytic cholangitis may precede development of the florid duct lesion or destructive lymphocytic cholangitis, and their clinical significance is unclear.[15,28–30] The proportion of patients with these less specific features who will eventually develop well-defined recurrent PBC is yet to be determined.

Laboratory analysis

The fate of antimitochondrial antibodies (AMA) after liver transplantation is not predictable. AMA levels may decline, remain elevated for the first year and disappear afterward, or remain unchanged. Even after disappearing, AMA may later become detectable again.[31] Therefore, serologic detection of AMA after transplant cannot be used to diagnose recurrent PBC.

The typical cholestatic picture observed in pretransplant PBC is not recognized in most patients with recurrent PBC. More often, only mild nonspecific liver biochemistries abnormalities are noticed at the time of diagnosis.[22,28] Elevation of serum alkaline phosphatase (ALP) is seen in roughly 50% of patients at the time of diagnosis of recurrent PBC.[5]

Epidemiology

The prevalence of recurrent PBC ranges between 9% and 35%.[5,6,14,15,17–19,22,30,32–34] Several factors influence the observed rate of recurrence, including whether protocol biopsies are obtained, length of follow-up period, diagnostic criteria used, pathologist's expertise, and the inherent sampling error associated with liver biopsies. As liver enzymes may remain normal for several years after histologic diagnosis of recurrence, recurrent PBC may be missed unless protocol biopsies are performed.[6]

The mean time to recurrence ranges between 1.6 and 6.5 years,[5,6,15,17–19,22,28,30,34,35] with a reported cumulative incidence rate between 21% and 37% at 10 years[4,5,18] and as high as 43% at 15 years.[5] Thus, the observed recurrence rate is higher with longer duration of follow-up.

A significantly higher rate of recurrence has been described among patients transplanted in the most recent era when compared with the prior decade, with 10-year cumulative recurrence rate of 55% to 70% versus 13% to 20%, respectively. This effect is likely the result of increased awareness of recurrent PBC as a clinical entity, as well as widespread use of tacrolimus as preferential immunosuppression since 1999.[5,18]

Predictors of Recurrence

Several groups have sought to identify predictors of PBC recurrence in the allograft (Table 1). Nevertheless, findings are conflicting. Both recipient and donor factors have been proposed to affect the rate of recurrence, including increased donor and recipient age,[4–6] increased warm ischemia time,[4] male recipient gender,[5] use of tacrolimus as the mainstay for immunosuppression,[5,6,18,19,32,33] and specific human leukocyte antigen (HLA) alleles in donor and recipient.[22] Alternatively, use of azathioprine may be associated with protection against recurrence.[15,17,19] Of interest, multiple studies suggest that recurrence is not only more frequent, but may also occur significantly earlier in patients receiving tacrolimus when compared with those on cyclosporine. However, whether or not tacrolimus increases the rate of recurrence is an ongoing debate. A systematic review by Gautam and colleagues[35] including 16 original studies with a total of 1241 patients transplanted for PBC, of whom 16% had recurrence, was able to demonstrate only a trend toward more recurrence with use

Table 1
Published studies evaluating predictors of PBC recurrence after liver transplantation

Authors, Year	Cohort of OLT for PBC, n	Histologic Recurrence, n (%)	Donor Risk Factors	Recipient Risk Factors	Immunosuppressant Associated with Recurrence	Graft Dysfunction, Death, and Re-OLT
Dmitrewski et al,[32] 1996	27	8 (29.6)	—	—	TAC	Not reported
Sanchez et al,[22] 2003	156	17 (10.9)	HLA A1, B57, B58, DR44, DR57, DR58	HLA B48	Trend toward more recurrence with TAC	2/17
Levitsky et al,[34] 2003	46	7 (15.2)	—	—	No difference	0/7
Khettry et al,[15] 2003	43	13 (30.2)	—	—	AZA protects	7/13
Neuberger et al,[19] 2004	485	114 (23)	—	—	TAC	Not reported
Guy et al,[33] 2005	48	17 (35.4)	DR3	—	TAC	Not reported
Jacob et al,[6] 2006	100	14 (14)	—	Older age	TAC	2/14
Charatcharoenwitthaya et al,[5] 2007	154	52 (33.7)	—	Male	TAC	2/52
Campsen et al,[14] 2009	70	18 (25.7)	Living donor	—	Longer time to recurrence with CyA	0/18
Montano-Loza et al,[18] 2010	108	28 (25.9)	—	—	CyA protects	Not reported
Manousou et al,[17] 2010	103	36 (34.9)	—	—	AZA protects	8/36

Abbreviations: AZA, azathioprine; CyA, cyclosporine A; OLT, orthotopic liver transplantation; TAC, tacrolimus.

of tacrolimus (30%) when compared with cyclosporine (23%; 95% confidence interval [CI] −7.03%–8.75%)].

PBC is also reported to recur in 10% to 50% of patients undergoing living donor liver transplantation (LDLT) for PBC; it has been proposed that the lower number of HLA-A, HLA-B, and HLA-DR mismatches between donor and recipient could increase the risk of recurrence in this population.[36–38]

Treatment

UDCA is widely used for the treatment of recurrent PBC.[4,5,22,33] Although no standard guideline exists, the well-documented efficacy in PBC and the fact that most cases of recurrence are diagnosed in the early stages make the use of UDCA very appealing. Indeed, Guy and colleagues[33] reported improvement in serum ALP in 75% of 16 patients with recurrent PBC treated with UDCA. Charatcharoenwitthaya and colleagues[5] also showed improvement of serum ALP in treated versus untreated patients with recurrent PBC, with 52% of treated patients actually normalizing the test. These investigators did not observe a significant difference in histologic progression between UDCA-treated and untreated patients; however, the proportion of cases with histologic progression was significantly lower among patients with biochemical response compared with their counterparts without response (27% vs 73%, $P = .02$). The appropriate dose to be used in the posttransplant setting has not yet been established.

Prognosis

Recurrent PBC has little impact on patient and graft outcomes, and is not associated with increased overall mortality even after extended periods of follow-up.[5,18] However, recurrent PBC may rarely evolve into graft failure, leading to death or retransplantation (see **Table 1**).[5,6,17,22] In this respect, Rowe and colleagues[39] assessed the impact of disease recurrence on long-term graft survival in a large cohort of patients undergoing liver transplantation in Birmingham, UK. Among patients transplanted for PBC, only 5.4% of all graft losses was attributable to recurrent disease. Furthermore, when compared with PBC, the highest risk of graft loss due to disease recurrence was seen in patients transplanted for hepatitis C virus (hazard ratio 2.1; 95% CI 1.5–3.0), PSC (hazard ratio 1.6; 95% CI 1.2–2.3), and AIH (hazard ratio 1.6; 95% CI 1.0–2.4). When graft dysfunction occurs, the median time from recurrent disease to graft loss is 7.8 years,[39] or a mean time of 6.7 years (range 22–181 months).[17]

Recommendations

In summary, histologic recurrence of PBC in the allograft is now a well-recognized complication, with a cumulative incidence approaching 40% at 10 years. Nevertheless, graft loss due to recurrent PBC is uncommon. Treatment with UDCA seems to improve liver biochemistries, but its overall impact on outcomes is yet to be determined.

As more definitive studies evaluating the influence of specific immunosuppressants in the rate of PBC recurrence are awaited, strong recommendations cannot be made. Furthermore, to fully appreciate the rate of recurrence and its impact on the natural history of disease, transplant centers should consider performing protocol liver biopsies, perhaps at 3 and 5 years after transplant.

PRIMARY SCLEROSING CHOLANGITIS

PSC is a chronic cholestatic liver disease characterized by inflammation and fibrotic obliteration of the intrahepatic and extrahepatic biliary tree.[40] To date, medical, endoscopic, and surgical therapies have failed to make an impact on disease progression, and OLT remains the only curative therapy for patients with end-stage liver disease from PSC. It is estimated that PSC accounts for approximately 4% to 5% of adult liver transplantations performed in Europe and the United States.[1,3] Posttransplant survival for patients with PSC at 1 year and 5 years have reached 90% and 80%, respectively, and 1-year and 5-year graft survival rates have ranged from 85% to 88% and approximately 80%, respectively.[3,8–10] The importance of recurrent PSC is becoming increasingly recognized as the posttransplant outcomes continue to improve and increased patient follow-up is available.

Diagnostic Criteria and Epidemiology

Diagnosing recurrent PSC can be very challenging, as there are no gold-standard diagnostic criteria and a variety of other conditions in the posttransplant setting, such as hepatic artery thrombosis/stenosis, allograft ABO incompatibility, reperfusion injury, chronic rejection, biliary tract infections, and anastomotic strictures can resemble the biliary strictures seen in recurrent PSC. Therefore, to diagnose recurrent PSC an effort to exclude other known causes of intrahepatic and extrahepatic biliary strictures is of utmost importance.

In 1988 Lerut and colleagues[41] reported one case of intrahepatic biliary stricture developing within 1 year after liver transplantation for PSC, where no other cause of biliary injury was identified, raising the suspicion of recurrent PSC. After that study several investigators reported an increased frequency of biliary strictures in patients undergoing OLT for PSC.[42–49]

In one study Graziadei and colleagues[50] investigated the recurrence of PSC by developing strict criteria and applying them in a cohort of 150 patients who underwent OLT for PSC at the Mayo Clinic. Thirty patients were excluded with other known causes of posttransplant biliary strictures. Of the 120 patients left for analysis, 24 (20%) patients were found to have either cholangiographic (22/24) or histologic (11/24) evidence of recurrent PSC, with 9 of 24 having both cholangiographic and histologic findings. The investigators also reported a significantly higher incidence of nonanastomotic biliary strictures, with a later onset as well as a higher incidence of hepatic histologic findings characteristic for PSC recurrence in the group of patients transplanted for PSC (150 patients) in comparison with a control group of 464 patients transplanted for non-PSC causes.

The diagnostic criteria used in the aforementioned study is currently the most widely accepted definition of recurrent PSC after OLT and, requires (**Table 2**): (1) a confirmed diagnosis of PSC before OLT, (2) cholangiography showing intrahepatic and/or extrahepatic biliary stricturing, beading, and irregularities at least more than 90 days following OLT, and/or (3) histologic findings of fibrous cholangitis and/or fibroobliterative lesions with or without ductopenia, biliary fibrosis, or biliary cirrhosis; in the absence of hepatic artery thrombosis/stenosis, chronic ductopenic rejection anastomotic strictures alone, nonanastomotic strictures before posttransplantation day 90, and ABO incompatibility between donor and recipient.[50] **Fig. 2** shows the histologic appearance of recurrent PSC.

The reported incidence of recurrent PSC has ranged from 10% to 25% (**Table 3**), with median time to recurrence ranging from 8 to 68 months in the published series using this more strict definition.[50–57] An even higher recurrence rate of 37% was reported by Vera and colleagues[49]; however, this study included strictures diagnosed less than 90 days posttransplantation.

In patients undergoing LDLT, recurrence rates as high as 60% have been reported, with transplant recipients of biological donors being at the highest risk of developing recurrent disease.[38,58–62]

Table 2
Diagnostic criteria for PBC, PSC, and AIH recurrence after OLT

	Presence of	Absence of
PBC AMA positivity is not helpful in diagnosing recurrent PBC	Histology Typical florid duct lesion (granulomatous cholangitis) or destructive cholangitis within a dense portal infiltrate OR Less specific: dense lymphoplasmacytic portal infiltrate or moderate lymphocytic cholangitis Serologic/Biochemical (not required for diagnosis) Mild nonspecific biochemical abnormalities Elevated alkaline phosphatase seen in about 50% of patients with recurrence	Acute cellular rejection
PSC[50] Confirmed PSC before transplantation is required for diagnosis of rPSC	Cholangiogram showing intra- and/or extrahepatic biliary stricturing, beading, and irregularities >90 days post-OLT AND/OR Histology showing fibrous cholangitis and/or fibroobliterative lesions with or without ductopenia, biliary fibrosis, or biliary cirrhosis	Hepatic artery thrombosis/stenosis Chronic ductopenic rejection Anastomotic strictures Nonanastomotic strictures before post-OLT day 90 ABO incompatibility Acute cellular rejection
AIH	Elevated transaminases Hypergammaglobulinemia Autoantibodies Consistent histology: Lobular and/or periportal hepatitis (lobular and interface necroinflammatory activity) Steroid responsiveness	Viral infection Drugs

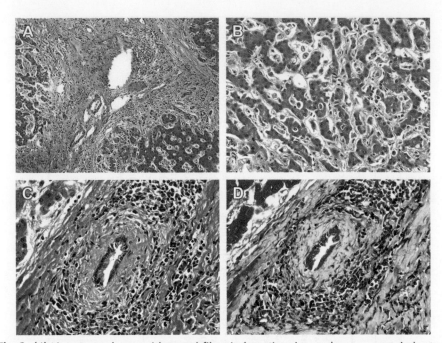

Fig. 2. (*A*) Liver parenchyma with septal fibrosis, hepatic veins, and unaccompanied artery branches indicating bile duct loss (H&E, original magnification ×200). (*B*) Canalicular and minimal intracellular cholestasis (H&E, original magnification ×400). (*C*) Septal bile ductal surrounded by dense hyaline collagen and mild lymphoplasmacytic infiltrate (H&E, original magnification ×600). (*D*) Periductal fibrosis confirmed by trichrome stain (original magnification ×600). (*Courtesy of* Dr Monica Garcia, Department of Pathology, University of Miami Miller School of Medicine.)

Bacterial cholangitis may be the dominant symptom,[53] but a large proportion of patients can be asymptomatic. An elevated ALP level greater than 250 IU/mL of 1 or more year's duration after liver transplantation for PSC should prompt evaluation for recurrent PSC.

Predictors of Recurrence

Several studies have tried to identify risk factors associated with posttransplant recurrence of PSC. The results in general have been heterogeneous, at least in part because of the small number of patients and diagnostic challenges in recurrent PSC.

Reported potential risk factors include recipient age,[44] male gender,[49] donor-recipient gender mismatch,[45] (HLA)-DRB1*08,[52] the presence of inflammatory bowel disease,[55] an intact colon before liver transplantation,[49,51] episodes of acute cellular rejection (ACR),[52,57] steroid-resistant ACR,[53] Orthoclone (OKT3) use for steroid-resistant ACR,[56] maintenance steroid therapy for greater than 3 months post-OLT,[55] cytomegalovirus (CMV) infection,[44] CMV mismatch,[57] diagnosis of cholangiocarcinoma before liver transplantation,[54] and the use of extended donor criteria grafts.[51]

Outcomes

The impact of PSC recurrence on the long-term outcomes of patients transplanted for PSC still needs to be better defined.

Table 3
Incidence, predictors, and outcomes of recurrent PSC in published series using the Mayo diagnostic criteria

Authors, Year	Cohort Size	Incidence, n (%)	Predictors of Recurrence	Outcomes of Recurrent PSC			
				Patient 5-y Survival (rPSC vs nrPSC)	Graft 5-y Survival (rPSC vs nrPSC)	Re-OLT	Median Follow-Up
Graziadei et al,[50] 1999	120	24 (20%)	None identified	Unchanged (86% vs 91%)	Unchanged (79% vs 82%)	2/24	55 mo (mean)
Kugelmas et al,[56] 2003	71	15 (21.1%)	OKT3 use	Unchanged (92% vs 86%)	NA	NA	14–91 mo (range)
Brandsaeter et al,[53] 2005	49	9 (18%)	Steroid-resistant rejection	NA	NA	0[a]	6.4 y
Campsen et al,[54] 2008	130	22 (16.9%)	CCA pre-OLT	45% without re-OLT	NA	7/22	66 mo (median)
Alexander et al,[52] 2008	69	7 (10%)	(HLA)-DRB1*08; ACR; steroid-resistant ACR	NA	NA	NA	50 mo (median)
Cholongitas et al,[55] 2008	53	7 (13.5%)	Steroids >3 mo post-OLT	Unchanged (85% and 76%)	NA	3/7	110 mo (median)
Alabraba et al,[51]	230	54 (23.5%)	Intact colon	Decreased in rPSC	NA	11/54	6.9 y
Moncrief et al,[57] 2010	59	15 (25%)	ACR; CMV mismatch	Unchanged	Unchanged	4/15	68 mo (median)

Abbreviations: ACR, acute cellular rejection; CCA, cholangiocarcinoma; CMV, cytomegalovirus; HLA, human leukocyte antigen; nrPSC, no recurrence of PSC; OKT3, Orthoclone; OLT, orthotopic liver transplantation; rPSC, recurrent PSC.
[a] Three patients were under evaluation for re-OLT.

As longer follow-up becomes available, increasing evidence points to an increased number of graft dysfunction and need for retransplantation related to recurrent PSC. Campsen and colleagues[54] reported that once a patient was diagnosed with recurrent disease, the median survival time without receiving a second transplant was 39.1 months. Although most published studies failed to show a significant decrease in patient survival in patients with recurrent disease (see **Table 3**),[50–57] one study reported that out of 263 liver transplants performed for PSC, 9% of the graft failures were attributable to recurrent PSC.[51]

Treatment

As for PSC in the native liver, treatment options are limited for recurrent PSC.[63] There is no supporting evidence that the use of UDCA is beneficial in treating or preventing recurrent PSC. Symptomatic biliary strictures and episodes of bacterial cholangitis are primarily treated with percutaneous and/or endoscopic approaches and antibiotic therapy.[54]

Patients with recurrent PSC who have repeated episodes of cholangitis, refractory jaundice, and evidence of end-stage liver disease with a high MELD (model for end-stage liver disease) score and complications of portal hypertension should be evaluated and listed for retransplantation.

Recommendations

Recurrent PSC is now increasingly recognized as an important cause of graft dysfunction after transplantation for PSC. Experts have tried to identify risk factors for recurrent disease; however, reported predictors in general have not been confirmed across the different studies. Current available evidence points toward an association of rejection and corticosteroid use with recurrence of PSC. The impact of recurrent PSC on long-term patient and graft survival still needs to be better defined. The implementation of more strict and uniform diagnostic criteria and multi-center studies with longer follow-up should help answer these important questions. Treatment of this condition relies mainly on relief of symptomatic biliary strictures, but no medical or endoscopic treatment has been able to alter the disease course, and patients with end-stage liver disease from recurrent PSC should be considered for retransplantation.

AUTOIMMUNE HEPATITIS

AIH is a chronic inflammatory liver disease characterized by interface hepatitis, hyper-gammaglobulinemia, circulating autoantibodies, and response to steroids. OLT represents the ultimate therapeutic option in AIH for up to 10% of patients who do not respond to medical therapy. AIH is an infrequent indication for OLT and accounts for 4% to 5% of OLT procedures performed for liver cirrhosis within Europe and the United States. Overall survival rates after transplantation for AIH are favorable, but worse than survival rates for PBC. The reported 5-year survival of European patients undergoing OLT for AIH is 73%.[12]

AIH recurrence is a well-recognized problem estimated to affect 23% of AIH transplanted recipients after a median interval of 26 months,[35] and the underlying mechanism of disease recurrence remains especulative.[64] The frequency of AIH recurrence increases with time after OLT,[65,66] and silent progression to cirrhosis is possible.[65,67] Although outcomes are favorable after treatment for recurrence, retransplantation is required in up to 18% (3/17) of the cases.[65,68] Long-term follow-up is needed to clarify the impact of recurrence on the graft.

Diagnosis

Diagnostic criteria

In the setting of liver transplantation, diagnosis of AIH recurrence can be particularly challenging, and better definition of diagnostic criteria is still needed.[35,69]

The scoring system used to diagnose AIH in the native liver cannot be used after OLT as some parameters such as the presence of elevated transaminases, hypergammaglobulinemia, autoantibodies, and the absence of other causes of chronic liver disease may persist after transplantation without necessarily implying recurrence. Furthermore, the presence of periportal hepatitis, with or without lobular hepatitis, can be a marker of recurrence but can also be nonspecific or represent other causes of graft damage.

Although standard criteria have not been developed, the American Association for the Study of Liver Diseases considers a combination of the following parameters as indicative of recurrent AIH in the absence of rejection or viral infection (see **Table 2**): (1) elevated serum levels of transaminases, (2) hypergammaglobulinemia or elevated immunoglobulin G (IgG) levels, (3) presence of autoantibodies, (4) consistent histologic features such as lobular and/or periportal hepatitis, and (5) steroid responsiveness.[1]

Histology

The classic histologic picture in AIH recurrence is a chronic inflammatory infiltrate with plasma cells, interface hepatitis (piecemeal necrosis), and bridging necrosis and fibrosis (**Fig. 3**).[69,70] Studies from centers performing routine protocol biopsies pointed

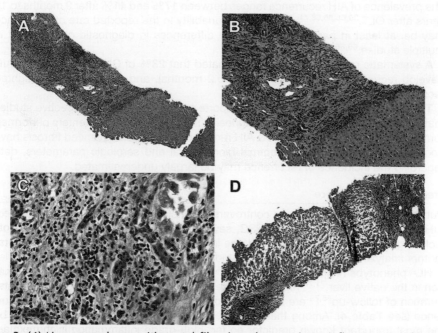

Fig. 3. (*A*) Liver parenchyma with septal fibrosis and a prominent inflammatory infiltrate (H&E, original magnification ×100). (*B*) Septal and interface inflammation. Note a bile duct adjacent to the artery and vein (H&E, original magnification ×200). (*C*) Lymphoplasmacytic infiltrate (H&E, original magnification ×600). (*D*) Bridging fibrosis confirmed by trichrome stain (original magnification ×100). (*Courtesy of* Dr Monica Garcia, Department of Pathology, University of Miami Miller School of Medicine.)

toward histopathology as the most appropriate diagnostic marker for recurrent AIH; furthermore, interface/portal hepatitis with lymphoplasmacytic infiltrate appears to precede laboratory and clinical evidence of AIH recurrence.[65,71] In a series of 17 patients, all 4 patients showing histologic recurrence of AIH as diagnosed by protocol biopsy performed 1 to 5 years after OLT also presented clinical and/or biochemical evidence of recurrent AIH within 10 years of OLT; 2 of these patients developed a severe form of recurrence requiring re-OLT despite immunosuppressive treatment.[65] Those patients showed consistent inflammatory features on liver biopsy despite liver biochemistries within normal range. In this regard, late protocol biopsies have been advocated because normal biochemical liver tests, normal gammaglobulin levels, and nonreactivity of autoantibodies may mask the recurrence of AIH.

Laboratory analyses

The role of autoantibodies in the diagnosis of AIH recurrence needs further evaluation, as few studies have addressed this issue. Autoantibodies titers have been shown to decrease shortly after OLT, followed by an increase 2 years later.[72] To date, two studies failed to demonstrate a correlation between the presence of autoantibodies and recurrence of AIH.[65,66] However, autoantibody titers exceeding levels detected before transplantation have been associated with AIH recurrence,[68] and autoantibodies against soluble liver antigen (SLA) have been found in patients with AIH recurrence.[65,66]

Epidemiology

The prevalence of AIH recurrence ranges between 17% and 41% after 9 months to 12 years after OLT.[39,65,66,68,71–78] The large variability in the reported rate of recurrence may be, at least in part, attributed to the differences in diagnostic criteria used in multiple studies.[65,66,68,71,74–76,78–83]

A systematic review of 13 studies estimated that 23% of OLT recipients with AIH develop recurrent disease (range 14.4–55.2 months), and the calculated weighted recurrence rate was 22%.[35]

Table 4 shows AIH recurrence rates reported in uncontrolled retrospective studies that included histologic criteria for diagnosis. In this regard, only 2 centers performed routine protocol biopsies.[65,71,72] As AIH recurrence and even advanced fibrosis have been shown in the context of normal biochemical and serologic parameters, data regarding the incidence of recurrence may be largely underestimated.

Predictors of Recurrence

Published series have produced controversial conclusions as regards risk factors for AIH recurrence. As for PBC and PSC, several factors influence these conclusions, including the diagnostic criteria used, the immunosuppression regimen, the different factors analyzed, and whether protocol biopsies are obtained.

HLA phenotype recipient and donor,[65,74,75] disease type,[78,79] severity of inflammation in the native liver,[71,77] high IgG before OLT,[77] level of immunosuppression, and duration of follow-up[65,73] are the risk factors more often associated with AIH recurrence (see **Table 4**). Among these, disease severity in the native liver seems to be the most important known predictor so far; high-grade inflammation in the explant was first reported as a strong predictor by Ayata and colleagues.[71] Moreover, a recent study confirmed this association between severity of inflammation in the native liver and high serum levels of IgG pre-OLT with AIH recurrence.[77]

Higher recurrence rates of AIH in HLA-DR3–positive transplant recipients have been suggested by some[65,74,75] but not all studies.[66,76] Similar controversy exists with

Table 4
AIH recurrence and cirrhosis/retransplantation due after liver transplantation

Authors, Year	N	Follow-Up, Months	AIH Recurrence	Median Recurrence Time, Months (Range)	Risk Factors	Cirrhosis or Graft Loss
Prados et al,[78] 1998	27	44	9/27 (33%)	30 (8–53)	Type 1	0
Milkiewicz et al,[75] 1999	47	29	13/47 (28%)	29 (6–63)	Donor DR3/recipient DR#	3
Ratziu et al,[72] 1999[a]	25	63	3/15 (20%)	24 (12–36)	—	2
Reich et al,[68] 2000	24	27	6/24 (25%)	15 (12–18)	—	4
Ayata et al,[71] 2000[a]	12	67	5/12 (41%)	4 (1–9)	Explant high-grade inflammation	2
Gonzalez-Koch et al,[74] 2001	41	27	7/41 (17%)	52	Recipient HLA DR3/DR4	0
Molmenti et al,[76] 2002	55	28	11/55 (20%)	—	—	0
Vogel et al,[66] 2004	28	24	9/28 (32%)	—	—	3
Duclos-Vallee et al,[65] 2003[a]	17	>120	7/17 (41%)	28 (7–60)	Severe recurrence/recipient HLA DR3	3
Montano-Loza et al,[77] 2009	46	79	11/46 (24%)	30 (9–144)	Explant moderate/severe inflammation high IgG before OLT	—
Campsen et al,[73] 2008	66	81	23/66 (35%)	51	—	0
Rowe et al,[39] 2008	103	61	28%[b]	17	—	5

Abbreviations: AIH, autoimmune hepatitis; HLA, human leukocyte antigen; OLT, orthotopic liver transplantation.
[a] Diagnosis based on histologic criteria.
[b] Based on a previous study from the same center.

respect to HLA phenotype mismatch between donor and recipient.[35] In contrast to previously reported data,[78] a recent study showed no prognostic role of AIH subtypes in recurrence after OLT.[66]

Acute rejection episodes are more frequent in AIH transplanted patients compared with other etiology, but do not influence the long-term patient and graft survival and are not related to recurrence.[66,76] Although some investigators have shown a difference in AIH recurrence according to the type of primary immunosuppression, a recent systematic review of 13 studies found no significant difference.[35,76,80]

Data regarding the practice of weaning patients off steroids are controversial, and most centers continue steroids at a low dose after OLT.[80] Recently, a large long-term follow-up study attempted withdrawing steroids in 50% of AIH transplanted patients. Recurrence rates increased over time to 35%, but were not related to steroid withdrawal, and all patients had a favorable outcome.[73] However, as for previous studies, protocol biopsies were not performed. Furthermore, reports of silent recurrence diagnosed by protocol biopsies and leading to severe late AIH recurrence (10 years or more)[65,77] suggest the need for continuous use of prednisone.

Treatment

The treatment of recurrent AIH is based on reintroduction of corticosteroids or more potent immunosuppression. Preferred regimens vary between centers. Increasing the dosage and maintaining patients on steroids, introducing azathioprine or mycophenolate, and switching cyclosporine to tacrolimus are some of the recommended approaches.[65]

Even though the treatment is effective in most cases, disease recurrence is still a significant cause of graft loss.[39,65,69] Thus to prevent recurrence, maintenance immunosuppressive therapy is thought to be important even in the setting of normal serum liver biochemistries.[65,69] This approach may be responsible for the recent decrease in AIH recurrence rate as suggested by some, but longer follow-up is needed to confirm the effect of continued corticosteroid therapy in this setting.[39]

Prognosis and Outcome

Most investigators agree that prognosis and outcome of recurrent AIH is quite favorable. Patients usually respond promptly after reinstatement or increase in immunosuppression. The clinical, biochemical, and histologic features usually resolve, even in patients with a severe presentation, but some patients may progress toward retransplantation.[39,65,66,75] While there are reports of progression to cirrhosis and re-OLT, the frequency of graft loss remains to be determined.

De Novo Autoimmune Hepatitis

De novo AIH is an uncommon cause of late graft dysfunction associated with serologic and histologic features of AIH in patients transplanted for indications other than AIH. First reported in the pediatric population in 1998 by Kerkar and colleagues,[84] de novo AIH has been described in both adult and child recipients, occurring in up to 5% of all OLT recipients[85] and usually presenting within 2 to 10 years after OLT.[86–88]

Although classic autoantibodies (antinuclear and antismooth muscle) are frequently present, an atypical liver/kidney microsome autoantibodies pattern on immunofluorescence has been characteristically associated with de novo AIH.[89–91] Those atypical antibodies have been related to several proteins[90] including one antibody type that seems to be directed against the cytosolic enzyme glutathione-S-transferase T1 (GSST1).[89] Anti-GSTT1 antibodies have been detected in null GSTT1 genotype patients receiving a graft from a GSTT1-positive genotype donor.[92] GSTT1 mismatch between the donor and recipient seems to be a prerequisite for the development of de novo AIH after OLT.[91,92] Salcedo and colleagues[85] recently showed anti-GSTT1 antibodies preceding de novo AIH; 74% (20/27) of patients with donor/recipient GSTT1 mismatch and anti-GSTT1 antibodies developed AIH de novo after a median follow-up of 26 months. Male donor gender, nonalcoholic etiology of original liver disease, and a high anti-GSTT1 titer ($\geq$640) were also independent risk factors for disease development.[85]

De novo AIH generally responds to conventional treatment for AIH (steroids and azathioprine).[93] However, it has been recognized as a significant cause of late allograft loss in undiagnosed and untreated patients.[85] In this sense, anti-GSTT1 antibodies may have a role in helping to identify a subset of patients at risk of developing de novo AIH after liver transplant.[85]

Recommendations

In summary, approximately 25% of patients transplanted for AIH may recur within 5 years post-OLT. The recurrence rate increases with time after OLT. Diagnosis of disease recurrence must include a combination of histologic features with increase in serum transaminases/IgG/autoantibodies as well as corticosteroid dependence. Treatment involves increasing immunosuppression, and is largely successful. Maintenance immunosuppressive therapy and protocol liver biopsies are supported by many experts in order to diagnose asymptomatic histologic recurrence, to prevent severe recurrence and the need for retransplantation. A long-term multicenter study is needed to address the impact of such an approach on disease recurrence and graft survival.

De novo AIH is a cause of late graft dysfunction, occurring in up to 5% of OLT recipients. It is characterized by histologic features of AIH and the presence of autoantibodies that can progress to graft failure if unrecognized and left untreated.

SUMMARY

Although the overall patient and graft survival of PBC, PSC, and AIH remains excellent, recurrence of these autoimmune diseases after liver transplantation is described in roughly 20% to 40% of patients. Efforts should be directed at identification of predictors of recurrence as well as early diagnosis. In this regard, protocol liver biopsies are of utmost importance especially for diagnosis of recurrent PBC and AIH, whereas recurrent PSC can also be diagnosed based on cholangiographic findings. Further studies are needed to better define appropriate immunosuppression and treatment recommendations.

REFERENCES

1. Duclos-Vallee JC, Sebagh M. Recurrence of autoimmune disease, primary sclerosing cholangitis, primary biliary cirrhosis, and autoimmune hepatitis after liver transplantation. Liver Transpl 2009;15(Suppl 2):S25–34.
2. Kuiper EM, Hansen BE, Metselaar HJ, et al. Trends in liver transplantation for primary biliary cirrhosis in the Netherlands 1988-2008. BMC Gastroenterol 2010;10:144.
3. LaRusso NF, Shneider BL, Black D, et al. Primary sclerosing cholangitis: summary of a workshop. Hepatology 2006;44(3):746–64.
4. Liermann Garcia RF, Evangelista Garcia C, McMaster P, et al. Transplantation for primary biliary cirrhosis: retrospective analysis of 400 patients in a single center. Hepatology 2001;33(1):22–7.

5. Charatcharoenwitthaya P, Pimentel S, Talwalkar JA, et al. Long-term survival and impact of ursodeoxycholic acid treatment for recurrent primary biliary cirrhosis after liver transplantation. Liver Transpl 2007;13(9):1236–45.
6. Jacob DA, Neumann UP, Bahra M, et al. Long-term follow-up after recurrence of primary biliary cirrhosis after liver transplantation in 100 patients. Clin Transplant 2006;20(2):211–20.
7. Mottershead M, Neuberger J. Transplantation in autoimmune liver diseases. World J Gastroenterol 2008;14(21):3388–95.
8. Graziadei IW, Wiesner RH, Marotta PJ, et al. Long-term results of patients undergoing liver transplantation for primary sclerosing cholangitis. Hepatology 1999; 30(5):1121–7.
9. Roberts MS, Angus DC, Bryce CL, et al. Survival after liver transplantation in the United States: a disease-specific analysis of the UNOS database. Liver Transpl 2004;10(7):886–97.
10. Wiesner RH. Liver transplantation for primary sclerosing cholangitis: timing, outcome, impact of inflammatory bowel disease and recurrence of disease. Best Pract Res Clin Gastroenterol 2001;15(4):667–80.
11. Adam R, McMaster P, O'Grady JG, et al. Evolution of liver transplantation in Europe: report of the European Liver Transplant Registry. Liver Transpl 2003;9(12):1231–43.
12. Schramm C, Bubenheim M, Adam R, et al. Primary liver transplantation for autoimmune hepatitis: a comparative analysis of the European Liver Transplant Registry. Liver Transpl 2010;16(4):461–9.
13. Poupon R. Primary biliary cirrhosis: a 2010 update. J Hepatol 2010;52(5):745–58.
14. Campsen J, Zimmerman M, Trotter J, et al. Liver transplantation for primary biliary cirrhosis: results of aggressive corticosteroid withdrawal. Transplant Proc 2009; 41(5):1707–12.
15. Khettry U, Anand N, Faul PN, et al. Liver transplantation for primary biliary cirrhosis: a long-term pathologic study. Liver Transpl 2003;9(1):87–96.
16. Maheshwari A, Yoo HY, Thuluvath PJ. Long-term outcome of liver transplantation in patients with PSC: a comparative analysis with PBC. Am J Gastroenterol 2004; 99(3):538–42.
17. Manousou P, Arvaniti V, Tsochatzis E, et al. Primary biliary cirrhosis after liver transplantation: influence of immunosuppression and human leukocyte antigen locus disparity. Liver Transpl 2010;16(1):64–73.
18. Montano-Loza AJ, Wasilenko S, Bintner J, et al. Cyclosporine A protects against primary biliary cirrhosis recurrence after liver transplantation. Am J Transplant 2010;10(4):852–8.
19. Neuberger J, Gunson B, Hubscher S, et al. Immunosuppression affects the rate of recurrent primary biliary cirrhosis after liver transplantation. Liver Transpl 2004; 10(4):488–91.
20. Rust C, Rau H, Gerbes AL, et al. Liver transplantation in primary biliary cirrhosis: risk assessment and 11-year follow-up. Digestion 2000;62(1):38–43.
21. Salguero O, Moreno JM, Seijas MC, et al. Recurrence of primary biliary cirrhosis after liver transplantation. Transplant Proc 2003;35(2):721–2.
22. Sanchez EQ, Levy MF, Goldstein RM, et al. The changing clinical presentation of recurrent primary biliary cirrhosis after liver transplantation. Transplantation 2003; 76(11):1583–8.
23. Tinmouth J, Tomlinson G, Heathcote EJ, et al. Benefit of transplantation in primary biliary cirrhosis between 1985-1997. Transplantation 2002;73(2):224–7.
24. Lee J, Belanger A, Doucette JT, et al. Transplantation trends in primary biliary cirrhosis. Clin Gastroenterol Hepatol 2007;5(11):1313–5.

25. Mendes FD, Kim WR, Pedersen R, et al. Mortality attributable to cholestatic liver disease in the United States. Hepatology 2008;47(4):1241–7.
26. Neuberger J, Portmann B, Macdougall BR, et al. Recurrence of primary biliary cirrhosis after liver transplantation. N Engl J Med 1982;306(1):1–4.
27. Neuberger J. Recurrent primary biliary cirrhosis. Liver Transpl 2003;9(6):539–46.
28. Sylvestre PB, Batts KP, Burgart LJ, et al. Recurrence of primary biliary cirrhosis after liver transplantation: histologic estimate of incidence and natural history. Liver Transpl 2003;9(10):1086–93.
29. Mells G, Mann C, Hubscher S, et al. Late protocol liver biopsies in the liver allograft: a neglected investigation? Liver Transpl 2009;15(8):931–8.
30. Sebagh M, Farges O, Dubel L, et al. Histological features predictive of recurrence of primary biliary cirrhosis after liver transplantation. Transplantation 1998;65(10): 1328–33.
31. Dubel L, Farges O, Bismuth H, et al. Kinetics of anti-M2 antibodies after liver transplantation for primary biliary cirrhosis. J Hepatol 1995;23(6):674–80.
32. Dmitrewski J, Hubscher SG, Mayer AD, et al. Recurrence of primary biliary cirrhosis in the liver allograft: the effect of immunosuppression. J Hepatol 1996; 24(3):253–7.
33. Guy JE, Qian P, Lowell JA, et al. Recurrent primary biliary cirrhosis: peritransplant factors and ursodeoxycholic acid treatment post-liver transplant. Liver Transpl 2005;11(10):1252–7.
34. Levitsky J, Hart J, Cohen SM, et al. The effect of immunosuppressive regimens on the recurrence of primary biliary cirrhosis after liver transplantation. Liver Transpl 2003;9(7):733–6.
35. Gautam M, Cheruvattath R, Balan V. Recurrence of autoimmune liver disease after liver transplantation: a systematic review. Liver Transpl 2006; 12(12):1813–24.
36. Hashimoto E, Taniai M, Yatsuji S, et al. Long-term clinical outcome of living-donor liver transplantation for primary biliary cirrhosis. Hepatol Res 2007;37(Suppl 3): S455–61.
37. Morioka D, Egawa H, Kasahara M, et al. Impact of human leukocyte antigen mismatching on outcomes of living donor liver transplantation for primary biliary cirrhosis. Liver Transpl 2007;13(1):80–90.
38. Yamagiwa S, Ichida T. Recurrence of primary biliary cirrhosis and primary sclerosing cholangitis after liver transplantation in Japan. Hepatol Res 2007; 37(Suppl 3):S449–54.
39. Rowe IA, Webb K, Gunson BK, et al. The impact of disease recurrence on graft survival following liver transplantation: a single centre experience. Transpl Int 2008;21(5):459–65.
40. Lee YM, Kaplan MM. Primary sclerosing cholangitis. N Engl J Med 1995;332(14): 924–33.
41. Lerut J, Demetris AJ, Stieber AC, et al. Intrahepatic bile duct strictures after human orthotopic liver transplantation. Recurrence of primary sclerosing cholangitis or unusual presentation of allograft rejection? Transpl Int 1988;1(3): 127–30.
42. Goss JA, Shackleton CR, Farmer DG, et al. Orthotopic liver transplantation for primary sclerosing cholangitis. A 12-year single center experience. Ann Surg 1997;225(5):472–81 [discussion: 481–3].
43. Harrison RF, Davies MH, Neuberger JM, et al. Fibrous and obliterative cholangitis in liver allografts: evidence of recurrent primary sclerosing cholangitis? Hepatology 1994;20(2):356–61.

44. Jeyarajah DR, Netto GJ, Lee SP, et al. Recurrent primary sclerosing cholangitis after orthotopic liver transplantation: is chronic rejection part of the disease process? Transplantation 1998;66(10):1300–6.
45. Khettry U, Keaveny A, Goldar-Najafi A, et al. Liver transplantation for primary sclerosing cholangitis: a long-term clinicopathologic study. Hum Pathol 2003; 34(11):1127–36.
46. Kubota T, Thomson A, Clouston AD, et al. Clinicopathologic findings of recurrent primary sclerosing cholangitis after orthotopic liver transplantation. J Hepatobiliary Pancreat Surg 1999;6(4):377–81.
47. Narumi S, Roberts JP, Emond JC, et al. Liver transplantation for sclerosing cholangitis. Hepatology 1995;22(2):451–7.
48. Sheng R, Campbell WL, Zajko AB, et al. Cholangiographic features of biliary strictures after liver transplantation for primary sclerosing cholangitis: evidence of recurrent disease. AJR Am J Roentgenol 1996;166(5):1109–13.
49. Vera A, Moledina S, Gunson B, et al. Risk factors for recurrence of primary sclerosing cholangitis of liver allograft. Lancet 2002;360(9349):1943–4.
50. Graziadei IW, Wiesner RH, Batts KP, et al. Recurrence of primary sclerosing cholangitis following liver transplantation. Hepatology 1999;29(4):1050–6.
51. Alabraba E, Nightingale P, Gunson B, et al. A re-evaluation of the risk factors for the recurrence of primary sclerosing cholangitis in liver allografts. Liver Transpl 2009;15(3):330–40.
52. Alexander J, Lord JD, Yeh MM, et al. Risk factors for recurrence of primary sclerosing cholangitis after liver transplantation. Liver Transpl 2008;14(2): 245–51.
53. Brandsaeter B, Schrumpf E, Bentdal O, et al. Recurrent primary sclerosing cholangitis after liver transplantation: a magnetic resonance cholangiography study with analyses of predictive factors. Liver Transpl 2005;11(11):1361–9.
54. Campsen J, Zimmerman MA, Trotter JF, et al. Clinically recurrent primary sclerosing cholangitis following liver transplantation: a time course. Liver Transpl 2008;14(2):181–5.
55. Cholongitas E, Shusang V, Papatheodoridis GV, et al. Risk factors for recurrence of primary sclerosing cholangitis after liver transplantation. Liver Transpl 2008; 14(2):138–43.
56. Kugelmas M, Spiegelman P, Osgood MJ, et al. Different immunosuppressive regimens and recurrence of primary sclerosing cholangitis after liver transplantation. Liver Transpl 2003;9(7):727–32.
57. Moncrief KJ, Savu A, Ma MM, et al. The natural history of inflammatory bowel disease and primary sclerosing cholangitis after liver transplantation—a single-centre experience. Can J Gastroenterol 2010;24(1):40–6.
58. Egawa H, Taira K, Teramukai S, et al. Risk factors for recurrence of primary sclerosing cholangitis after living donor liver transplantation: a single center experience. Dig Dis Sci 2009;54(6):1347–54.
59. Graziadei IW. Live donor liver transplantation for primary sclerosing cholangitis: is disease recurrence increased? Curr Opin Gastroenterol 2011;27(3): 301–5.
60. Haga H, Miyagawa-Hayashino A, Taira K, et al. Histological recurrence of autoimmune liver diseases after living-donor liver transplantation. Hepatol Res 2007; 37(Suppl 3):S463–9.
61. Kashyap R, Mantry P, Sharma R, et al. Comparative analysis of outcomes in living and deceased donor liver transplants for primary sclerosing cholangitis. J Gastrointest Surg 2009;13(8):1480–6.

62. Tamura S, Sugawara Y, Kaneko J, et al. Recurrence of primary sclerosing cholangitis after living donor liver transplantation. Liver Int 2007;27(1):86–94.
63. Chapman R, Fevery J, Kalloo A, et al. Diagnosis and management of primary sclerosing cholangitis. Hepatology 2010;51(2):660–78.
64. Czaja AJ. Recurrent autoimmune hepatitis after liver transplantation: a disease continuum or a fresh start? Liver Transpl 2009;15(10):1169–71.
65. Duclos-Vallee JC, Sebagh M, Rifai K, et al. A 10 year follow up study of patients transplanted for autoimmune hepatitis: histological recurrence precedes clinical and biochemical recurrence. Gut 2003;52(6):893–7.
66. Vogel A, Heinrich E, Bahr MJ, et al. Long-term outcome of liver transplantation for autoimmune hepatitis. Clin Transplant 2004;18(1):62–9.
67. Yao H, Michitaka K, Tokumoto Y, et al. Recurrence of autoimmune hepatitis after liver transplantation without elevation of alanine aminotransferase. World J Gastroenterol 2007;13(10):1618–21.
68. Reich DJ, Fiel I, Guarrera JV, et al. Liver transplantation for autoimmune hepatitis. Hepatology 2000;32(4 Pt 1):693–700.
69. Neuberger J. Transplantation for autoimmune hepatitis. Semin Liver Dis 2002; 22(4):379–86.
70. Neuberger J, Portmann B, Calne R, et al. Recurrence of autoimmune chronic active hepatitis following orthotopic liver grafting. Transplantation 1984;37(4): 363–5.
71. Ayata G, Gordon FD, Lewis WD, et al. Liver transplantation for autoimmune hepatitis: a long-term pathologic study. Hepatology 2000;32(2):185–92.
72. Ratziu V, Samuel D, Sebagh M, et al. Long-term follow-up after liver transplantation for autoimmune hepatitis: evidence of recurrence of primary disease. J Hepatol 1999;30(1):131–41.
73. Campsen J, Zimmerman MA, Trotter JF, et al. Liver transplantation for autoimmune hepatitis and the success of aggressive corticosteroid withdrawal. Liver Transpl 2008;14(9):1281–6.
74. Gonzalez-Koch A, Czaja AJ, Carpenter HA, et al. Recurrent autoimmune hepatitis after orthotopic liver transplantation. Liver Transpl 2001;7(4):302–10.
75. Milkiewicz P, Hubscher SG, Skiba G, et al. Recurrence of autoimmune hepatitis after liver transplantation. Transplantation 1999;68(2):253–6.
76. Molmenti EP, Netto GJ, Murray NG, et al. Incidence and recurrence of autoimmune/alloimmune hepatitis in liver transplant recipients. Liver Transpl 2002; 8(6):519–26.
77. Montano-Loza AJ, Mason AL, Ma M, et al. Risk factors for recurrence of autoimmune hepatitis after liver transplantation. Liver Transpl 2009;15(10):1254–61.
78. Prados E, Cuervas-Mons V, de la Mata M, et al. Outcome of autoimmune hepatitis after liver transplantation. Transplantation 1998;66(12):1645–50.
79. Cattan P, Berney T, Conti F, et al. Outcome of orthotopic liver transplantation in autoimmune hepatitis according to subtypes. Transpl Int 2002;15(1): 34–8.
80. Heffron TG, Smallwood GA, Oakley B, et al. Autoimmune hepatitis following liver transplantation: relationship to recurrent disease and steroid weaning. Transplant Proc 2002;34(8):3311–2.
81. Narumi S, Hakamada K, Sasaki M, et al. Liver transplantation for autoimmune hepatitis: rejection and recurrence. Transplant Proc 1999;31(5):1955–6.
82. Wright HL, Bou-Abboud CF, Hassanein T, et al. Disease recurrence and rejection following liver transplantation for autoimmune chronic active liver disease. Transplantation 1992;53(1):136–9.

83. Yusoff IF, House AK, De Boer WB, et al. Disease recurrence after liver transplantation in Western Australia. J Gastroenterol Hepatol 2002;17(2):203–7.
84. Kerkar N, Hadzic N, Davies ET, et al. De-novo autoimmune hepatitis after liver transplantation. Lancet 1998;351(9100):409–13.
85. Salcedo M, Rodriguez-Mahou M, Rodriguez-Sainz C, et al. Risk factors for developing de novo autoimmune hepatitis associated with anti-glutathione S-transferase T1 antibodies after liver transplantation. Liver Transpl 2009;15(5):530–9.
86. Gupta P, Hart J, Millis JM, et al. De novo hepatitis with autoimmune antibodies and atypical histology: a rare cause of late graft dysfunction after pediatric liver transplantation. Transplantation 2001;71(5):664–8.
87. Heneghan MA, Portmann BC, Norris SM, et al. Graft dysfunction mimicking autoimmune hepatitis following liver transplantation in adults. Hepatology 2001;34(3):464–70.
88. Hernandez HM, Kovarik P, Whitington PF, et al. Autoimmune hepatitis as a late complication of liver transplantation. J Pediatr Gastroenterol Nutr 2001;32(2):131–6.
89. Aguilera I, Wichmann I, Sousa JM, et al. Antibodies against glutathione S-transferase T1 (GSTT1) in patients with de novo immune hepatitis following liver transplantation. Clin Exp Immunol 2001;126(3):535–9.
90. Huguet S, Vinh J, Johanet C, et al. Identification by proteomic tool of atypical anti-liver/kidney microsome autoantibodies targets in de novo autoimmune hepatitis after liver transplantation. Ann N Y Acad Sci 2007;1109:345–57.
91. Rodriguez-Mahou M, Salcedo M, Fernandez-Cruz E, et al. Antibodies against glutathione S-transferase T1 (GSTT1) in patients with GSTT1 null genotype as prognostic marker: long-term follow-up after liver transplantation. Transplantation 2007;83(8):1126–9.
92. Aguilera I, Sousa JM, Gavilan F, et al. Glutathione S-transferase T1 mismatch constitutes a risk factor for de novo immune hepatitis after liver transplantation. Liver Transpl 2004;10(9):1166–72.
93. Salcedo M, Vaquero J, Banares R, et al. Response to steroids in de novo autoimmune hepatitis after liver transplantation. Hepatology 2002;35(2):349–56.

Extended Donors in Liver Transplantation

Theresa R. Harring, MD[a,*], Christine A. O'Mahony, MD[a,b],
John A. Goss, MD[a,b]

KEYWORDS

- Extended criteria donor • Marginal donor • Liver transplant
- Deceased after cardiac death • Advanced age • Steatosis

The use of extended donors has been studied extensively by the transplant community over the past years. As the waiting list expands for orthotopic liver transplant (OLT), transplant teams are searching for new ways to increase the donor pool. According to the United Network of Organ Sharing/Organ Procurement and Transplantation Network (UNOS/OPTN) database, there are 16,141 patients on the liver transplant list.[1] In 2010, 6124 OLTs were performed.[1] In the same year, 1445 patients died while on the waiting list and 1221 patients were removed because they were too sick to transplant.[1] Less than 40% of the patients of the waiting list eventually receive a liver, and almost 10% die while waiting. It is obvious from these figures that there is a paucity of organs compared with the need for transplantation. One of the ways to augment the donor pool is through use of allografts previously believed to be untransplantable. Although the definition of extended donor has not been thoroughly established, most agree that it conveys either a higher risk of physiologic dysfunction or a higher risk of transmission of disease.

Extended donors can be separated into 2 groups: donor-related and surgical technique-related issues. Donor-related issues include deceased after cardiac death (DCD), advanced donor age, increased cold ischemia time (CIT), ABO incompatibility, steatosis, previous malignancy in the donor, hepatitis C virus (HCV) infection, human T-cell lymphotrophic virus type I/II (HTLV-I/II) infection, other active infections, and Centers for Disease Control and Prevention (CDC) high-risk donors. These extended criteria can generally be accepted or denied by the transplant team during evaluation of the allograft. Surgical technique-related issues of extended donors include split liver transplantation and living donor liver transplantation (LDLT). Both of these methods provide the recipient with an allograft when a whole cadaveric organ is unavailable.

The authors have nothing to disclose.
[a] Michael E. DeBakey Department of Surgery, Baylor College of Medicine, One Baylor Plaza, Suite #404D, Houston, TX 77030, USA
[b] Division of Abdominal Transplantation, Michael E. DeBakey Department of Surgery, The Liver Center, Baylor College of Medicine, 1709 Dryden Street, Suite #1500, Houston, TX 77030, USA
* Corresponding author.
E-mail address: th147867@bcm.edu

Clin Liver Dis 15 (2011) 879–900
doi:10.1016/j.cld.2011.08.006
1089-3261/11/$ – see front matter © 2011 Elsevier Inc. All rights reserved.
liver.theclinics.com

DONOR-RELATED ISSUES
DCD

One source of potential liver donors is DCD donors, previously known as nonheart-beating donors. These donors present specific challenges because they have the potential to significantly increase the risk of ischemia to the allograft. One option that has been developed and used by the transplantation community is the idea of controlled DCD procurement in which life support is withdrawn in the operating room to minimize additional ischemic time. The use of DCD donors has increased steadily and now accounts for 5% of OLT.[2] Moreover, the number of liver transplant centers using DCD allografts has also increased.[2] By incorporating DCD donors into the transplantation program, some have seen increased numbers of transplants by 8% and have expected increases up to 25%.[3]

Multiple articles have been written in the medical literature examining the feasibility of these donors compared with traditional deceased after brain death (DBD) donors. Several single-center studies have been documented with large differences in survivals between DCD and DBD allografts (**Table 1**). Some studies report favorable results with use of DCD allografts, with patient and allograft survivals up to 100% and 100% at 1 year, 89.5% and 68.4% at 3 years, and 89.5% and 63.2% at 5 years, respectively[4–7]; although others report significantly reduced patient and allograft survival, down to 68% and 70% patient survival at 3 and 5 years, respectively, and down to 56% allograft survival at 3 and 5 years.[3,6] According to studies examining national data from UNOS/OPTN or Scientific Registry of Transplant Recipient (SRTR) databases, DCD allograft recipients have overall worse patient and allograft survival, down to 60% allograft survival at 3 years[2,8–10]; however, it seems they do not fare significantly worse when compared with DBD donors less than 60 years of age or split liver allografts.[10]

The most common complications with the use of DCD allografts seem to be caused by the threat of prolonged ischemia. Higher incidences of primary nonfunction up to 12%, and biliary complications as high as 60%, including significantly increased

Table 1
DCD allografts transplanted: series reported in the medical literature

Author	Foley et al[3]	Nguyen et al[4]	Detry et al[5]	de Vera et al[6]	Mateo et al[8]	Merion et al[9]	Doshi and Hunsicker[10]
Number of transplants	36	19	13	141	367[a]	472[b]	345[a]
Patient survival (%)							
1 y	80	89.5	100	79	–	–	–
3 y	68	89.5	–	–	–	–	77
5 y	–	89.5	–	70	–	–	–
Allograft survival (%)							
1 y	67	73.7	100	69	71	70.1	–
3 y	56	68.4	–	–	60	60.5	65
5 y	–	63.2	–	56	–	–	–

[a] Authors used UNOS/OPTN database.
[b] Authors used SRTR database.

bile duct injury, biliary stricture, and ischemic cholangiopathy rates, in DCD allograft recipients have been documented.[3,6,7,11] In contrast, others report low incidences of these complications comparable with other types of allografts.[4,5] Others state that their rates of primary nonfunction have been virtually eliminated after the institution of practice protocols related to procurement.[3] In addition, some single-center studies have reported increased retransplantation rates as high as 19.4% in recipients of DCD allografts, supposedly because of the above complications.[3,6] This increase in retransplant rates has been confirmed by several national database studies.[10] Enhanced post-OLT therapeutic interventions, including improved technical ability of endoscopic retrograde cholangiopancreatography, have been suggested as a way to decrease the occurrence of biliary complications, thereby increasing the usefulness of DCD allografts.[6] Moreover, Mateo and colleagues[8] suggests that with improving surgical technique and with more experience using DCD allografts, we may expect patient and graft survivals to approach those of standard allografts.

In contrast, some studies recommend cautious use of DCD allografts, including using special criteria to decide if DCD allograft should be allocated to a certain patient. These criteria include low-risk recipients including HCV-negative patients, patients with a low Model for End-stage Liver Disease (MELD) score, and stable patients with hepatocellular carcinoma; DCD donor age less than 50 years; body mass index (calculated as weight in kilograms divided by the square of height in meters) less than 35; recipient age younger than 50 years; warm ischemia time less than 30 minutes; and CIT less than 9 hours.[3–8,12] Moreover, 1 study examining the UNOS database showed that low-risk recipients who received low-risk DCD allografts had comparable graft survival rates with DBD allograft recipients.[8] Overall, this mimics the consensus of the medical literature that with special consideration, DCD allografts can be used with similar patient and allograft survivals compared with DBD.

Advanced Donor Age

As life expectancy overall increases, the age of potential donors also increases. However, there is no age limit that is considered universally as advanced within the transplant community. The liver seems to resist aging possibly because of the functional reserve, regenerative capacity, and the dual blood supply of the liver.[13]

Multiple single-center studies in the medical literature describe their own experience with advanced age (**Table 2**). Some Investigators report favorable results,[14–21] yet others report the cautious use of these allografts.[22–26] Many investigators agree on the need for especially low CIT when transplanting these allografts and minimizing other donor risk factors such as steatosis.[13–15,18–20,23,27,28] Several centers have even defined criteria on which to accept an allograft from an advanced age donor. These criteria include absence of hemodynamic instability, normal liver function tests, no steatosis on visual examination or less than 30% by biopsy, and regular appearance on inspection by procuring surgeon.[15,18,20–22,27]

In contrast, 1 study using UNOS/OPTN data showed significantly worse patient and allograft outcomes when using allografts from donors aged 80 years or more compared with allografts from donors aged less than 60 years.[13] Even in studies for living donor liver transplants, younger donor age has proven benefits on graft and patient survivals.[29] One investigator states that advanced age should be considered a calculated risk during evaluation of the donor and recipient and should be weighed against other risks.[29]

Despite the willingness of many surgeons to use allografts from advanced age donors, most investigators agree that advanced age donors produce significantly decreased patient and graft survival in recipients with HCV.[14,21,28,30,31] Moreover,

Table 2
Advanced donor age allografts transplanted: series reported in the medical literature

Author	Rauchfuss et al[14]	Singhal et al[13]	Zapletal et al[15]	Petridis et al[22]	Emre et al[17]	Washburn et al[23]	Romero et al[27]	Grazi et al[18]	Grande et al[19]	Ravaioli et al[28]
Number of transplants	54	4200	5	10	36	29	4	36	40	89
Age of donors (y)	≥65	60–79	≥80	≥80	≥70	≥60	≥80	≥70	>60	≥60
Patient survival (%)										
1 y	77.8	83.8	100	80	91	58.6	100	77.4	82	–
3 y	–	71.8	–	40	–	–	–	–	–	–
Allograft survival (%)										
1 y	75.9	77.4	100	70	85	44.8	66	73.3	77	71
3 y	–	64.2	–	20	–	–	–	–	–	54

several studies confirmed that advanced donor age was an independent predictor of graft failure in patients undergoing OLT for HCV.[28,32]

The overall consensus with regards to advanced donor age is to not exclude advanced age donors based solely on age especially with the current allograft shortage. If the allograft is considered suitable after evaluation, an advanced age allograft may be appropriate for transplantation, especially for a recipient who may otherwise be waiting longer for a perfect allograft.

Increased CIT

Increased CIT, longer than 10 to 12 hours, has been shown to negatively affect the graft outcome, with significant effects on graft loss and primary nonfunction rate with increasing levels of CIT.[33,34] Although the exact mechanism is still unknown, CIT is believed to affect the allograft by contributing to ischemia and reperfusion injury; therefore, minimizing CIT is crucial to the success of every OLT. Moreover, especially when dealing with allografts with other suboptimal characteristics, some have proposed even more stringent guidelines for consideration of CIT.[33] Compared with other factors discussed that affect the donor allograft, CIT can be controlled and minimized by the transplant surgery team, thereby increasing the chances for successful long-term allograft outcomes.

ABO Incompatibility

There is little in the medical literature about the effects of ABO incompatibility on OLT. OLT historically requires only ABO matching and not HLA matching. However, because of recent innovations in pediatric heart transplants with ABO-incompatible allografts,[35–41] and the suggestion that pediatric, and especially infantile, immune systems may be so naive to be able to accept an ABO-incompatible allograft,[42] this concept has been applied to liver transplantation. One single-center study examined the ABO-incompatibility effects in adult LDLTs.[43] The investigators concluded that their success was in part because of their use of a novel regimen including portal vein infusion therapy and rituximab prophylaxis.[43] One study that examined the UNOS database found no significant difference in allograft loss with the use of ABO-incompatible livers compared with ABO-compatible livers in pediatric recipients.[42] These investigators concluded that ABO-incompatible allografts may be used when an ABO-compatible allograft cannot be procured, especially with the difficulties of finding an appropriate size-matched and age-matched liver allograft in the pediatric population.[42] In contrast, a different review from our own institution did not corroborate these results (Harring TR, Guiteau JJ, Nguyen NT, et al. Are ABO-incompatible liver transplants a durable option in infants? Abstract accepted for presentation at AASLD, 2010, unpublished data). Therefore, without additional evidence to the contrary, ABO-incompatible liver allografts are not recommended unless used in emergency situations for pediatric recipients.

Steatosis

Many donor livers are discarded during evaluation because of steatosis, or fatty liver. As the epidemic of obesity continues within developed countries, it is projected that even more steatosis will be encountered during evaluation of donor liver allografts. The prevalence within developed countries of steatosis ranges between 10% and 30% of the population and increases with the incidence of overweight or obese populations, because the major risk factors for steatosis include obesity, insulin resistance, and excess alcohol intake.[44,45] Because steatosis is so prevalent, the transplant community benefits from extra evaluation of these livers to see if they may be suitable for transplantation.

Two types of steatosis are recognized: microvesicular, in which there are multiple small fat vacuoles within the hepatocyte; and macrovesicular, in which there is 1 fat vacuole that replaces most of the cytoplasm of the hepatocyte and displaces the nucleus. Macrovesicular steatosis is subdivided into grades: low (5%–15%), mild (16%–30%), moderate (31%–60%), and severe (>60%). Macrovesicular steatosis is more commonly associated with unfavorable post-OLT allograft and patient outcomes. The grade of macrovesicular steatosis, determined by biopsy, may be the important factor as to which steatotic allografts lead to primary nonfunction or primary dysfunction. Adding to the debate is the fact that fatty liver changes may be reversed with lifestyle changes, or may progress to fibrosis and cirrhosis.

Part of the problem with using steatotic liver allografts is the fact that biopsy is necessary to evaluate the grade severity. Severe macrosteatosis can be macroscopically seen by the procurement team, but microscopic examination is necessary to see low to moderate grades of steatosis. One study looked at explanted liver allografts deemed untransplantable because of steatosis to further evaluate whether the grafts could have been used in transplantation.[46] By examining 36 explanted liver specimens, the researchers concluded that radiographic studies are not specific for steatosis, more frequent microscopic evaluation is necessary during organ evaluation, and that biopsies must be gathered from 2 different parts of the liver.[46] Overall they found that 16.7% of the discarded liver allografts could have potentially been used in transplantation, thereby increasing the donor pool.[46]

One single-center study examined the use of liver allografts according to moderate (<30%) or moderate to severe (≥30%) steatosis.[47] This study found 4-month and 5-year graft survival rates were 87% and 68% in the moderate steatosis category and 77% and 58% in the moderate to severe steatosis category, respectively.[47] These investigators also found that the degree of steatosis was not independently associated with long-term outcome on multivariate analysis.[47] The investigators concluded that there is no major effect of moderate to severe steatosis on overall long-term allograft survival, and even stated that feared complication rates may have been incorrectly attributed to steatosis.[47] They reported that allografts with steatosis can be transplanted with good results; however, they recommend against using an allograft combining steatosis with another extended criterion, including the use of a steatotic allograft for LDLT or split liver transplantation.[47]

A different single-center study examined transplanting allografts with low to moderate steatosis into patients younger than 70 years of age and with MELD scores less than 27.[48] Of a total of 35 allografts with steatosis that were evaluated by this group, 43% were discarded and 57% were transplanted based on severity of macrovesicular steatosis, with a 6-month graft survival of 80%.[48] These investigators also recommend against the use of steatotic allografts in recipients with other risk factors for primary nonfunction or primary dysfunction.[48] They concluded that liver allografts with low to moderate steatosis can safely be used in patients in stable condition, with no additional risk factors, age less than 70 years, and MELD less than 27.[48]

According to the available data in the medical literature, the use of certain steatotic allografts, especially those with low or moderate steatosis, must be considered as an important source of organs; therefore, regular donor biopsies should be used by the procurement team to allow more of these acceptable allografts into the donor pool.

Previous Malignancy

The risk of malignancy after transplantation can fall into 1 of 3 categories: the use of allografts from donors with previous malignancy, the transplantation of a recipient with previous malignancy, and the risk of de novo malignancy in the transplant recipient. Immunosuppression is believed to be a risk factor alone in the acquisition of malignancy after OLT. Several studies have strived to determine the exact risk of malignancy after transplantation. The range of de novo cancer risk ranges in the literature from 3.1% to 55%.[49–52] One study reports that 1 of every 6 liver transplant patients is expected to develop a malignancy by 20 years after OLT, a 2.6-fold increase over the general population.[49] With regard to extended criteria donors, the question becomes whether donors with a history of malignancy are acceptable to use for transplantation.

Generally, patients with a history of previous malignancy are not eligible for organ donation. The medical literature has multiple case reports of incidental transmission of high-grade malignancies from the donor allograft into the recipient with generally unfavorable outcomes.[53–57] The general treatment of these aggressive tumors includes cessation of or decreased immunosuppression and explantation of the allograft if the malignancy is not metastatic and immediate retransplantation. A UNOS/OPTN database report on allograft use from donors with a previous history of malignancy shows a cancer-free interval of greater than 5 years for most recipients of these allografts.[58] These investigators state that the possible increased risk of developing a malignancy from the donor should be weighed carefully against the real risk of dying on the waitlist.[58]

Another question arises with the use of donors with central nervous system (CNS) malignancies. The blood-brain barrier is believed to prevent transmission of CNS tumors to the recipient. Some investigators argue that violation of the barrier, including ventriculoperitoneal shunts and extensive craniotomies, increases the risk of tumor dissemination and transmission.[59–62] One author even states that high-grade CNS tumors and cerebellar lesions add even more risk.[59] When screened appropriately, 1 single-center series reported no difference in survival between recipients of allografts from donors with CNS tumors and recipients of allografts without CNS tumors, concluding that allografts from these donors can be used safely.[60] Although the true risk remains unknown, the risk of cancer transmission from donors with CNS malignancies has been reported to be between 0% and 23%.[59,60,63,64]

Donors with a previous history of malignancy must be evaluated on a case-by-case basis. Patients with a history of malignancy outside the CNS should not be used for transplantation unless extraneous circumstances dictate that the recipient needs an immediate organ. On the other hand, certain patients with previous CNS tumors may be acceptable for organ donation. Overall, the risk of tumor transmission must be weighed against the immediate need for an allograft.

HCV-positive Donors

A different situation the transplant team must consider is what to do when an HCV-positive graft becomes available. The concern is for transmission of a different or more virulent strain of HCV into an immunocompromised host[65,66]; however, these fears have not been validated in the medical literature.

There have been multiple reports of transmission of HCV by OLT,[67–69] along with considerable studies into the effects of transplanting HCV-positive allografts into HCV-positive recipients.[65,66,70–73] Multiple single-center series have been reported showing favorable results with HCV-positive recipients receiving HCV-positive allografts (**Table 3**).[66,71–74] In all of these studies, survival rates were not statistically different compared with those recipients receiving an HCV-negative allograft.[66,71–74] One study even discovered that the HCV recurrence rate was lower in HCV-positive recipients with an HCV-positive allograft compared with those who received an HCV-negative allograft, thereby finding a benefit to transplanting HCV-positive

Table 3
HCV-positive allografts transplanted: series reported in the medical literature

Author	Vargas et al[65]	Ghobrial et al[70]	Velidedeoglu et al[71]	Saab et al[72]	Torres et al[73]
Number of transplants	23	59	13	59	8
Patient survival (%)					
1 y	89	85	–	76	75
3 y	–	–	–	–	75
5 y	72	70	–	64	–
Allograft survival (%)					
1 y	–	73	69.2	74	75
3 y	–	–	69.2	–	75
5 y	–	63	–	58	–

allografts.[73] The conclusion from all these studies is that HCV-positive allografts free from fibrosis or severe inflammation are a safe option for HCV-positive recipients,[72,73,75] because patient and graft survival rates are not significantly different from those patients who receive a liver from an HCV-negative donor.

In several analyses of the UNOS/OPTN database, the survival of HCV-positive allografts was studied.[65,70,72] The investigators found that most HCV-positive allografts went to recipients who were also HCV-positive, and that recipients of HCV-positive allografts tended to be older, men, not White, and had hepatocellular carcinoma.[70] A different review showed that donor HCV status was not an independent predictor of decreased graft survival.[72] Most importantly, they reported that there was no statistical difference in 5-year survival in HCV-positive recipients when they received HCV-positive or HCV-negative allografts, concluding that use of HCV-positive allografts for HCV-positive recipients is comparable in outcome with use of HCV-negative allografts for long-term survival.[70,72] One study even showed that 2-year patient survival was significantly increased when an HCV-positive recipient received an HCV-positive allograft versus an HCV-negative allograft (90% vs 77% [$P = .01$], respectively).[65]

A different report studied the recipient opinion on accepting an HCV-positive allograft, indicating that the recipients themselves may be the largest obstacle to the use of HCV-positive allografts.[76] These investigators showed that only a few patients, 18%, with HCV willingly accept an HCV-positive allograft.[76] The investigators also reported a clear correlation with acceptance of an HCV-positive allograft and time spent on the waiting list. Yet, even after waiting longer than 6 months for a standard liver allograft, only 35% of the HCV-positive patients stated that they would accept an HCV-positive allograft.[76]

Overall, it has been shown that OLT using an HCV-positive allograft into an HCV-positive recipient is safe and leads to long-term survival outcomes comparable with the use of HCV-negative allografts. However, the procurement team should consider donor biopsy to evaluate these HCV-positive allografts, because any allograft with fibrosis or severe inflammation should not be used for transplantation.

HTLV-I/II Infection

HTLV-I and HTLV-II were the first identified human retroviruses. The prevalence is lower than the human immunodeficiency virus (HIV), with an estimated 0.05% to

0.1% of the United States population being carriers. Higher prevalence up to 30% is associated with endemic areas, specifically, South America, Asia, Africa, and the Caribbean. Transmission of HTLV-I/II is through breastfeeding, sexual contact, and exposure to contaminated blood. HTLV-I is implicated in the development of HTLV-associated myelopathy or tropical spastic paraparesis and adult T-cell leukemia. HTLV-II has not been linked to any disease. HTLV-I/II testing is no longer part of the workup of most donors, partly because of the low seroprevalence in the United States.

HTLV-I/II-positive allografts may be suitable for use in select OLT recipients. In a single-center study, the presence of positive serologies, including HTLV-I/II, did not affect early allograft failure, or patient or allograft survival at 90 days, 1, or 2 years.[77] In a case series from New York, 5 HTLV-I-positive allografts were used in OLT: 3 were false-positives, 1 true-positive was placed in a patient with concurrent HIV/HCV infection who died at 12 months as a result of recurrent HCV, and 1 true-positive was allocated to a patient with concurrent HIV/hepatitis B virus infection who was reported to be healthy at 18 months after OLT.[78] After examination of the UNOS/OPTN database, 9 HTLV-I/II-positive livers were used for OLT but none of the recipients developed HTLV-I/II-related disease during a median follow-up of 11.9 months.[79] Another examination of UNOS/OPTN data found similar results, with no statistically significant difference in patient and allograft survivals between HTLV-I/II-positive and HTLV-I/II-negative allografts used during OLT.[80]

In contrast, according to a case report from Spain, HTLV-I infection from a liver allograft causing associated myelopathy has proved devastating.[81–84] This group has written several papers on the warnings of using HTLV-I/II-positive allografts for hepatic and renal transplantations, suggesting that immunocompromised status may increase the risk of developing HTLV-I/II-associated myelopathy.[81–84]

A single-center study in Japan, where HTLV-I/II is endemic, showed that only 3 of 8 HTLV-I/II-positive patients before transplant (37.5%) developed adult T-cell leukemia after OLT.[85] This study further proved that the HTLV-I/II strain present in the recipient before transplantation was the same strain causing the leukemia.[85] In a single-center series from Kentucky, the investigators reported that 5 HTLV-I-positive patients received OLT and none developed myelopathy or leukemia.[80] These studies together suggest that HTLV-I/II does present a small but real increased risk, especially when combined with immunosuppression, to develop an associated myelopathy or adult T-cell leukemia.

Because of the relatively low prevalence of HTLV-I/II in the United States, and despite the possible devastating consequences of HTLV-I/II-related disease, HTLV-I/II-positive allografts should be considered an option for donation for certain recipients. Some patients may benefit from the use of these allografts, especially those with an urgent need of transplant, older patients, and those with known HTLV-I/II infection.[79,80] However, even with the low chance of acquiring a disease from HTLV-I/II transmission, recipients of HTLV-I/II-positive allografts should receive heightened screening after OLT.[78–81]

Active Infections

Of particular concern in the recently transplanted and immunocompromised patient is transmission of bacterial, viral, or fungal infection. Because donors are screened carefully, the concern of transmitting infection from the donor to the recipient is theoretically minimized; however, there remain sporadic case reports of rare donor-transmitted life-threatening infections during OLT.[86–97] The question to the transplant community becomes how to screen donors for these infections without wasting organs as potential recipients are dying on the waitlist.[98]

One study compared 2 groups of recipients with regard to infection: those who received an allograft from a donor with infection versus from a donor without infection.[99] The study showed that donors with infection had significantly longer intensive care unit (ICU) admission, higher incidences of cardiopulmonary resuscitation and episodes of hypotension, more inotropic medication administration, and higher aspartate aminotransferase, alanine aminotransferase, and blood urea nitrogen levels.[99] Multivariate analysis showed that ICU admission of 7 days or longer, previous cardiopulmonary resuscitation, and inotropic agent medication administration were independent predictors of potential donor infection.[99] However, despite these findings, the investigators failed to show a significant difference in recipient ICU admission days, or 1-week or 1-month mortality in recipients of allografts from donors with infection.[99] This finding suggests that although donor infection remains an important consideration during evaluation, the transplant team need not necessarily exclude a donor based solely on possible bacterial infection transmission.

Several studies outline survival after OLT using allografts from donors diagnosed with bacterial meningitis. One study of 34 transplants states that all recipients received appropriate prophylactic, broad-spectrum antibiotics after transplantation to prevent transmission of infection.[100] This study reports overall patient and allograft survival at 1, 6, 12, and 60 months of 79%, 76%, 72%, and 72% and 77%, 70%, 65%, and 65%, respectively.[100] These investigators also compared these survival rates with a matched control group and found no significant differences in patient or allograft survivals or postoperative infectious complications caused by meningeal pathogens.[100] These investigators state that they accept donors with bacterial meningitis to expand their donor pool providing the donor has received appropriate antibiotic treatment and is hemodynamically stable.[100] Another study outlines the transplantation of 6 liver allografts from donors whose cause of death was bacterial meningitis or acute bacterial epiglottitis.[101] These investigators reported a graft survival of 75%, with 1 recipient dying after OLT because of graft rejection.[101] They conclude that certain clinically infected donors can be used safely for OLT.[101] Another report supports these observations, because the organisms that most commonly cause bacterial meningitis are especially susceptible to low temperatures during organ procurement and storage.[102] However, these investigators caution that any patient with sustained bacteremia, infection with an unknown agent, or with concern for metastatic infection should not be used in organ donation.[102]

Case reports and single-center series in the medical literature also describe rare causes of infection in the post-OLT patient. Even in an endemic area for histoplasmosis, 1 large single-center study reports an incidence of 1 case out of 746 OLTs performed.[86] These researchers comment that although histoplasmosis can cause disseminated and deadly disease in immunocompromised posttransplant patients, the overall incidence remains low and prognosis seems good.[86] One case report describes a transmitted *Strongyloides* infection from the donor into an OLT recipient.[87] These investigators suggest a modification of pretransplant screening to include imported infections, especially in countries with a high rate of immigration.[87] Several case reports describe transmission of West Nile virus (WNV) through OLT with varying results.[88,91,92] Some investigators recommend early therapy, reduction of immunosuppression, and careful following to ensure that the WNV infection does not spread to the recipient's CNS.[88] Another case report describes the transmission of aspergillosis from a donor used in multiple recipients because the donor's death was presumed incorrectly, and was discovered to be caused by disseminated aspergillosis 3 weeks after her death.[89] These investigators argue that a donor should be accepted only if the donor cause of death is known without doubt.[89] Another case report describes OLT with a donor with known *Naegleria fowleri* infection.[90] The recipient of the allograft had no evidence of infection or complications at follow-up.[90] These investigators carefully state that this infection, which is known to remain in the CNS and not spread to other organs, does not preclude donation.[90]

Careful donor screening and selection should protect the recipient from undue exposure of infectious agents. Increased screening in endemic areas should be mandated, and donor cause of death should be known before procurement. When infection is limited to the CNS and transmission to a recipient is highly unlikely, organs may be allocated from these donors as long as recipients are aware of the infection risk.

CDC High-risk Donors

Transmission of HIV and HCV continues to be of concern in the transplant community. Because organ shortage continues to be a problem, many centers must contemplate using allografts from high-risk donors, weighing the risk of transmission of a potentially fatal disease versus the decompensation or death of the recipient on the waiting list.

Although screening for blood-borne pathogens has improved with our understanding of the disease, there is still a risk for transmission during solid organ transplantation. Case reports outline this continued risk with poor outcomes in immunocompromised post-OLT patients.[103,104] Infection through transplantation likely occurs because of multiple blood transfusions before evaluation or because of organ donation during the window period for the infection.[67,105]

The CDC have stated that persons with certain criteria should be excluded from donation unless the risk to the recipient of not receiving the transplant outweighs the risk of HIV transmission and disease.[106] These exclusionary criteria include men who have had sex with a man within 5 years; persons who report nonmedical intravenous, intramuscular, or subcutaneous injection of drugs within 5 years; persons with hemophilia or related clotting disorders who have received human-derived clotting factor concentrations; men and women who have engaged in sex in exchange for money or drugs within 5 years; persons who have had sex within a year with any person described in this list or with a person known or suspected to have HIV infection; persons who have been exposed within the year to known or suspected HIV-infected blood through percutaneous inoculation or through contact with an open wound, nonintact skin, or mucous membranes; or inmates of correctional systems.[106]

Although we will likely never be able to make the transmission risk of blood-borne pathogens such as HIV and HCV zero, the transplant team must individually weigh the risks of using a donor for each recipient, and include these risks in the surgical consent before transplantation. Moreover, if a disease has been acquired through transplantation, open communication about the transmission with the recipient and the recipient's family is necessary.

SURGICAL TECHNIQUE-RELATED ISSUES
Split Liver Transplantation

Split liver donation, in which 1 allograft is split into 2 transplantable allografts, is another method to expand the donor pool. This method was first introduced as a way to decrease mortality of pediatric patients on the waiting list, but it has now been adapted for adult transplantation as well. Most commonly, the liver is split into 1 graft for a pediatric recipient and 1 graft for an adult patient; however, increasing evidence supports the use of both grafts being implanted into size-appropriate adults.

Several factors influence the decision of whether a liver is suitable for splitting, including cause of death, length of stay in the ICU, amount of inotropic support, vascular and biliary anatomic considerations, quality of the allograft as evidenced by liver function tests and presence of steatosis, age of the donor, and CIT.[107–111] However, even outside these limitations and with splitting of allografts beyond optimal criteria, acceptable survival rates can be achieved.[112] With regards to these considerations and possible limitations, many argue that good-quality cadaveric livers should be considered paired organs and that liver-splitting programs should be mandatory to decrease the organ shortage.[107,111] Implementing a mandatory splitting program has been projected to increase the number of available allografts by 20% to 30%.[107,113]

According to several studies, survival rates after split liver transplants are acceptable.[107–110,112–115] Several studies including multiple matched-pair analyses and the largest matched-pair analysis in the literature with 165 pairs found no significant differences in 3-month, 6-month, 1-year, 3-year, and 5-year patient or allograft survivals when comparing split liver transplantations with whole liver transplantations (Table 4).[107–109,114,115] Moreover, these investigators found no statistical difference in rejection rates, biliary complications, primary poor function, primary nonfunction, or retransplantation rates in the split liver transplant recipients versus the whole liver transplant recipients.[107–110,113,114] Several studies even highlighted that overall patient and graft survival can remain high, even when an allograft is split for use in 2 adults.[110,111,113,116]

Split liver transplantation can be a great source to increase allografts; however, special caution must be used. Splitting techniques require technical precision, and only some liver allografts may be appropriate for splitting. Special attention should be paid to the fact that survival rates increase as a center gains more experience in this technically difficult type of transplant.[112]

Living Donors

Another way to increase the liver allograft pool is for transplant centers to incorporate LDLTs. Many institutions, including our own, no longer consider LDLT as an extended criterion; an improved term reflecting the use of these nonstandard allografts may be expanded. Nevertheless, this type of transplantation remains ethically charged, because the transplant team must take into account the safety of the donor. This risk to the donor must be carefully weighed against the risk of the recipient's mortality by staying on the waiting list. This dilemma directly contradicts the ethical concept of nonmalficence, or "do no harm".[117] One author states that it is a daunting task for the transplant community to establish acceptable mortality and morbidity when the baseline risk of the donor is zero without donation.[118] Moreover, this author also suggests that true informed consent is impossible, because donors cannot fully comprehend the possible complications.[118] Therefore, preserving the health of the donor and not allowing donation from a suboptimal candidate should be the most important priority of the transplant team.[117]

The number of LDLTs peaked in 2001 with 411 LDLTs and has since then declined, with only 198 LDLTs performed in 2007.[119,120] This situation is believed to be the result of several factors, including better use of other extended criteria allografts and the concern of donor complications.[118]

Several investigators conclude that LDLT is a feasible option with comparable survival rates with that of cadaveric donation,[118,121,122] although one states that adult outcomes are significantly worse than pediatric outcomes (Table 5).[123] Many also state that paramount to a successful program is strict selection of living donors, reasonable choice of graft type, intensive postoperative surveillance, and improvement of surgical techniques.[121,122] During evaluation for donation for an adult recipient, one must consider patient size, age, disease process and manifestations, and

Table 4
Split liver transplantations: series reported in the medical literature

Author	Broering et al[107]	Spada et al[108]	Decoster et al[112]	Baccarani et al[114]	Wilms et al[109]	Gundlach et al[116]	Azoulay et al[111]	Yersiz et al[115]
Number of transplants	40	15	22	14	70	4	30	165[a]
Patient survival (%)								
3 mo	92.5	90	–	–	84.3	100	–	–
6 mo	–	–	–	–	–	100	–	79
1 y	87.5	86	84	83	–	–	74.2/87.5[a]	78
3 y	–	79	84	73	–	–	–	75
5 y	–	–	56	73	82.8	–	–	–
Allograft survival (%)								
3 mo	87.5	89	–	–	75.7	100	–	–
6 mo	–	–	–	–	–	100	–	72
1 y	77.4	84	79	73	–	–	–	68
3 y	–	75	79	73	–	–	–	64
5 y	–	–	64	73	74.3	–	–	–

[a] Right allograft/left allograft.

Table 5
LDLTs: series reported in the medical literature

Author	Olthoff et al[119]	Hwang et al[121]	Shimazu and Kitajima[122]	Goldstein et al[123]
Number of transplants	385	1000	63	45
Pediatric patient survival (%)				
1 y	–	–	–	91
2 y	–	87.5	–	–
5 y	–	84.8	83.1	–
Adult patient survival (%)				
1 y	89	–	–	74
2 y	–	86.6	–	–
5 y	–	83.2	79.2	–
Pediatric allograft survival (%)				
1 y	–	–	–	91
Adult allograft survival (%)				
1 y	81	–	–	65

urgency of transplant.[123] LDLT seems especially plausible for patients with hepatocellular carcinoma, who may particularly benefit from an earlier transplant compared with a long wait time with likely progression of disease.[118]

Along with donor safety is the concern for allowing a large enough allograft in the recipient and providing enough residual volume for the donor. Generally, safe donation is only possible if at least 30% of residual liver volume is left in the donor. Several surgical techniques have evolved allowing different types of allografts, including left lobe allograft, right lobe allograft, and extended right lobe allograft. Several studies showed that the type of living donor liver graft is important to the complication rate in the donors.[123,124] Right or extended right hepatectomy, donor age greater than 40 years, and prolonged operative time more than 400 minutes have been proved as independent risk factors for biliary complications in donors.[124] One of these studies also experienced donor death caused by previously undiagnosed nonalcoholic steatohepatitis.[124] These researchers concluded that right and extended right lobe donation have significantly more complications compared with other allograft donations.[124]

A large consortium study named the Adult-to-Adult Living Donor Liver Transplantation Cohort Study (A2ALL) organized 9 liver transplant centers to follow patients receiving an adult LDLT to better understand specific LDLT risks.[119,120] This study reported patient and allograft survival at 90 days and 1 year of 94% and 89%, and 87% and 81%, respectively.[119] These investigators found that recipient and donor age, CIT, diagnosis of HCV, diagnosis of hepatocellular carcinoma, higher serum creatinine level, preoperative medical condition, and center experience were associated with an independent risk of patient mortality and allograft failure.[119,120] Center experience of 20 cases or less was associated with an 83% higher risk of allograft failure.[119]

Another study from the A2ALL group focused on donor morbidity.[125] These investigators found that most donors (62%) did not suffer complications from LDLT; however, donor complication rate remained high (38%).[125] Biliary complications and incisional hernia were the most frequent causes of morbidity in donors, occurring in 10% and 5% of cases, respectively.[125] A total of 3 donor deaths associated with LDLT have been reported in the United States according to A2ALL: 1 patient died of infection and multiorgan system failure during the initial hospitalization, 1 patient died of drug overdose, and the other patient committed suicide.[117,125] Along with 2 other recent living donor deaths in 2010, the donor mortality associated with LDLT is between 0.5% and 1%.[117,125]

Recipient morbidity is also common with LDLT. Biliary complications seem to also be the most common complication, occurring in 20% to 30% of LDLT, with bile leaks most frequently.[117] Hepatic artery thrombosis and septic complications, especially in patients with decompensated cirrhosis, also occur more frequently in LDLT as opposed to cadaveric donation.[117]

A study on transplant surgeons' perspectives gave more insight into living donor liver donations.[126] Of surgeons, 72% agreed that transplant programs have a duty to their patients to offer adult LDLT and 63% agreed that the success of LDLT leads to expanded indications for liver transplantation.[126] With regard to ethical implications of LDLT, 77% agreed that placing a donor's life at risk creates a moral dilemma; however, 58% believed that the increasing number of deaths on the waiting list justified the risk to the donor.[126]

As with split liver transplantation, LDLT can provide an excellent resource to transplant centers wishing to increase their allograft pool. Yet, the transplant community must be willing to accept certain factors. LDLT causes the transplant team to care for 2 patients, balancing the risk to a healthy donor with no baseline risk, with the survival of the liver patient who desperately needs an allograft. Furthermore, LDLT requires surgical precision to delicately remove enough liver parenchyma from the donor for the recipient to survive and leave enough behind for the donor to recover successfully. Large centers have been successful, as shown by the review of medical literature, but smaller centers may require additional resources to have similar outcomes.

SUMMARY

With the current supply and demand discrepancy of liver allografts, the transplant team must decide how and when to use extended donors. There are ethical implications to using extended donors that the transplant team must weigh carefully: do you sacrifice the individual patient by using a suboptimal allograft, thereby decreasing waitlist time and benefitting the whole transplant population, or do you maintain optimal transplantation specifications so that the individual patient has improved results but many others die while waiting for an organ? Should you endanger recipients in overall better condition, such as patients with lower MELD scores and younger patients, who can tolerate a lengthy waitlist, or should you transplant them with an extended donor allograft because they are likely to better tolerate a lesser-quality allograft? If an extended donor allograft fails, does the recipient automatically receive a standard cadaveric allograft, even although the same patient may not have qualified for a standard allograft for many more months or years? Often these types of questions are not answered easily, especially when there are personal connections to individual recipients. Moreover, when a recipient fails because of organ dysfunction, the transplant team must assume complete responsibility. Therefore, the use of extended donors is not a simple solution based on broad recommendations. Each transplant center must decide on their allocation procedures to best fit their recipient population. Only in this type of environment can certain extended donor allografts be used safely.

REFERENCES

1. The United Network for Organ Sharing/Organ Procurement and Transplantation Network. Available at: http://optn.transplant.hrsa.gov. Accessed March 21, 2011.

2. Berg CL, Steffick DE, Edwards EB, et al. Liver and Intestine Transplantation in the United States 1998-2007. Am J Transplant 2009;9(2):907–31.
3. Foley DP, Fernandez LA, Leverson G, et al. Donation after cardiac death: the University of Wisconsin experience with liver transplantation. Ann Surg 2005; 242(5):724–31.
4. Nguyen JH, Bonatti H, Dickson RC, et al. Long-term outcomes of donation after cardiac death liver allografts from a single center. Clin Transplant 2009;23: 168–73.
5. Detry O, Seydel B, Delbouille MH, et al. Liver transplant donation after cardiac death: experience at the University of Liege. Transplant Proc 2009;41:582–4.
6. de Vera ME, Lopez-Solis R, Dvorchik I, et al. Liver transplantation using donation after cardiac death donors: long-term follow-up from a single center. Am J Transplant 2009;9:773–81.
7. Chan EY, Olson LC, Kisthard JA, et al. Ischemic cholangiopathy following liver transplantation from donation after cardiac death donors. Liver Transpl 2008; 14:604–10.
8. Mateo R, Cho Y, Singh G, et al. Risk factors for graft survival after liver transplantation from donation after cardiac death donors: an analysis of OPTN/UNOS data. Am J Transplant 2006;6:791–6.
9. Merion RM, Pelletier SJ, Goodrich N, et al. Donation after cardiac death as a strategy to increase deceased donor liver availability. Ann Surg 2006; 244(4):555–62.
10. Doshi MD, Hunsicker LG. Short- and long-term outcomes with the use of kidneys and livers donated after cardiac death. Am J Transplant 2007;7:122–9.
11. Maheshwari A, Maley W, Li Z, et al. Biliary complications and outcomes of liver transplantation from donors after cardiac death. Liver Transpl 2007;13:1645–53.
12. Yagci G, Fernandez LA, Knechtle SJ, et al. The impact of donor variables on the outcome of orthotopic liver transplantation for hepatitis C. Transplant Proc 2008; 40:219–23.
13. Singhal A, Sezginsoy B, Ghuloom AE, et al. Orthotopic liver transplant using allografts from geriatric population in the United States: is there any age limit? Exp Clin Transplant 2010;8(3):196–201.
14. Rauchfuss F, Voigt R, Dittmar Y, et al. Liver transplantation utilizing old donor organs: a German Single-Center Experience. Transplant Proc 2010;42:175–7.
15. Zapletal CH, Faust D, Wullstein C, et al. Does the liver ever age? Results of liver transplantation with donors above 80 years of age. Transplant Proc 2005;37:1182–5.
16. Cascales-Campos PA, Romero PR, Gonzalez R, et al. Improving the waiting list by using 75-year-old donors for recipients with hepatocellular carcinoma. Transplant Proc 2010;42:627–30.
17. Emre S, Schwartz ME, Altaca G, et al. Safe use of hepatic allografts from donors older than 70 years. Transplantation 1996;62(1):62–5.
18. Grazi GL, Cescon M, Ravaioli M, et al. A revised consideration on the use of very aged donors for liver transplantation. Am J Transplant 2001;1:61–8.
19. Grande L, Rull A, Rimola A, et al. Outcome of patients undergoing orthotopic liver transplantation with elderly donors (over 60 years). Transplant Proc 1997; 29:3289–90.
20. Nardo B, Masetti M, Urbani L, et al. Liver transplantation from donors aged 80 years and over: pushing the limit. Am J Transplant 2004;4:1139–47.
21. Cescon M, Grazi GL, Ercolani G, et al. Long-term survival of recipients of liver grafts from donors older than 80 years: is it achievable? Liver Transpl 2003; 9(11):1174–80.

22. Petridis I, Gruttadauria S, Nadalin S, et al. Liver transplantation using donors older than 80 years: a single-center experience. Transplant Proc 2008;40: 1976–8.
23. Washburn WK, Johnson LB, Lewis WD, et al. Graft function and outcome of older (> or = 60 years) donor livers. Transplantation 1996;61(7):1062–6.
24. Busquets J, Xiol X, Figueras J, et al. The impact of donor age on liver transplantation: influence of donor age on early liver function and on subsequent patient and graft survival. Transplantation 2001;71(12):1765–71.
25. Marino IR, Doyle HR, Doria C, et al. Outcome of liver transplantation using donors 60 to 79 years of age. Transplant Proc 1995;27(1):1184–5.
26. Hoofnagle JH, Lombardero M, Zetterman RK, et al. Donor age and outcome of liver transplantation. Hepatology 1996;24(1):89–96.
27. Romero CJ, Gonzalez EM, Ruiz FC, et al. Use of octogenarian livers safely expands the donor pool. Transplantation 1999;68(4):572–5.
28. Ravaioli M, Grazi GL, Cescon M, et al. Liver transplantations with donors aged 60 years and above: the low liver damage strategy. Transpl Int 2009;22:423–33.
29. Ikegami T, Nishizaki T, Yanaga K, et al. The impact of donor age on living donor liver transplantation. Transplantation 2000;70(12):1703–7.
30. Tallon-Aguilar L, Molina-Garcia D, Barrera-Pulido, et al. Influence of donor age on survival in liver transplantation due to hepatitis C virus. Transplant Proc 2008;40:2968–70.
31. Perez-Daga JA, Ramirez-Plaza C, Suarez MA, et al. Impact of donor age on the results of liver transplantation in hepatitis C virus-positive recipients. Transplant Proc 2008;40:2959–61.
32. Condron SL, Heneghan MA, Patel K, et al. Effect of donor age on survival of liver transplant recipients with hepatitis C virus infection. Transplantation 2005;80(1): 145–8.
33. Totsuka E, Fung JJ, Lee MC, et al. Influence of cold ischemia time and graft transport distance on postoperative outcome in human liver transplantation. Surg Today 2002;32:792–9.
34. Furukawa H, Todo S, Imventarza O, et al. Effect of cold ischemia time on the early outcome of human hepatic allografts preserved with UW solution. Transplantation 1991;51(5):1000–4.
35. Dipchand AI, Pollock BarZiv SM, Manlhiot C, et al. Equivalent outcomes for pediatric heart transplantation recipients: ABO-blood group incompatible versus ABO-compatible. Am J Transplant 2010;10:389–97.
36. Everitt MD, Donaldson AE, Casper TC, et al. Effect of ABO-incompatible listing on infant heart transplant waitlist outcomes: analysis of the United Network for Organ Sharing (UNOS) database. J Heart Lung Transplant 2009; 28:1254–60.
37. Almond CS, Gauvreau K, Thiagarajan RR, et al. Impact of ABO-incompatible listing on wait-list outcomes among infants listed for heart transplantation in the United States: a propensity analysis. Circulation 2010;121:1926–33.
38. Saczkowski R, Dacey C, Bernier PL. Does ABO-incompatible and ABO-compatible neonatal heart transplant have equivalent survival? Interact Cardiovasc Thorac Surg 2010;10:1026–33.
39. Urschel S, Campbell PM, Meyer SR, et al. Absence of donor-specific anti-HLA antibodies after ABO-incompatible heart transplantation in infancy: altered immunity or age? Am J Transplant 2010;10:149–56.
40. Gambino A, Torregrossa G, Cozzi E, et al. ABO-incompatible heart transplantation: crossing the immunological barrier. J Cardiovasc Med 2008;9:854–7.

41. Patel ND, Weiss ES, Scheel J, et al. ABO-incompatible heart transplantation in infants: analysis of the united network for organ sharing database. J Heart Lung Transplant 2008;27:1085–9.
42. Stewart ZA, Locke JE, Montgomery RA, et al. ABO-incompatible deceased donor liver transplantation in the United States: a national registry analysis. Liver Transpl 2009;15:883–93.
43. Tanabe M, Kawachi S, Obara H, et al. Current progress in ABO-incompatible liver transplantation. Eur J Clin Invest 2010;40(10):943–9.
44. Preiss D, Sattar N. Non-alcoholic fatty liver disease: an overview of prevalence, diagnosis, pathogenesis and treatment considerations. Clin Sci 2008;115: 141–50.
45. Farrell GC, Larter CZ. Nonalcoholic fatty liver disease: from steatosis to cirrhosis. Hepatology 2006;43:S99–112.
46. Rey JW, Wirges U, Dienes HP, et al. Hepatic steatosis in organ donors: disparity between surgery and histology? Transplant Proc 2009;41:2557–60.
47. Angele MK, Rentsch M, Hartl WH, et al. Effect of graft steatosis on liver function and organ survival after liver transplantation. Am J Surg 2008;195:214–20.
48. Avolio AW, Frongillo F, Nicolotti N, et al. Successful use of extended criteria donor grafts with low to moderate steatosis in patients with model for end-stage liver disease scores below 27. Transplant Proc 2009;41:208–12.
49. Aberg F, Pukkala E, Hockerstedt K, et al. Risk of malignant neoplasms after liver transplantation: a population-based study. Liver Transpl 2008;14:1428–36.
50. Haagsma EB, Hagens VE, Schaapveld M, et al. Increased cancer risk after liver transplantation: a population-based study. J Hepatol 2001;34:84–91.
51. Saigal S, Norris S, Srinivasan P, et al. Successful outcome of orthotopic liver transplantation in patients with preexisting malignant states. Liver Transpl 2001;7(1):11–5.
52. Benten D, Sterneck M, Panse J, et al. Low recurrence of preexisting extrahepatic malignancies after liver transplantation. Liver Transpl 2008;14:789–98.
53. Ortiz JA, Manzarbeitia C, Noto KA, et al. Extended survival by urgent liver re-transplantation after using a first graft with metastasis from initially unrecognized donor sarcoma. Am J Transplant 2005;5:1559–61.
54. Kim JK, Carmody IC, Cohen AJ, et al. Donor transmission of malignant melanoma to a liver graft recipient: case report and literature review. Clin Transplant 2009;23:571–4.
55. Foltys D, Linkerman A, Heumann A, et al. Organ recipients suffering from undifferentiated neuroendocrine small-cell carcinoma of donor origin: a case report. Transplant Proc 2009;41:2639–42.
56. Braun-Parvez L, Charlin E, Caillard S, et al. Gestational choriocarcinoma transmission following multiorgan donation. Am J Transplant 2010;10:2541–6.
57. Vernadakis S, Poetsch M, Weber F, et al. Donor origin de novo HCC in a noncirrhotic liver allograft 3 years after liver transplantation. Transpl Int 2010;23:341–3.
58. Kauffman HM, Cherikh WS, McBride MA, et al. Deceased donors with a past history of malignancy: an organ procurement and transplantation network/united network for organ sharing update. Transplantation 2007;84(2):272–4.
59. Buell JF, Trofe J, Sethuraman G, et al. Donors with central nervous system malignancies: are they truly safe? Transplantation 2003;76(2):340–3.
60. Kashyap R, Ryan C, Sharma R, et al. Liver grafts from donors with central nervous system tumors: a single-center perspective. Liver Transpl 2009;15:1204–8.
61. Detry O. Liver graft procurement in donors with central nervous system cancers. Liver Transpl 2010;16:914–5.

62. Penn I. Questions about the use of organ donors with tumors of the central nervous system. Transplantation 2000;70(1):249–50.
63. Kaufman HM, McBride MA, Delmonico FL. First report of the United Network for Organ Sharing Transplant Tumor Registry: donors with a history of cancer. Transplantation 2000;70(12):1747–51.
64. Kauffman HM, McBride MA, Cheikh WS, et al. Transplant tumor registry: donors with central nervous system tumors. Tranplantation 2002;73(4):579–82.
65. Marroquin CE, Marino G, Kuo PC, et al. Transplantation of hepatitis C-positive livers in hepatitis C-positive patients is equivalent to transplanting hepatitis C-negative livers. Liver Transpl 2001;7(9):762–8.
66. Vargas HE, Laskus T, Wang LF, et al. Outcome of liver transplantation in hepatitis C virus-infected patients who received hepatitis C virus-infected grafts. Gastroenterology 1999;117:149–53.
67. Ahn J, Cohen SM. Transmission of human immunodeficiency virus and hepatitis C virus through liver transplantation. Liver Transpl 2008;14:1603–8.
68. Gruttadauria S, Pagano D, Petridis I, et al. Hepatitis C virus infection in a living-related liver donor. Am J Transplant 2010;10:191.
69. Pereira BJ, Milford EL, Kirkman RL, et al. Transmission of hepatitis C virus by organ transplantation. N Engl J Med 1991;325:454–60.
70. Northup PG, Argo CK, Nguyen DT, et al. Liver allografts from hepatitis C positive donors can offer good outcomes in hepatitis C positive recipients: a US National Transplant Registry analysis. Transpl Int 2010;23:1038–44.
71. Ghobrial RM, Steadman R, Gornbein J, et al. A 10-year experience of liver transplantation for hepatitis C: analysis of factors determining outcome in over 500 patients. Ann Surg 2001;234(3):384–94.
72. Velidedeoglu E, Desai NM, Campos L, et al. The outcome of liver grafts procured from hepatitis C-positive donors. Transplantation 2002;73(4):582–7.
73. Saab S, Ghobrial RM, Ibrahim AB, et al. Hepatitis C positive grafts may be used in orthotopic liver transplantation: a matched analysis. Am J Transplant 2003;3:1167–72.
74. Torres M, Weppler D, Reddy KR, et al. Use of hepatitis C-infected donors for hepatitis C-positive OLT recipients. Gastroenterology 1999;117:1253–61.
75. Berenguer M. Risk of extended criteria donors in hepatitis C virus-positive recipients. Liver Transpl 2008;14:S45–50.
76. Martinez-Alarcon L, Rios A, Ramirez P, et al. Would patients with hepatitis C virus on the waiting list for a liver transplant accept a hepatitis C-positive organ? Transpl Infect Dis 2009;11:475–6.
77. Tector AJ, Mangus RS, Chestovich P, et al. Use of extended criteria livers decreases wait time for liver transplantation without adversely impacting post-transplant survival. Ann Surg 2006;244(3):439–50.
78. Alkofer B, Samstein B, Guarrera JV, et al. Extended-donor criteria liver allografts. Semin Liver Dis 2006;26:221–3.
79. Angelis M, Cooper JT, Freeman RB. Impact of donor infections on outcome of orthotopic liver transplantation. Liver Transpl 2003;9(5):451–62.
80. Marvin MR, Brock GN, Kwarteng K, et al. Increasing utilization of human T-cell lymphotropic virus (+) donors in liver transplantation: is it safe? Transplantation 2009;87(8):1180–90.
81. Zarranz JJ, Rouco I, Gomez-Esteban JC. Human T lymphotropic virus type I (HTLV-I) associated myelopathy acquired through a liver transplant. J Neurol Neurosurg Psychiatry 2001;71:817–24.

82. Zarranz-Imirizaldu JJ, Gomez-Esteban JC, Rouco-Axpe I, et al. Post-transplantation HTLV-I myelopathy in three recipients from a single donor. J Neurol Neurosurg Psychiatry 2003;74:1080–4.

83. Toro C, Rodes B, Poveda E, et al. Rapid development of subacute myelopathy in three organ transplant recipients after transmission of human T-cell lymphotropic virus type I from a single donor. Transplantation 2003;75(1):102–4.

84. Gonzalez-Perez MP, Munoz-Juarez L, Cardenas-Cardenas F, et al. Human T-cell leukemia virus type I infection in various recipients of transplants from the same donor. Transplantation 2003;75(7):1006–11.

85. Kawano N, Shimoda K, Ishikawa F, et al. Adult T-cell leukemia development from a human T-cell leukemia virus type I carrier after a living-donor liver transplantation. Transplantation 2006;82(6):840–3.

86. Cuellar-Rodriguez J, Avery RK, Lard M, et al. Histoplasmosis in solid organ transplant recipients: 10 years of experience at a large transplant center in an endemic area. Clin Infect Dis 2009;49:710–6.

87. Rodriguez-Hernandez MJ, Ruiz-Perez-Pipaon M, Canas E, et al. *Strongyloides stercoralis* hyperinfection transmitted by liver allograft in a transplant recipient. Am J Transplant 2009;9:2637–40.

88. Morelli MC, Sambri V, Grazi GL, et al. Absence of neuroinvasive disease in a liver transplant recipient who acquired West Nile virus (WNV) infection from the organ donor and who received WNV antibodies prophylactically. Clin Infect Dis 2010; 51(4):e34–7.

89. Mueller NJ, Weisser M, Fehr T, et al. Donor-derived aspergillosis from use of a solid organ recipient as a multiorgan donor. Transpl Infect Dis 2010;12:54–9.

90. Bennett WM, Nespral JF, Rosson MW, et al. Use of organs for transplantation from a donor with primary meningoencephalitis due to *Naegleria fowleri*. Am J Transplant 2008;8:1334–5.

91. Iwamoto M, Jernigan DB, Guasch A, et al. Transmission of West Nile virus from an organ donor to four transplant recipients. N Engl J Med 2003;348:2196–203.

92. West Nile Virus infections in organ transplant recipients–New York and Pennsylvania, August-September 2005. Centers for Disease Control and Prevention. MMWR Recomm Rep 2005;54(40):1021–3.

93. Srinivasan A, Burton EC, Kuehnert MJ, et al. Transmission of rabies virus from an organ donor to four transplant recipients. N Engl J Med 2005;352:1103–11.

94. Rabies in patients who received organ transplants in Germany. CDR Wkly (Online) 2005;15. News.

95. Fischer SA, Graham MB, Kuehnert MJ, et al. Transmission of lymphocytic choriomeningitis virus by organ transplantation. N Engl J Med 2006;354:2235–49.

96. Palacios G, Druce J, Du L, et al. A new arenavirus in a cluster of fatal transplant-associated disease. N Engl J Med 2008;358:991–8.

97. Baddley JW, Schain DC, Gupte AA, et al. Transmission of *Cryptococcus neoformans* by organ transplantation. Clin Infect Dis 2011;52(4):e94–8.

98. Kusne S. Regarding unexpected severe and life-threatening donor-transmitted viral infections and use of high-risk behavior donors. Liver Transpl 2008;14: 1564–8.

99. Wu TJ, Lee CF, Chou HS, et al. Suspect the donor with potential infection in the adult deceased donor liver transplantation. Transplant Proc 2008;40:2486–8.

100. Satoi S, Bramhall SR, Solomon M, et al. The use of liver grafts from donors with bacterial meningitis. Transplantation 2001;72(6):1108–13.

101. Little DM, Farrell JG, Cunningham PM, et al. Donor sepsis is not a contraindication to cadaveric organ donation. QJM 1997;90:641–2.

102. Issa NC, Patel R. Potential for expansion of the donor pool using liver allografts from donors with bacterial meningitis. Liver Transpl 2002;8(10):977–9.
103. Simonds RJ, Holmberg SD, Hurwitz RL, et al. Transmission of human immuno-deficiency virus type 1 from a seronegative organ and tissue donor. N Engl J Med 1992;326(11):726–32.
104. Epidemiologic Notes and Reports Human Immunodeficiency Virus Infection Transmitted From on Organ Donor Screened for HIV Antibody – North Carolina. Centers for Disease Control and Prevention. MMWR Recomm Rep 1987;36(20): 306–8.
105. Ison MG, Friedewald JJ. Transmission of human immunodeficiency virus and hepatitis C virus through liver transplantation. Liver Transpl 2009;15:561.
106. Guidelines for preventing transmission of human immunodeficiency virus through transplantation of human tissue and organs. Centers for Disease Control and Prevention. MMWR Recomm Rep 1994;43(RR-8):1–17.
107. Broering DC, Topp S, Schaefer U, et al. Split liver transplantation and risk to the adult recipient: analysis using matched pairs. J Am Coll Surg 2002;195: 648–57.
108. Spada M, Cescon M, Aluffi A, et al. Use of extended right grafts from in situ split livers in adult liver transplantation: a comparison with whole-liver transplants. Transplant Proc 2005;37:1164–6.
109. Wilms C, Walter J, Kaptein M, et al. Long-term outcome of split liver transplan-tation using right extended grafts in adulthood: a matched pair analysis. Ann Surg 2006;244(6):865–73.
110. Cescon M, Grazi GL, Ravaioli M, et al. Conventional split liver transplantation for two adult recipients: a recent experience in a single European center. Transplan-tation 2009;88:1117–22.
111. Azoulay D, Castaing D, Adam R, et al. Split-liver transplantation for two adult recipients: feasibility and long-term outcomes. Ann Surg 2001;233(4):565–74.
112. Decoster EL, Troisi R, Sainz-Barriga M, et al. Improved results for adult split liver transplantation with extended right lobe grafts: could we enhance its applica-tion? Transplant Proc 2009;41:3404–6.
113. Humar A, Ramcharan T, Sielaff TD, et al. Split liver transplantation for two adult recipients: an initial experience. Am J Transplant 2001;1:366–72.
114. Baccarani U, Adani GL, Risaliti A, et al. Long-term results of in situ split-liver transplantation. Transplant Proc 2005;37:2592–4.
115. Yersiz H, Renz JF, Farmer DG, et al. One hundred in situ split-liver transplanta-tions: a single-center experience. Ann Surg 2003;238(4):496–507.
116. Gundlach M, Broering D, Topp S, et al. Split-cava technique: liver splitting for two adult recipients. Liver Transpl 2000;6(6):703–6.
117. Shiffman ML, Brown RS, Olthoff KM, et al. Living donor liver transplantation: summary of a conference at The National Institutes of Health. Liver Transpl 2002;8(2):174–88.
118. Olsen SK, Brown RS. Live donor liver transplantation: current status. Curr Gas-troenterol Rep 2008;10:36–42.
119. Olthoff KM, Merion RM, Ghobrial RM, et al. Outcomes of 385 adult-to-adult living donor liver transplant recipients: a report from the A2ALL Consortium. Ann Surg 2005;242(3):314–25.
120. Olthoff KM, Abecassis MM, Emond JC, et al. Outcomes for adult living donor transplantation: comparison of the Adult-to-adult Living Donor Liver Transplan-tation Cohort Study and the national experience. Liver Transpl 2011;17(7): 789–97.

121. Hwang S, Lee SG, Lee YJ, et al. Lessons learned from 1,000 living donor liver transplantations in a single center: how to make living donations safe. Liver Transpl 2006;12:920–7.
122. Shimazu M, Kitajima M. Living donor liver transplantation with special reference to ABO-incompatible grafts and small-for-size grafts. World J Surg 2004;28:2–7.
123. Goldstein MJ, Salame E, Kapur S, et al. Analysis of failure in living donor liver transplantation: differential outcomes in children and adults. World J Surg 2003;27:356–64.
124. Iida T, Ogura Y, Oike F, et al. Surgery-related morbidity in living donors for liver transplantation. Transplantation 2010;89(10):1276–82.
125. Ghobrial RM, Freise CE, Trotter JF, et al. Donor morbidity after living donation for liver transplantation. Gastroenterology 2008;135:468–76.
126. Cotler SJ, Cotler S, Gambera M, et al. Adult living donor liver transplantation: perspectives from 100 liver transplant surgeons. Liver Transpl 2003;9(6): 637–44.

Index

Note: Page numbers of article titles are in **boldface** type.

United States Postal Service

Statement of Ownership, Management, and Circulation
(All Periodicals Publications Except Requestor Publications)

1. Publication Title	2. Publication Number								3. Filing Date
Clinics in Liver Disease	0	1	6	-	7	5	4		9/16/11

4. Issue Frequency	5. Number of Issues Published Annually	6. Annual Subscription Price
Feb, May, Aug, Nov	4	$251.00

7. Complete Mailing Address of Known Office of Publication *(Not printer) (Street, city, county, state, and ZIP+4®)*

Elsevier Inc.
360 Park Avenue South
New York, NY 10010-1710

Contact Person
Stephen Bushing
Telephone (Include area code)
215-239-3688

8. Complete Mailing Address of Headquarters or General Business Office of Publisher *(Not printer)*

Elsevier Inc., 360 Park Avenue South, New York, NY 10010-1710

9. Full Names and Complete Mailing Addresses of Publisher, Editor, and Managing Editor *(Do not leave blank)*

Publisher *(Name and complete mailing address)*

Kim Murphy, Elsevier, Inc., 1600 John F. Kennedy Blvd. Suite 1800, Philadelphia, PA 19103-2899

Editor *(Name and complete mailing address)*

Kerry Holland, Elsevier, Inc., 1600 John F. Kennedy Blvd. Suite 1800, Philadelphia, PA 19103-2899

Managing Editor *(Name and complete mailing address)*

Sarah Barth, Elsevier, Inc., 1600 John F. Kennedy Blvd. Suite 1800, Philadelphia, PA 19103-2899

10. Owner *(Do not leave blank. If the publication is owned by a corporation, give the name and address of the corporation immediately followed by the names and addresses of all stockholders owning or holding 1 percent or more of the total amount of stock. If not owned by a corporation, give the names and addresses of the individual owners. If owned by a partnership or other unincorporated firm, give its name and address as well as those of each individual owner. If the publication is published by a nonprofit organization, give its name and address.)*

Full Name	Complete Mailing Address
Wholly owned subsidiary of	4520 East-West Highway
Reed/Elsevier, US Holdings	Bethesda, MD 20814

11. Known Bondholders, Mortgagees, and Other Security Holders Owning or Holding 1 Percent or More of Total Amount of Bonds, Mortgages, or Other Securities. If none, check box ▸ ☐ None

Full Name	Complete Mailing Address
N/A	

12. Tax Status *(For completion by nonprofit organizations authorized to mail at nonprofit rates) (Check one)*
The purpose, function, and nonprofit status of this organization and the exempt status for federal income tax purposes:
☐ Has Not Changed During Preceding 12 Months
☐ Has Changed During Preceding 12 Months *(Publisher must submit explanation of change with this statement)*

PS Form 3526, September 2007 (Page 1 of 3 (Instructions Page 3) PSN 7530-01-000-9931 PRIVACY NOTICE: See our Privacy policy in www.usps.com

13. Publication Title		14. Issue Date for Circulation Data Below
Clinics in Liver Disease		August 2011

15. Extent and Nature of Circulation			Average No. Copies Each Issue During Preceding 12 Months	No. Copies of Single Issue Published Nearest to Filing Date
a. Total Number of Copies *(Net press run)*			781	704
b. Paid Circulation (By Mail and Outside the Mail)	(1)	Mailed Outside-County Paid Subscriptions Stated on PS Form 3541. *(Include paid distribution above nominal rate, advertiser's proof copies, and exchange copies)*	215	188
	(2)	Mailed In-County Paid Subscriptions Stated on PS Form 3541 *(Include paid distribution above nominal rate, advertiser's proof copies, and exchange copies)*		
	(3)	Paid Distribution Outside the Mails Including Sales Through Dealers and Carriers, Street Vendors, Counter Sales, and Other Paid Distribution Outside USPS®	120	119
	(4)	Paid Distribution by Other Classes Mailed Through the USPS (e.g. First-Class Mail®)		
c. Total Paid Distribution *(Sum of 15b (1), (2), (3), and (4))*		▸	335	307
d. Free or Nominal Rate Distribution (By Mail and Outside the Mail)	(1)	Free or Nominal Rate Outside-County Copies Included on PS Form 3541	67	63
	(2)	Free or Nominal Rate In-County Copies Included on PS Form 3541		
	(3)	Free or Nominal Rate Copies Mailed at Other Classes Through the USPS (e.g. First-Class Mail)		
	(4)	Free or Nominal Rate Distribution Outside the Mail (Carriers or other means)		
e. Total Free or Nominal Rate Distribution *(Sum of 15d (1), (2), (3) and (4))*		▸	67	63
f. Total Distribution *(Sum of 15c and 15e)*		▸	402	370
g. Copies not Distributed *(See instructions to publishers #4 (page #3))*		▸	379	334
h. Total *(Sum of 15f and g)*		▸	781	704
i. Percent Paid (15c divided by 15f times 100)			83.33%	82.97%

16. Publication of Statement of Ownership

☐ If the publication is a general publication, publication of this statement is required. Will be printed in the **November 2011** issue of this publication. ☐ Publication not required

17. Signature and Title of Editor, Publisher, Business Manager, or Owner

Stephen R. Bushing | Date

Stephen R. Bushing –Inventory/Distribution Coordinator | September 16, 2011

I certify that all information furnished on this form is true and complete. I understand that anyone who furnishes false or misleading information on this form or who omits material or information requested on the form may be subject to criminal sanctions (including fines and imprisonment) and/or civil sanctions (including civil penalties).

PS Form 3526, September 2007 (Page 2 of 3)

Moving?

Make sure your subscription moves with you!

To notify us of your new address, find your **Clinics Account Number** (located on your mailing label above your name), and contact customer service at:

Email: journalscustomerservice-usa@elsevier.com

800-654-2452 (subscribers in the U.S. & Canada)
314-447-8871 (subscribers outside of the U.S. & Canada)

Fax number: 314-447-8029

Elsevier Health Sciences Division
Subscription Customer Service
3251 Riverport Lane
Maryland Heights, MO 63043

*To ensure uninterrupted delivery of your subscription, please notify us at least 4 weeks in advance of move.

Printed and bound by CPI Group (UK) Ltd, Croydon, CR0 4YY

03/10/2024

01040455-0006